Counseling Adults
in Transition

Nancy K. Schlossberg, EdD, is a full professor at the University of Maryland, College Park, in the Department of Counseling and Personnel Services, College of Education, and Director of the Center of Human Services Development. She received her doctorate in education degree from Teachers College, Columbia University, in counseling. She served on the faculties of Wayne State University, Howard University, and Pratt Institute, and was the first woman executive at the American Council on Education (ACE), where she established the Office of Women in Higher Education. Dr. Schlossberg is currently a Senior Fellow at ACE's Center on Adult Learning.

Dr. Schlossberg's awards include: Fellow of three divisions of the American Psychological Association (APA), Fellow of the Gerontological Association, the 1983 APA G. Stanley Hall Lecturer on Adult Development, Distinguished Scholar at the University of Maryland (1983). She was named as one of the Eminent Women in Psychology by the American Psychological Association and listed in *Who's Who of American Women* in 1993. In addition, Dr. Schlossberg has received highest honors and awards from the following national organizations: The National Career Development Association, American College Personnel Association, the National Association for Women in Education, and the American Society for Training and Development.

Elinor B. Waters, EdD, is an associate professor in the School of Education and Human Services at Oakland University in Rochester, Michigan. She received her doctoral degree in counseling from Wayne State University. She has worked for the Michigan Civil Rights Commissions, the Fels Research Institute, the Merrill-Palmer Institute and the University of the West Indies.

Dr. Waters is a former president of the Association for Adult Development and Aging, and a past chair—and current member—of the Board of Directors of the National Board for Certified Counselors. She is a member of the leadership council of the Mental Health and Aging Network of the American Society on Aging and the Health and Long Term Care Advisory Committee of the American Association of Retired Persons.

Jane Goodman, PhD, is an assistant professor of counseling in the Department of Leadership and Counseling, College of Education, Eastern Michigan University, Ypsilanti, Michigan. She received her doctorate degrees in Guidance and Counseling from Wayne State University, Detroit. She formerly worked as a consultant and trainer for the Continuum Center, Oakland University, Rochester, Michigan. She was the 1994–95 President of the National Career Development Association.

Dr. Goodman's awards include Group Worker of the Year Award from the Michigan Association for Specialists in Group Work and Champion of Career Development from the Michigan Career Development Association.

Counseling Adults in Transition

Linking Practice With Theory

Second Edition

Nancy K. Schlossberg, EdD
Elinor B. Waters, EdD
Jane Goodman, PhD

 SPRINGER PUBLISHING COMPANY

Springer Publishing Company, Inc.
536 Broadway
New York, NY 10012–3955

Cover design by Tom Yabut
Production Editor: Pam Ritzer

95 96 97 98 99 / 5 4 3 2 1

Library of Congress Cataloging-in-Publication Data

Schlossberg, Nancy K., 1929–
  Counseling adults in transition : linking practice with theory /
Nancy K. Schlossberg, Elinor B. Waters, Jane Goodman. — 2nd ed.
    p. cm.
  Includes bibliographical references and index.
  ISBN 0-8261-4231-1
  1. Counseling. 2. Adulthood. 3. Middle age—Psychological
aspects. 4. Middle aged person—Counseling of. I. Waters, Elinor
B. II. Goodman, Jane, 1942– . III. Title.
BF637.C6S325 1995
158'.3—dc20   95-7294
                                                        CIP

Printed in the United States of America

We have all, in the past decade, lost our last parent. Their deaths made us the older generation, a major transition. To all of our parents, we dedicate this book.

N.K.S.
E.B.W.
J.G.

Contents

Preface to Second Edition   ix
Acknowledgments   xiii

Part I What Do We Need To Know?
Introduction   1
1 Adult Development Theories   3
2 The Transition Framework   25
3 Factors That Influence Transitions   47

Part II What Are We Likely To Hear?
Introduction   79
4 Individual Transitions   81
5 Relationship Transitions   107
6 Work Transitions   139

Part III What Can We Do With What We Know And Hear?
Introduction   167
7 Individual Counseling   169
8 Group Counseling   203
9 Consultation, Program Development, And Advocacy   241

Afterword   269
References   273
Index   299

Preface to Second Edition

This book discusses what, as a counselor to adults in transition, you need to know, are apt to hear, and can do to help your clients. To begin, let us consider the kinds of questions and concerns adults bring to helping professionals, paraprofessionals, and friends:

- We both retired last year. For me it was easy; for my wife it was unbearable.
- What advice can you give someone whose lover is going through an unbelievable crisis?
- My last five years have drained me. My father died after a long, painful bout with cancer. My mother and mother-in-law both live near me and want things all the time. I've had a hysterectomy; my husband a prostatectomy. My son was involved in drugs last year. I'm pulled in all directions—and often I'm angry.
- When Tom was in the factory working all day, I expected him to be tired at night. Now he's been laid off, and he lies around the house all day. I can't stand it.
- I wish being a football star could go on forever. I also wish I didn't have to face what to do after it's over.
- I'm contemplating early retirement, but my job has lots of status and I'm afraid if I retire I'll lose all my sense of identity and power. Yet I've had two heart attacks, I need to care for my sick wife, and really, I'm bored with many of my work-related activities.
- Why me? The kids are finally grown and doing well. We've had two years of marriage counseling, and are getting along better than ever. And now, all of a sudden, I have cancer.

- My husband is facing a job threat; my children are preadolescent; and I'm conflicted about my own career.
- My wife has been loyal, a good mother, a good wife. But I'm bored with her. Do I stay and resign myself to a dull, sexless life? Do I continue having affairs? Or do I free myself and start over?
- As head of a major institution I assumed when I retired that I'd be the elder statesman. When the phone stopped ringing, when my wife and I started arguing and bumping into each other, I realized I was in the midst of a major crisis.

These concerns relate to how adults explore, understand, and cope with what is happening in their lives. Add to these the "what ifs" and "if onlys," the cries of more and more adult men and women of all ages and walks of life who have made basic decisions about education, career, and lifestyle and feel there is no turning back: "What if I had known earlier that women could be women as well as engineers?" "If only I had completed high school!"

Also add to these the questions asking "Where is . . . ," "Is there . . . ," and "What are . . ."—questions that may indicate little immediate psychic pain and turmoil but are equally urgent to the individual seeking to achieve full development: "Where is there a school with part-time training in tailoring?" "Is there an opportunity for women morticians?" "What are the options for someone with my abilities or disabilities?"

How can we as counselors help adults address these very real concerns? In the preface to the first edition of this book, Nancy wrote: "For many years I have been intrigued with how adults develop. This interest has led me to study how adults deal with the ordinary and extraordinary process of living, and how to help them do it." Elly and Jane joined Nancy to write this substantially new edition because we all share that same curiosity, along with a passion to help adults manage the ups, downs, and turning points in their lives.

As a part of that commitment we have counseled individuals and groups, trained professional and paraprofessional counselors, consulted with a variety of profit and non-profit organizations, and been active in professional associations which further the practice of adult counseling. This book is part of our ongoing effort to reach people who can positively intervene in the lives of adults grappling with changes.

Our goal is to help counselors acquire the knowledge, skills, and attitudes that will enable them to work more effectively with their adult clients. Whether we are working with the unemployed, newly appointed middle management, displaced homemakers, returning learners, abused women, recovering alcoholics, divorced persons, or caregivers of dementia patients, our goals are the same—through counseling and other interventions, to help people become more self-aware, more in control of their reactions to life, more empowered, and more able to use strategies that will get them where they want to go. Toward that end we have divided this book into three parts: (a) what we need to know, (b) what we are likely to hear, and (c) what we can do with what we know and hear in counseling adults in transition.

The first part, "What Do We Need to Know?" serves as a backdrop or base for the other two. It includes a review of the major theories of adult development, an explanation of the transition framework, and a discussion of the factors that influence how adults negotiate transitions. The transition model explicated here enumerates four major areas which affect how clients cope with transitions. Those areas, called the 4 S's, are Situation, Self, Supports, and Strategies. Throughout the rest of the book we look for ways to help clients assess their resources for coping and increase the balance of resources to deficits in each of these areas.

The second part, "What We are Likely to Hear?" provides readers with an opportunity to listen to the voices of adults in transition. Combining case studies and relevant literature, we discuss a variety of events and non-events that cause adults to seek counseling. We also consider recurring themes confronting adults facing individual, relationship, and work transitions. Throughout their lives, most adults face a number of transitions, and they change their interests, goals, and values as a result of those experiences. Nevertheless, it is still possible to trace themes that recur in their lives, themes that crop up again and again—though in slightly altered forms and at different times in the life span. The organization of this section, like the lives of adults in transition, is not neat and tidy. Just as various parts of a person's life interact and overlap, so do the chapters of this section in the book.

The third part, "What Can We Do with What We Know and Hear?" focuses on interventions. Here we suggest a number of strategies for counselors to use to help adults increase their resources for coping with transitions. We look first at individual counseling, and suggest ways to use the transition model in conjunction with basic counseling skills and knowledge of adult development. In the chapter on group counseling, we consider the variety of groups available to people facing individual, relationship, and work transitions. In the last chapter, we go beyond face-to-face interventions and discuss activities such as consulting and advocacy.

In writing this book, we have tried to present material from both the client and counselor points of view, for after all counseling is an interaction and a collaboration. Writing this book has also been a collaboration of three people who have studied together, worked together, and played together. Our lives have overlapped in many ways, and even though writing this book has been hard work, the result reflects our shared commitment to the field of adult counseling and our joy in working together.

NANCY K. SCHLOSSBERG
ELINOR B. WATERS
JANE GOODMAN
October, 1994

Acknowledgments

We wish to thank our respective universities: The University of Maryland, College Park; Oakland University; and Eastern Michigan University; our editors Mary Grace Luke and Harry Wagner; our assistants Kate Burdick, Barbara Karvonen, Sally Nulph, and Lori Pierce, as well as our secretaries, Betty Bowers and Lisa Hill. We also wish to thank all of the clients whose transitions helped further our understanding of the process, and the students whose comments helped us reconceptualize this second edition.

Part I
WHAT DO WE NEED TO KNOW?

INTRODUCTION

To set the stage for what counselors need to know, the reader is introduced to an overview of adult development theories. These illustrate the different ways adult behavior can be explained. Some believe adults can change at will, others that they can change only if the environment changes. Some theorists assume that changes are inevitable and part of the developmental process, while still others theorize that the transitions one initiates and weathers make the difference in adult behavior.

Once the larger landscape showing these different perspectives is in place, the reader is introduced to the transition perspective in great detail. This includes examining the transition process itself, and the factors that make a difference as clients go through this process.

This first part provides the cognitive framework for practitioners so that they can understand adults in a more comprehensive manner. The knowledge about adult development and transitions provides counselors and other helpers with the necessary background so they can enable clients to manage transitions more creatively.

1

Adult Development Theories

Adults need to explore, understand, and cope with what is happening in their lives. As counselors, we basically try to help them achieve these ends. We help them increase, or at least maintain, their capacity for love, work, and play—goals often talked about in terms of increased competency, maturity, mental health, or some similar catch-all phrase. Theorists, whose work we will discuss later in this chapter, often talk about adults' capacity to continually invest in life, the ability to respond autonomously, and the flexibility to cope with the "hassles" of life. Indeed, Smelser and Erikson (1980) organized a book around the themes of work and love in adulthood, based on Freud's definition of maturity as the "capacity to love and work."

How can we, as counselors, best help adults understand, explore, and cope? What will enable us to most effectively assist adults as they change the situations—or the meaning of the situations—that need to be changed in their lives? How can we find the best way to support them in handling the stresses that accompany the changes?

One of the best ways of achieving these goals is to connect a knowledge of adult development perspectives to our already acquired helping skills. The more we as counselors and other practitioners know about normal adult development, the more effective we can make our responses and programs. Connecting a theoretical knowledge base to our practical counseling skills helps us to be more creative, more tuned in, more connected to the "normal" adults we try to help.

Before we can focus on a framework for using adult development knowledge (see Chapters 2 and 3), we present an overview of four major theoretical perspectives: contextual, developmental, life span, and transition. This chapter serves as the foundation upon which the transition framework is based.

3

THEORETICAL APPROACHES TO UNDERSTANDING ADULTHOOD

All of us are theorists. We are continually making assumptions about whether or not we can change ourselves, partners, children, parents, or friends. The assumptions we make reflect our theories about adult behavior. In this chapter, we will compare the way different theorists explain adult behavior. Although we believe that transition theories offer the most useful framework, it is important to realize that they grow out of and include insights from the work of many others.

A theory is a set of abstract principles that can be used to predict facts and to organize them within a particular body of knowledge. A theory of adult development would thus suggest how cognition, personality, and other characteristics might change over an adult's life course. Ideally, theory should allow one to go beyond prediction to explain development, and should offer new ideas about how events not currently understood (like memory decline in old age) are related to things already understood.

The study of adulthood, however, has not yet produced such rigorous or ideal theories; current theories offer interesting but essentially untested predictions about the course of adult life. In our review of theoretical approaches, we place the four "perspectives" on adult development on a continuum according to the degree to which they encompass predictability or variability in the life course. Although these conceptual perspectives are discussed separately here, in actuality they overlap, interact, and build upon one another (Fassinger & Schlossberg, 1992).

The Contextual Perspective

The first perspective on our continuum—the contextual perspective— views adulthood primarily in relation to the context within which it occurs. For example, although dated, the study of bakery workers in France (Bertaux, 1982) illustrated the importance of context. According to this study, the individual life stories of the bakers and their wives were a direct result of the structure and nature of the work world in which they participated. Most bakery workers were "at their jobs at least six nights a week, at least nine hours per night (from 3:00 A.M., or earlier, to noon)." This meant that whether "they were from rural or urban backgrounds, Catholic or agnostic, fat or thin, married or single, "they worked at least 54 hours a week. As Bertaux stated, this fact:

> determined most of the rest of their lives: . . . weekly time budget, family life . . . health (which declines after age 40 because of long hours and working in front of an oven), [and] activities outside work . . . For bakery workers there is no reading, no participation in cultural activities, no movies; for, as they say, because of the chronic lack of sleep they tend to fall asleep "as soon as the lights are off." (p. 133)

This pattern of living, this same life story recurred over and over, "as a direct consequence of the structure of relations of production" (p. 134). Bertaux's position is relevant to those working with adults because it suggests ways to help people identify the social factors that may lie at the root of some of their personal problems.

Environment also has an impact on such transition problems as the popularly accepted "midlife crisis." Researchers like Rosenbaum (1979) and Kanter (1977) first challenged the popular view attributing the midlife crisis to an individual's confrontation with aging. They suggested an alternate view that focused on the impact of organizations on individuals. Rosenbaum plotted the pattern of a cohort's promotional mobility from 1962 to 1975 and studied the relation between promotion and age, controlling for sex, race, education, and level in the hierarchy. He found that promotion chances increased gradually for those without bachelor's degrees until age 35 or 40, and then gradually declined. Promotion chances for those with bachelor's degrees, however, reached a peak of over 60% at about age 35 and then declined abruptly to less than 20% five to ten years later. Thus, Rosenbaum concluded that the promotion selection system tended to withdraw active consideration from those with bachelor's degrees after age 40. Such precipitous decreases in people's chances for promotion are likely to be traumatic and, therefore, conducive to the psychological reactions that are often attributed to midcareer or midlife crisis. Kanter corroborated Rosenbaum's position. She postulated that people's problems stem basically from organizational structures rather than from intrapsychic issues. She "locates a large measure of the responsibility for the behaviors people engage in at work and their fate inside organizations in the structure of the work systems themselves" (p. 10).

Occupational environment factors affecting personality and learning capacity were also identified by Kohn (1980). Twelve dimensions significantly affect psychological functioning when all other pertinent factors are statistically controlled. The most important of these dimensions is substantive complexity, which may be defined as "the degree to which the work, in its very substance, requires thought and independent judgment" (p. 197). Individuals whose work is substantively complex demonstrate stronger intellectual functioning over time.

Some recent theorists have begun to examine the impact of context on individual lives in an even broader perspective, namely, the state. Mayer and Schoepflin (1989), for example, presented an interesting analysis of the way in which the state, through legislation, social programs, and economic regulation, provides a general framework for the individual life course. They maintained that the state sets the boundaries for entry into and exit out of the educational system, marriage, occupational structure, and even illness and disability, effectively turning these personal transitions into public life events. In their view the need for efficient administration of the legal, social, and economic order leads to more rigid age stratification, weakened social bonds, and an external rather than individually created order throughout life. They were concerned that the institutional order determining much of the social fabric of our lives may lead increasingly to the irrelevance of the person and his/her biographical contexts. This in turn may cause people to become passive rather than active in planning the course of their lives.

Another view of the impact of context comes from Hagestad and Neugarten (1985). They stated that cultures have different age systems that "comprise norms which regulate status and role occupancy across the span of life. For the individual, such norms provide a scheduled set of transitions . . . they create a sense of what lies ahead" (p. 3). Nearly all cultures celebrate rites of passage for birth, puberty, marriage, death, and other predictable punctuation marks of the life course. Many of these changes in social identity lead to "new social roles, rights, and obligations" (Hagestad & Neugarten, 1985). Hagestad (1986), for example, outlined the way changing demographics have led to increased multigenerational sharing of lives and dramatic changes in the structure and demands of the family.

A full understanding of these transitions in the life course requires an examination of cultural age norms and age constraints as well as consideration of three kinds of time: individual, family, and historical (Hareven, 1992). For instance, a decision to have a baby appears to be an individual couple's decision; yet the decision is dependent on the social and demographic factors operating in the couple's culture at a particular time.

As an example of the impact of historical time on adult transitions, Hiner (1985) compared the differences in Colonial and present-day responses to the death of one's child. He noted that high infant mortality rates during the 18th century had a profound impact on the character and duration of married life, particularly for women, who literally spent all of their adulthood bearing and raising children. Marriages were more frequent and of shorter duration, and the loss of a child was an expected reality of adult life. Hiner contrasted this with today's ideologies, which idealize long-term partnerships and fewer children. Loss of a child is an unexpected and particularly traumatic experience.

Neugarten and Neugarten (1987) emphasized that in order to understand a particular life history, one must view it in its appropriate historical context. Clearly, as historical times change, social prescriptions for age-appropriate behavior also may change. For example, people are living longer, and the postparental period has consequently lengthened considerably. At the same time, economic maturity for many young people is being delayed while a larger proportion of them attend college and go on to graduate or professional schools. Patterns for women have also changed radically, with most women now combining work and child-rearing. In some families child-rearing practices are changing as fathers slowly begin to share responsibility with their working wives.

These kinds of historical trends have a definite impact on the chronological and social norms for age-appropriate behavior, norms that appear to be blurring and loosening up in today's society (Neugarten & Neugarten, 1987). In adulthood, there seems to be little biological necessity for such norms; the most dramatic biological change after puberty is menopause, which itself has become surrounded by many emotional myths. Research, however, suggests that responses to menopause are closely tied to other midlife events (such as children leaving home), which in turn are very much influenced by environmental, cultural, and historical contexts.

This blurring of age-defined roles and tasks, often referred to as the "fluid life cycle," represents flexibility and freedom for many. Others, however—some of whom may appear in counselors' offices—find it difficult to adjust their timetables. For example, some young men and women may feel inadequate if they have not met their achievement and family goals by the age of 35, even though they are likely to live into their 80s. When people maintain traditionally defined internal timetables that are at odds with their actual situations, they are susceptible to anxiety and conflict (Neugarten & Neugarten, 1987).

Additionally, in a pluralistic society such as ours, subgroups may have their own age-normative systems. Factors such as race, socioeconomic status, disability, sexual orientation, and geographic location may determine differences in age-defined behavior (Hagestad & Neugarten, 1985). For example, the length of the "coming out" process for gay people (Fassinger, 1991) may delay the establishment of permanent relationships and the creation of families. Similarly, occupational prejudice and discrimination may impede and delay career attainment for specific minority groups. These variations become especially obvious when we attempt to apply general normative theories to our intervention efforts.

It is evident then that a body of literature is now accumulating in which researchers explain behavior by analyzing the social context in which it occurs. Regardless of the focus of investigative attention, the result is to examine individuals by also accounting for the sociological and ecological factors that affect them. As counselors, we must be aware of this school of adult development. Where appropriate, it can help us to recommend interventions designed to change the environment of clients or to alter the way clients cope with their environment.

The Developmental Perspective

The second perspective on the continuum, the developmental perspective, emphasizes the sequential nature of adult development and is the one most familiar to the lay public. Stage theories of development can be categorized into three types: those based on age; those based on the resolution of specific, crucial issues; and those—called domain-specific theories—that are related to the unfolding of ethical and moral, cognitive, ego, or various kinds of identity development. Again, it should be noted that overlap exists among these types, although they are presented here separately.

Development based on age. Levinson (1986) focused on relatively universal, age-linked developmental periods that unfold in an orderly sequence. Stable (structure-building) periods alternate with transitional (structure-changing) periods.

In 1969 Levinson began a longitudinal study with a group of 40 men, aged 35 to 45, who represented a wide variety of occupational and social characteristics. Levinson and his associates explored in depth six distinct periods, each closely linked to age. Extended and subsequent research has refined these six stages as follows:

1. Early Adult Transition or Leaving the Family (ages 16–20);
2. Entering the Adult World (ages 21–29);
3. Settling Down (ages 30–34);
4. Becoming One's Own Person (ages 35–39);
5. Midlife Transition (ages 40–42); and
6. Restabilization (ages 43–50).

Each period is characterized by its own developmental tasks. For instance, during the Settling Down period an individual is concerned with establishing a place in society (that is, affirming one's own integrity and becoming a full-fledged adult) and with advancing toward one's goals.

Levinson's formulations, which allow for individual variation, nonetheless emphasized an underlying sequential order and similarity. His findings showed "relatively low variability in the age at which every period begins and ends," and his later research (Levinson, 1989) suggested that the hypothesized patterns operate in women's lives as well. A review of four dissertation studies investigating the applicability of Levinson's theory to women's lives (Roberts & Newton, 1987), however, indicated limited support for the theory.

In these studies, women were found to progress through the same developmental periods at roughly the same ages as had men in Levinson's work. However, despite similarity in the timing of the periods and the nature of the developmental tasks, both the strategies for addressing the tasks and the outcomes were different for the women in these samples. The authors discussed the "split dreams" reported by these women, involving a generalized image of work and family rather than a specific image of self-in-occupational-role, as lending a tentative, provisional, and conflicted quality to women's lives throughout much of early adulthood and into middle age. The fact that women's choices were continually influenced by inner conflict entailed specific results: a sense of dissatisfaction with both family and career, requiring greater time and experiencing more difficulty in establishing an occupation, forming fewer mentor relationships, and a recurring perception of husbands as obstacles to their development. Thus, the life structures of these women appeared less stable than those of their male counterparts in

Levinson's studies because of the greater complexity in the dreams they attempted to integrate into their lives and the obstacles they encountered in doing so. This leads to a greater variety in the "seasons" of women's lives where the timing of family events plays a far more critical role than age-related changes. Findings such as these reflect a pattern consistent in empirical work on women's development—a shift away from age-based determinants of behavior stemming from the greater diversity of roles held by women relative to men and the increased complexity in living out those roles.

Several studies have shown how ethnic background interacts with Levenson's stages. Ross (1984), in a study of Mexican immigrants, found that subjects followed the general sequence hypothesized by Levinson, but differed dramatically in attained education (which influenced occupational choices), mentoring (with family members filling this role), occupational goals (with focus on providing security and independence), family (with strong ties to extended family), and transition (with transition to a new culture overshadowing later life transitions). In studies of Levinson's model as applied to African Americans, Ruffin (1989) and Gooden (1989) found mixed support. Ruffin's study of African American professional women found that racial identity strongly influenced the developmental phases, with the formation of intimacy especially salient during early adulthood, support for occupational goals sought in family and friendship networks rather than "mentors," and achievement aspirations related to becoming successful in a White world.

Gooden's research on professional and working class African American men found limitations in Levinson's theory with regard to both race and socioeconomic status. The school teachers in his study, for example, fit Levinson's theory better than did the "street men." Gooden also discussed the impact of victimization in the early lives of African American men in terms of difficulties in finding mentors, developing the capacity for intimate, long-term relationships, and forming and sustaining "the dream" in a context of limited opportunity and numerous obstacles. Gooden (1989) noted that African American adult development must be viewed in a context of "how individuals encounter and respond to social opportunities and restrictions in their efforts at forming a viable life" (p. 88)—a reminder of the strong impact of race and class in the life course. It would seem that theories of racial identity should be incorporated into age-related conceptualizations such as Levinson's if we are to understand the lives of racially diverse groups of adults. In this respect contextual and stage theories clearly interact.

Development based on the resolution of specific, crucial issues. Another view of adult development is that human beings pass through an invariable sequence of developmental stages that are not necessarily linked exactly with chronological age. Some people move through the stages faster than do others, and some people may become arrested at one stage and never successfully move on. Erikson (1950), for instance, postulated a well-known eight-stage progression in psychosocial development, each characterized by a crucial issue that must be successfully resolved before an individual can move on. The adult stages involve the issues of identity (vs. role diffusion), intimacy (vs. isolation), generativity (vs. stagnation), and ego integrity (vs. despair).

Erikson's work provided the backdrop for Vaillant's (1977) analysis of advantaged men in a 40-year longitudinal study of Harvard students. Vaillant added an additional stage, labeled "career consolidation." He also found that those men who were able to achieve intimacy were then able to deal effectively with their careers, which in turn led to the achievement of generativity and integrity. In Vaillant's (1982) longitudinal study of inner city men interviewed in 1940 and again in 1976, he found the same progression through Erikson's stages, although the external circumstances and details of life looked very different.

Erikson's work has also provided a context for the well-known "identity status" research (Josselson, 1987) that classified individuals into categories based on their identities. In a longitudinal study of 34 women, Josselson (1987) concluded that the different pathways women follow in their identity development tell more about women than merely examining their social roles. In other words, what is relevant is not whether a woman is a mother, a worker, a single parent, or childless, but rather the way in which the woman separates from family and anchors or commits to the adult world. Although there is no pure type, Josselson identified four general categories (or statuses) of women:

- Foreclosures are those women who stick with their families' expectations. These women often adopt their parents' standards and follow their career direction;
- Identity achievers are those who have tested new waters, are forging their own identities, and keep focusing on the future. These women are more concerned with their own view of themselves than the foreclosures who are more concerned with their parents' expectation;
- Moratoriums are those who struggle to make commitments but

have not found the right niche. While open to choice, they fear
too many options. They are struggling to find their own identity;
- Identity diffusions are those who are drifting and avoiding an
identity. This group has the most difficulty forming stable relationships. They are the most troubled.

Josselson asserted that women's development is tied to "relational
connections" (p. 169), and that women's identity achievement depends
on a process of differentiation within attachment—a process Josselson
termed "anchoring." Whether in the work, family, or social area, the
central aspect of identity for women appears to be the self-in-relation
rather than the self standing alone.

Domain-specific development. Another group of stage theorists view individuals as moving through domain-specific sequences of
stages. Each domain is characterized by a qualitative difference in the
way people view the world within that particular domain.

Based on extensive interviews with women, Belenky, Clinchy,
Goldberger, and Tarule (1986) postulated a developmental progression
by which women view the world:

1. silence, a voiceless position in which all knowledge is subject
   to external authority;
2. received knowledge, in which the individual can receive and
   reproduce but not create knowledge;
3. subjective knowledge, in which knowledge is personal and private, subjectively known or intuited;
4. procedural knowledge, in which there is investment in objective procedures for obtaining and communicating knowledge;
   and
5. constructed knowledge, in which knowledge is seen as contextual, objective, and subjective strategies are valued, and the individual can see herself as a creator of knowledge.

Loevinger (1993) described a sequence of ego development in several stages. At the earliest self-protective stage, individuals conform, follow rules, and think in stereotypes; at a higher stage, individuals develop
increasing self-awareness and the capacity to think in terms of alterna-

tives, exceptions, and multiple possibilities; most mature is the autonomous stage, in which adults make commitments, tolerate ambiguities,
and incorporate opposites. Because people are at different stages of development, adults facing similar transition problems will process those
experiences differently—some in a simplistic way, others in a more complex, autonomous manner.

Kohlberg (1970) developed a well-known sequence of stages of
moral development similar to Loevinger's ego progression. In
Kohlberg's scheme, people move from being motivated to obey rules
by fear of punishment, to conforming to society, to being internally prin-
cipled and autonomous. Gilligan (1988) asserted that there are qualitative differences in the way men and women process and interpret the
world, and challenged Kohlberg's moral development theory on two
grounds: procedural and substantive.

Procedurally, Kohlberg's studies focused on men, but the results
were applied to both men and women. Substantively, Gilligan argued
that different issues are central in women's moral development: the issues of attachment, responsibility, caring, and interdependence. A
woman's moral development proceeds from concern for survival, to concern for responsibility and not hurting others, to seeing herself as mer-
iting care equally with others. Gilligan asserted that the view of
adulthood needs remapping, to show that caring and interdependence
are central to human experience.

Somewhat related to moral development are stages of spiritual faith
development, one of which was proposed by Fowler (1981). Fowler's
seven stages embrace the formal structural-developmental models proposed by Kohlberg and Piaget but differ in their emphasis on emotions,
feelings, and imagination. Fowler's stages move from the symbolic images of childhood, to the critical reflection, personal responsibility,
awareness of paradox and polarity, and selfless devotion that aware adults
are capable of experiencing.

In all of these limited-domain theories, development is viewed as
a progression from the simple to the complex. The movement is projected as going from an external orientation (the individual is dependent on the authority or judgment of others) to an inner orientation
(an individual takes responsibility for the consequences of his/her own
actions), from absolutism and dogmatism to increasing tolerance for
ambiguity and uncertainty, from a tendency to perceive those outside
one's own immediate group in stereotypic terms to increasing awareness of individual differences and greater empathy with others, and from

a strong posture of group conformity to a mature focus on interdependence with others.

One area of limited-domain theories gaining increasing attention involves "identity development theories" referring to one's membership in a particular (often societally oppressed) group. In explicit recognition that identity is a "social psychological concept" (Deaux, 1993)—that is, largely socially determined—these models are especially important in counseling. Identity theories aid both clients and professionals in understanding, predicting, and normalizing experiences, as well as in identifying difficulties that may stem from developmental processes and tasks (Fassinger, 1991). In addition, they help members of oppressed groups identify and articulate their needs and responses vis-a-vis their own group as well as the larger culture, and they aid counselors in sorting out issues that arise in the therapeutic relationship.

One group of such theories is related to racial/ethnic identity development. Initial work in this area focused on the development of activism and racial identification of African Americans in the political upheaval of the 1960s. Later work (Helms, 1985, 1990) focused on extending this work to counseling situations. Models of the racial identity have also been applied to Asians and Hispanics (Sue & Sue, 1990; Szapocznik & Kurtines, 1993).

Helms (1985) pointed out that all of these racial identity models posit from three to five stages and propose an on-going conflict between one's internal views of two groups—one's own and that of the dominant culture. These models also assume that the identity transformation process is set in motion by a social movement that makes it possible for minority group members to rebel against socialization experiences and seek new ways of being. Assumptions that underlie these models include:

1. The notion of biculturality;
2. the idea that minority groups develop model personality patterns in response to white racism;
3. the belief that some styles of identity resolution are healthier than others;
4. the sense that these stages are distinguishable and can be assessed;
5. the assumption that affective, cognitive, and behavioral elements are involved;

6. and the conviction that cultural identification affects both intra-
    and inter-cultural interaction (Helms, 1985).

Most of these models begin with a lack of awareness of one's racial identity, even denigrating one's own culture and idealizing white
culture. The next stages involve confrontation with the reality of oppression, subsequent immersion in one's racial group, and rejection of the
dominant white group. The final stages involve the internalization of
identity, increased self-esteem, and interpersonal relationships which are
not restricted by race or social group membership. As Helms pointed
out, these theories are essentially cognitive theories, with identity transformation dependent on a combination of personal readiness, prior
cultural socialization experiences, and educational experiences.

As our field becomes increasingly aware of other oppressed groups,
efforts to extend these models have led to generic models of the cultural identification process. Models of women's identity (Peck, 1986),
feminist identity (Downing & Rousch, 1985), and gay identity (McCarn
& Fassinger, 1991) have been developed, several of them built on the
earlier models of racial identification. There are significant differences,
however. Racial minority identity development involves changing attitudes toward the meaning of an apparent identity and typically occurs
within the context of potential family and community support. Other
kinds of identity development (gay and feminist identity, for example)
involve a new awareness and articulation of a personal identity that is
often not supported in one's environment.

Fassinger (1991) observed that gay identity development often involves the confrontation of both external and internalized oppression.
It occurs over and over in situations where an individual's sexual orientation is ambiguous, and frequently involves a context of overt prejudice, lack of family support, and few if any role models. Gays of many
racial/ethnic groups also risk potential loss of their primary racial community. Integrating the experience of people who struggle with marginality and biculturalism into our clinical work challenges us as
counselors and can transform and enrich our understanding of human
behavior.

In summary, developmental theories cover many areas, but have
in common the assumption that people's development—whether cognitive, moral, spiritual, ethnic, or psychological—progresses through
predictable stages.

The Life-Span Perspective

The third perspective on our continuum—the life-span perspective—focuses on individuality and issues of continuity and change. Some theorists see continuity among individuals over the course of life; others see so many individual pathways that variability becomes the cornerstone of adulthood. Kagan (1980), for example, wondered why social scientists have invested so much effort in a search for stability and continuity. He questioned the premise that information about a growing child is sufficient to explain his or her life course. In examining conclusions about a Berkeley longitudinal study in which 166 people were observed from birth through adulthood, he noted: "When the subjects were seen at age 30, 12 years after their previous interviews, the researchers were shocked by the inaccuracy of their expectations. They were wrong in two-thirds of the cases, mainly because they had overestimated the damaging effects of early troubles" (1980, p. 64). Counselors who are aware of this can caution adults against using early problems as a rationale for being "stuck" and not taking responsibility for their actions as adults.

Neugarten (1982) also emphasized variability, which she called individual fanning out. She pointed out, for example, that 10-year-olds are more similar to each other than are 60-year-olds, and stated:

> Perhaps the most consistent finding to emerge from the study of aging is that people grow old in very different ways. [There are] . . . striking variations between successive groups who reach old age . . . between ethnic . . . urban and rural, and . . . socioeconomic groups. This is to say nothing of the idiosyncratic sequences that widen the divergence among individuals. The result is that 60-year-olds or 80-year-olds are extremely heterogeneous groups. (1982, p. 6)

Pearlin (1982), in his work on strain and coping, echoed Neugarten's emphasis on individuality and variation. He maintained that human variety is as rich as people's historic conditions and current circumstances, and that even within the same cohort, the impact of conditions may differ because of variations in coping responses. Thus, in his view it was untenable to speak of either ages or life stages as though undifferentiated people were following a uniform life course. Pearlin and Lieberman (1979) found that the adult experience differs according to whether an individual is a man or woman, member of a minority or a majority group, young or old, rich or poor, healthy or ill.

Pearlin also argued that one life phase or event should not be overly dramatized, and cited the "midlife crisis" as a case in point. It is known that crises can occur at any period and that, in fact, young adults have more strains on them than do other age groups. Yet the media and some writers continue to dramatize a crisis in midlife, the inevitability of which is not corroborated by hard data. Pearlin's caution applies to any theoretical perspective; overemphasizing any particular life event, period, or transition (like retirement or the birth of a child) risks categorizing people as if they were all the same.

Brim and Kagan (1980) championed a life-span development approach. Their view opposed stage theories, because "stages cast development as unidirectional, hierarchical, sequenced in time, cumulative, and irreversible—ideas that are not supported by commanding evidence" (p. 13). Life-span theorists identify life events as markers, milestones, or transition points, that play a pivotal role in individual development, giving shape and direction to the various aspects of each individual's life.

Whitbourne (1985) was another theorist who addressed coping and adaptation over the life-span. She saw adaptation as the result of a continuous evaluation of life experiences rather than reactions to discrete events. An individual's life-span construct is subject to change as the individual meets experiences that contradict it or are totally incongruent with it. For instance, the act of coping itself may result in an altered life story as individuals distort the meaning of events toward the maintenance of their self-esteem. Coping may also alter an individual's aspiration levels toward greater congruence with his/her environment when it is clear that failure to achieve aspirations does not stem from the individual's inadequacy. Thus, in this model, the adaptation process takes on different configurations depending on whether an event is consistent or inconsistent with an individual scenario.

Another area in which a life-span transitional approach offers promise is that of death and dying. Kastenbaum (1985) criticized stage theories of dying (e.g., Kübler-Ross, 1969) as not empirically valid and inadequate in their emphasis on predicting phases of response to immediate crisis. He argued that ideas of futurity and death are important from middle childhood on, well before advanced age or the close prospect of death are encountered. Presenting historical information as well as empirical research, Kastenbaum explored the increasing discrepancy between social expectations and immediate reality as an individual ages. He asserted that our attitudes toward the elderly may represent a special case of equity theory in which we ascribe certain psychological or spiritual qualities to the aged and dying to compensate for their failing health, lowered status, and imminent demise. Kastenbaum maintains that if aging individuals are to maintain a sense of continuity and selfhood over their entire life-span, they must learn ways to manage transitions around death and loss.

Theories of individual development also need to be seen in the light of gender differences, an area of burgeoning research in the past several decades. Although detailed discussion is beyond the scope of this chapter, differences in behavior and maturity that are ascribed to men and women are often the most striking differences among individuals. We return to Gilligan's (1988) work. Based on her findings that responsibility and care are central to her subjects' lives, she saw interdependence as a critical component of adult development. The view of the heroic individual marching up a sequence of stages and ladders is no longer adequate but must be replaced by a view of the individual renegotiating interdependence in ever-changing circles of attachment.

In a widely cited study on differences between women and men, Fiske and Chiriboga (1990) found that the women in their sample generally had less positive self-images than did the men, felt less in control of their lives, and were less likely to plan for transitions. At the same time, their affective lives were richer and more complex, and they had a greater tolerance for ambiguity. Men anticipated placing more value on expressive and interpersonal goals as they grew older, whereas women expected to direct their interests outward and to become more concerned with contributing to society and doing good in the world. The "crisscrossing trajectories" of men and women at successive stages reflect different types of developmental changes, as well as different scheduling. Gutmann supported these notions in his cross-cultural study of older men and women (1987).

The Transition Perspective

The fourth theoretical perspective in adulthood—the transition perspective—focuses on life events entailing change. Fiske and Chiriboga (1990) conducted a longitudinal study of what they labeled "ordinary people"— four groups of men and women in San Francisco: 1) graduating high

school seniors, 2) newlyweds, 3) middle-aged parents, and 4) preretirement couples, each group obviously on the threshold of a major transition at the start of the study. These individuals were interviewed five
times over a twelve-year period. The overriding question—how do adults
change over time—was answered in a number of ways. They found that
the groups differed considerably in their general outlook on life, the
stresses they faced, and their attitudes toward those stresses. The researchers concluded that it is less important to know that a person is
40 years old than it is to know that a person is 40, has adolescent children, is recently divorced, is about to retire, and so on. Men facing retirement, for example, encounter many of the same problems whether
they retire at age 50, 60, or 70. Newly partnered individuals of any age
are engaged in similar tasks of bonding, discovery, and negotiation. In
short, transitions are more important than chronological age for understanding and evaluating an individual's behavior.

Schlossberg (e.g., 1981, 1991) presented a transitional model that
incorporated both anticipated transitions—the scheduled, expected
events that are likely to occur for the individual and that can be anticipated and rehearsed—and unanticipated transitions—the nonscheduled
events that are not predictable. This model, described in detail in Chapters 2 and 3, is the cornerstone of this book.

The cognitive appraisal model emphasizes a transactional process
by which individuals adapt to events by viewing them as subjective phe-
nomena that impact on their psychological well-being (Lazarus &
Folkman, 1984). This model assumes that an individual appraises the
significance of an event for its possible impact on his/her well-being,
determines what personal and social resources are available for dealing with the event and what the consequences are likely to be, and re-
assesses both the situation and his/her responses after action has been
taken. The coping modes adopted can be instrumental (changing the
environment) or palliative (minimizing individual distress).

APPLYING THE THEORETICAL PERSPECTIVES

Table 1.1 illustrates that counselors' theoretical perspectives do, in fact,
influence (1) their assessments of an individual's behavior; and (2) their
plans for intervention.

Let's take the following two cases: one, a white, midlife male, the
other, a lesbian woman giving birth to a baby.

Table 1.1 The Adult Experience: Perspectives and Concepts

Contextual	Developmental	Life Span	Transitional
Rosenbaum • Career mobility results from organization structure • Midlife crisis, a sociological phenomenon Kanter • Individual progress determined by opportunity structure Kohn • Intellectual capacity dependent on substantive complexity at work Neugarten and Neugarten • Cultures provide age systems and age norms • Fluid life cycle today Hareven • Importance of historical period in setting norms and constraints	**Age** Levinson • Invariant sequence of developmental stages • Life structure, dream, mentor **Resolution of Issues** Erikson; Gooden; Josselson • Unfolding of life and resolving of inner issues • Identified hierarchical stages • Different issues for women, for African Americans **Domain Specific** Loevinger; Kohlberg; Belenky; Gilligan • Hierarchical sequence in ego development, moral development, intellectual development • Different ways of knowing for men and women Gilligan; Fassinger • Critique of models based on white males and applied to other groups Fowler • Faith follows a sequential pattern Cross; Helm • Models of racial identity	Neugarten • Individual variations • Fanning out • Fluid life span Vaillant • Early trauma not predictive of later behavior Pearlin and Lieberman • Variability • Differential distribution of strains by sex, age, different patterns of coping Brim; Kagan • Perspective, not theory • Opposed to life stages • Study impact of events and mediating variables	Lowenthal (Fiske); Chiriboga • Stage, not age • Coping with transitions: balance of resources to deficits • Sex differences Pearlin; Lazarus • Coping, not life events, is central issue • Classification of life strains and coping responses Kastenbaum • Face issues of loss and death Schlossberg • Balance of resources to deficits

Case of the Midlife Male

Well, I really don't—I really don't know where to begin. I don't know what I am going to say to you. My name is Stan and I'm 40 years old. I just got this feeling that I'm kind of just dead-end, you know? I got a job, it's all right, but there is no future. And I see younger men getting ahead of me. Here I have a house, a mortgage, I don't have the freedom to move as they do, but yet I get passed over for promotions. I got a good job, but it is going nowhere; it's just absolutely becoming part of my life that I don't like. I come to work, I do my job, I go home—there's no challenge. It's just kind of humdrum, I've done it many times before. But if I saw someplace I could move, someplace I could go, someplace I could get ahead, do some of the things I really wanted to do when I started in this organization. That's what I want. I don't know whether you are the person to help me or not, but it's just getting to me. I don't know where to turn. I don't know what I can do with my life at this particular juncture. The kids are getting older, I'm becoming less necessary there; you look at this organization, I'm becoming less necessary here. It's not much fun working here anymore, not much fun working, work is not what it used to be. I think I've got a lot to offer, I just don't know where I can go with it. Do you understand what I am saying, can you help me? I've just got to do something. I've got to move, got to grow.

It is possible to look at Stan's crisis from each of the perspectives discussed in this chapter and outlined in Table 1.1.

Those using the contextual perspective might describe Stan's crisis as a result of the organizational context. Instead of viewing his "midlife crisis" as a confrontation with aging, they might view his situation as a direct result of the impact of his work environment on him. He feels frustrated at not receiving promotions; this frustration is realistic since the promotion selection system in his company is probably focusing more on younger employees. His dismay resulted from options being closed, his crisis resulted from the cultural vision he held of younger men being promoted over him.

The other contexts that help explain Stan's crisis are social, family, and historical contexts. The social context says that men are expected to be promoted if they are worthy; Stan may feel a lack of self-worth because he is not being promoted. His family may be totally financially dependent on him; this context might make him feel stuck in a situation that is not fulfilling for him. The historical context may involve the idea that men are expected to stay with one company, climb the corporate ladder, and be the sole family supporter.

The intervention models suggested by contextual counselors might focus on changing either the context of Stan's work or changing Stan's reactions to his contexts.

Developmental counselors might ascribe his crisis to normal developmental unfolding. As a white male, Stan can be easily placed into one of the developmental theory's stages. For example, according to Levinson, Stan is typical of men at midlife who are faced with the discrepancy between their goals and the realities of their lives. According to Gould, people of all ages can feel "stuck" and this seems to fit Stan's situation and his reaction to it. The developmental perspective would see Stan's experience as quite normal in the progression of life. Developmentalists might choose to explain this to Stan in an effort to normalize his experience. Intervention efforts would probably be short-term, focused on helping Stan to progress through this developmental stage into a more comfortable phase of his development.

The life-span theorists might see Stan as very much an individual whose life is unfolding in unique ways. These theorists would argue against fitting Stan into one of the above-mentioned theories. Instead they would regard Stan's life as unique and evaluate it accordingly. This means that intervention might focus on Stan's job situation, or his family environment, or his personal feelings of restlessness; however, none of these would be from the perspective of a formal theory, rather they would involve a creative approach to Stan's individual set of issues.

Those who ascribe to the transition framework would re-examine Stan's personal and work transitions, by assessing his resources for coping, and helping him expand his coping repertoire.

Case of The Lesbian Mother

My name is Sue and I'm 30 years old. I am so excited but scared at the same time. I've always wanted to have a baby, and I can't believe I'm finally pregnant. My partner, Lisa, and I have talked about having children ever since we started our relationship. When my ex-husband and I split up, I almost gave up my dream of having a baby—but now I'm going to have one. How exciting! But it's also scary. My parents don't even know about Lisa and me yet—how are they going to react to my pregnancy? And what do I tell my boss? Of course, he knows I'm divorced and I think he suspects I'm a lesbian, but won't this raise even more questions? What if I lose my job? I want this baby to have a happy and healthy family life—

what if kids tease him or her about having two moms instead of a mom and a dad? Am I making a mistake? No, I can't be.

Contextualists would see Sue's situation in the context of her job, her family, and other social or historical contexts. Her job context may include an unsupportive boss and work environment; her family context may include expectations that she remarry, negative opinions of her lifestyle, or it may prove supportive—this context is currently unknown but seems anxiety-provoking. The historical context dictates that babies be born to married men and women, and Sue's social context likely says the same, although she may have support from friends and/or the gay community. Again, contextual intervention would focus on either changing her work context or changing her reactions to the whole situation.

The developmental theorists would conceptualize Sue's case from one of several developmental perspectives. She is entering the age period, according to Levinson, of Settling Down. As a woman, this also incorporates inner conflict concerning family and career—conflict Sue does seem to be experiencing. A stage perspective theorist might put Sue in Erikson's intimacy versus isolation stage or the theorist might agree with Josselson that women's development is tied to "relational connections" so that Sue's stages of development depend on her identity in terms of her relation with others. Finally, the identity development theories would be most relevant here, especially those particular to lesbians, in order to identify the difficulties Sue may be encountering. Development intervention would center on helping Sue see the normality of her concerns about the anticipated difficulties, and providing support as she progresses through this developmental period.

Life-span theorists would approach Sue's case as unique, and examine her situation without trying to fit it into a formal theory. Therefore, intervention will vary based on the individual counselor's analysis of Sue's situation (DeVault Lahey, 1993).

Transition theorists would look at Sue's resources for coping with this transition into motherhood and the possible transition of "coming out" as a lesbian to her family and/or employer. Another important focus for transition theorists involves helping Sue help her family. Transitional intervention will focus on identifying sources of support and strengthening Sue's resources.

CONCLUSION

Examining our theories is important because it helps us clarify our views and assumptions about adult development. Our aim here was to provide a quick overview of different theories and to set the stage for showing how theory affects practice. As we develop the transition perspective, we will see how all the theories described so far feed into it, making it an eclectic theory that looks at context, development, and life-span.

2

The Transition Framework

Adults are individuals—some are healthy, some unhealthy; some sexually alive, others uninterested; some happy, some sad; some productive, others disintegrating; some coping, some collapsing. The transition framework presented in this book incorporates the notion of variability while at the same time assuring counselors and helpers that they need not approach each situation anew. Certain assumptions based on adult development theory and the helping skills influence the framework presented in this book:

- Adults in transition are often confused and in need of assistance. Often they can identify the issues that trouble them—they are "burned out," getting divorced, forced to change jobs, discriminated against. These issues in turn, often relate to their ability to love, work, and play. When they are able to explore the issue more fully, understand the underlying meaning, and develop a plan, they are more likely to be able to cope effectively and resolve the problem.
- Friends, co-workers, and professional and paraprofessional helpers *can* learn about issues of major concern to most adults; they can listen to the adult in transition in a way that facilitates exploration; they can provide a framework for the adult to better understand his/her situation; and, finally, they can influence the adult to cope more creatively.
- To help adults explore, understand, and cope, helpers need to increase their communications skills, their counseling skills, and their knowledge of adult development. In short, helpers need to be able to weave their skills and knowledge at each phase of

25

the helping process—whether it is exploring why the individual can or cannot love, work, or play; understanding the underlying reason for the issue; or developing strategies to cope more effectively with life.

OVERVIEW OF THE TRANSITION MODEL

The transition model provides a systematic framework for counselors, psychologists, social workers, and other helpers as they listen to the many stories—each one unique—of colleagues, friends, and clients. The transitions differ, the individuals differ, but the structure for understanding individuals in transition is stable.

The transition model has three major parts:

- Approaching Transitions: Transition Identification and Transition Process
- Taking Stock of Coping Resources: The 4 S System
- Taking Charge: Strengthening Resources

Approaching Transitions identifies the nature of the transition and provides an understanding of which perspective is best for dealing with it. Transition Identification asks what change is impending? A new baby, a job change, a personal change, a relationship change? Is it anticipated, unanticipated, or a non-event? Knowing more about it, and being able to describe it, helps get the discussion moving about what is troubling or challenginging a client. Even more important than the mere identification of the change is the specifying of the degree to which the particular transition changes the client's life. For instance, three people describing a similar transition—job loss—are not talking about the same event. To understand its significance, the counselor needs to see how the job loss has changed each individual's roles, relationships, routines, and assumptions.

The Transition Process locates where the adult is in the transition. Did the client just learn of the impending job loss? Is the person in the first week after the job loss? Or is it a year after the loss? Reactions to any transition change over time depending on whether one is *moving in, through,* or *out of* the transition.

Taking Stock of Coping Resources—The 4 S System—provides a way to identify the potential resources someone has to cope with the

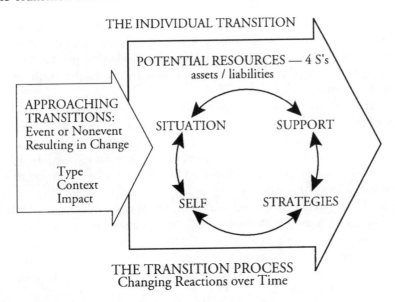

THE INDIVIDUAL TRANSITION

POTENTIAL RESOURCES — 4 S's
assets / liabilities

APPROACHING
TRANSITIONS:
Event or Nonevent
Resulting in Change

Type
Context
Impact

SITUATION   SUPPORT

SELF   STRATEGIES

THE TRANSITION PROCESS
Changing Reactions over Time

FIGURE 2.1 The individual in transition.

transition. The 4 S's refer to the person's **S**ituation, **S**elf, **S**upport, and **S**trategies. No matter where one is in the transition process, no matter what the transition is, one deals with it differently depending on these 4 S's.

Taking Charge: Strengthening Resources demonstrates the use of new strategies. Even though some transitions are out of our control, we can control the way we manage them—we can strengthen our resources, our 4 S's.

Figure 2.1, The Indiviual in Transition, depicts the model. Part 1, Approaching Transitions—the Transition Identification and The Transition Process—is detailed in this chapter. Taking Stock of The Coping Resources, The 4 S System, is described in Chapter 3. The rest of this book, particularly chapters 7, 8, and 9, describes the many ways counselors can help people "take charge."

APPROACHING TRANSITIONS

A transition, broadly, is any event, or non-event, that results in changed relationships, routines, assumptions, and roles. Transitions often require new patterns of behavior, but we prefer not to use the term "crisis" because of its negative connotations. A transition may well be a life event that involves gains as well as losses. Moreover, "crisis" implies a dramatic event, and we need also to be concerned with less high-profile events as well as non-events.

Transitions include not only obvious life changes (such as high school graduation, job entry, marriage, birth of the first child, bereavement) but also subtle changes (such as the loss of career aspirations or the non-occurrence of anticipated events, such as an expected job promotion that never comes through). Thus an event or a non-event can be a transition if it results in change.

Parkes (1971) proposed the term, *psychosocial transition,* which he defined as a change that necessitates "the abandonment of one set of assumptions and the development of a fresh set to enable the individual to cope with the new altered life space" (p. 103). The term *transition* is also preferred by other authorities. According to Spierer, a transition is any change that has:

> important consequences for human behavior . . . These transitions may be due to biological, sociological, environmental, historical, or other phenomena. They may have consequences that are evident now or are manifested at some future date (and thus have "sleeper effects"). They may be evident to friends and to society (going bald, becoming rich, losing a job) or remain unnoticed—although still dramatic—such as losing one's career aspirations. They may be sudden or, more likely, cumulative, as is true for example, of some diseases." (Spierer, 1977, p. 6)

A transition is not so much a matter of change as of the individual's own perception of the change. For our definition, a transition is a transition only if it is so defined by the person experiencing it. If, for example, menopause does not have much impact on a particular woman, and does not change her set of assumptions or her relationships, then, in our view, it cannot be regarded as a psychosocial transition (though, of course, it is a biological change). If, however, another woman experiences menopause as an event that marks her passage from youth to old age or from sexuality to nonsexuality, it does constitute a transition for her. For yet another woman who sees it as freedom from the necessity of using birth control, it is also a transition, albeit a positive one.

Types of Transitions

The first step in approaching a transition is to identify the type of transition that has happened or is happening: Was it anticipated or unanticipated?, or is it a non-event?

Anticipated transitions. These transitions comprise those normative "gains and losses or major alterations of roles that predictably occur in the course of the unfolding life cycle" (Pearlin & Lieberman, 1979, p. 220). These expected events include marriage, the birth of a first child, a child leaving home, starting a first job, and retiring.

Unanticipated transitions. These transitions comprise the "nonscheduled events" that are "not predictable." These usually "involve crises, eruptive circumstances, and other unexpected occurrences that are not the consequence of life-cycle transitions" (Pearlin, 1980, p. 179). "Events of this type in the occupational arena include being fired, laid off, or demoted; having to give up work because of illness . . . being promoted, and leaving one job for a better one. Divorce, separation . . . premature death of a spouse, . . . illness or death of a child represent such events in the parental arena" (p. 180).

Brim and Ryff (1980) made another useful distinction between events that have a high probability of occurrence in the life of the individual (getting married, starting work, having a child, retiring) and those which are improbable and happen to comparatively few people (inheriting a fortune, being convicted of a crime, having one's home destroyed by an earthquake or flood). Brim asserted that we need to "search for hidden unnamed events" because the more events we can identify, the better people can be prepared to deal with them through anticipatory socialization. During the 1993 floods in the Midwest, people all over the country began to discuss what possessions they would save given only three hours notice.

Non-event transitions. These transitions are the ones an individual had *expected* but which did not occur, thereby altering his or her life—the marriage that never occurred, the promotion that never materialized, the child who was never born, the cancer that did not metastasize. For example, a couple who had counted on having children may finally, in their mid-forties, realize that this will not occur. The realization that the expected transition did not and will never occur alters the way they see themselves and might well alter the way they behave. Generally, four types of non-events can be identified: personal, ripple, resultant, and delayed.

Personal non-events refer to individual aspirations and might include not having a baby, not being promoted, or never marrying. A person who has been in the same job for 20 years might present an example of nothing happening externally, yet everything changing internally— that is, the person's assumptions about competency and identity are gradually shaken.

Ripple non-events refer to the unfulfilled expectations of someone close to us, which, in turn, alters our own roles, relationships, and assumptions. In an interview, the parents of two young adults describe their children to friends as "just fine." Yet they are upset because neither child is married. The parents are in their late 60s and are not the grandparents or in-laws they expected to be. What is not happening to the adult children means that certain expected events are not happening to the parents. As we examine such disappointments more closely, we see that a non-event for one individual may ripple significantly into another's life.

Resultant non-events begin with an event that leads to a non-event. Take the example of the mother who gives birth to a child with a severe disability. From this traumatic event may come the resultant non-event of never being able to have another child, for physical, financial, or emotional reasons. Or consider a rejection from medical school: the resultant non-event, of course, is not becoming a physician. The events themselves have a beginning and an end. Not being a physician can last a lifetime.

Delayed non-event transitions are characterized as those, like marriage, that still might happen. Thus, an event or non-event can be somewhat planned, somewhat unplanned. It may be more useful for us to think of these transitions—anticipated, unanticipated, non-event—as being on a change–no-change continuum rather than as discrete entities. In other words, the issue is how much they have altered one's life.

It would be interesting to find out how the same person copes with anticipated, unanticipated, and non-event transitions. George and Siegler wrote, "We . . . hypothesize that imposed, unexpected, and negative events, as well as those that involve a high degree of change, will be more stressful and more likely to lead to negative outcomes than those that are chosen, expected, positive, and involve little behavioral disruption" (1981, p.29).

To summarize types of transitions: Retirement when the plant closes may be unanticipated, although for many retirement is anticipated. For those forced by economic necessity to continue working (and who are able to find work), retirement is a wished-for but non-occurring non-event. Retirement may also be a worry which supercedes all other issues. Thus it is not the transition itself that determines its meaning for the individual; rather it is whether the transition is expected, unexpected, or never occurring. Clearly, one person may be thrilled at a non-event (such as rediagnosis of no cancer) but another may be very sad with the realization that a promotion is not ever likely.

Several other points about types of transitions need to be mentioned. These points involve the concepts of relativity, context, and impact.

Relativity. An anticipated change for one person—going to college—might be unanticipated for another. For example, a school janitor who had always wanted to go to college anticipated never having that opportunity. On the day the last child graduated from the college, the family presented the father/janitor with an application blank filled out for the state university. He completed several years of college and was, at our last interview, an emergency substitute teacher. A non-event for one person—not getting married—can be a planned decision for another and not a transition at all.

As mentioned, the same event has different meanings for different individuals. George and Siegler (1981) interviewed 100 adults over age 50 asking them to identify the best and worst events of the past year, as well as of their whole lives. For one person retirement was "the best," for another "the worst." For some it was planned; for others unexpected.

Lazarus and Folkman (1984) defined transition as a transaction between the individual and environment. The individual's appraisal of the transition is key. Does the individual see it as positive, negative, or benign? One person might define retirement as positive, a challenge, an opportunity. Another might see it as the next step before dying, the end of a productive life. One's appraisal will clearly influence how one feels and copes with the transition or non-event.

Context

The relationship of the individual to the event or non-event resulting in change is central to our understanding of transitions. Does the primary event start with the individual (his or her illness) or with some other person (his or her boss's illness)? Is the transition personal (the individual has lost his or her job) or interpersonal (the individual has had a disagreement with his or her employer)? Or is the transition involved with the public or the community (does the individual feel disgraced by having to go on unemployment)?

Often if something is happening to an individual, he/she can mobilize resources and affect the transition process positively. But if something is happening to someone else—doom impending for an adult child—the individual often can only sit by, suffer, and offer support. We need to note that many feel the tragedies and excitements happening to their children as if they were happening to themselves.

What is the arena in which the transition occurs? Pearlin, working with others, wrote: "The problems of everyday life" are identified as the "persistent life strains that people encounter as they act as parents, jobholders, and breadwinners (Pearlin & Schooler, 1978, p. 3).

The researchers identified key strains in the areas of occupation, marriage, and parent roles by interviewing 100 people in an unstructured manner and then developing a structured interview with 2300 people between the ages of 18 and 65 living in the Chicago area. Further, they showed the differential impact of life strains on different segments of the population (Pearlin & Lieberman, 1979). This useful way of viewing various arenas of life—occupation, marriage, parenthood—in terms of unexpected "non-normative events" and expected normative and persistent problems can be extended to other arenas, such as economics, health, and education. Of course, what starts out as personal and economic—lack of income through the job loss—can also affect family relationships and precipitate other transitions.

To summarize context in transitions: Our own retirement, our spouse's retirement, and the local mayor's retirement all produce reactions. The primary setting for the retirement transition also affects our reactions. The transition may involve the self, friends, family, work, health, or economics. In the George and Siegler (1981) study, individuals chose their best and worst life experiences. Most of these experiences resided in the family setting, followed by self and work. Worst life events were typically in the health setting, followed by family and self. Retirement can be a "best" experience if it makes possible a long-desired trip, or it may be a "worst" experience if it is necessitated by ill health.

Impact

For an individual undergoing a transition, it is not the event or non-event that is most important but its impact, that is, the degree to which the transition alters one's daily life. Thus, when an event—a partner's business transfer involving a geographical move—creates problems for an individual, we need to look not only at the type and context but also at the impact of the event on the individual's relationships, routines, assumptions about self and the world, and roles. We may assume that the more the transition alters the individual's life, the more coping resources it requires, and the longer it will take for assimilation or adaptation. More empirical work must be done on events that happen to someone else but have impact on the individual we are trying to help. We need to distinguish those whose life patterns are changing because of others' transitions rather than their own.

One way of examining the impact of a transition is to assess the degree of difference between the pre-transition and the post-transition environments. Lieberman (1975), studying four groups of old people who made radical changes in living arrangements, concluded that the intensity of stress experienced depended not upon the individual's subjective interpretation of the change in living arrangements (whether it was welcomed or feared, whether regarded as a change for the better or the worse), but rather:

> ... upon the degree to which an individual is required to make new adaptations associated with environmental change . . . The greater the difference between the Time 1 life space and the Time 2 life space, the higher the degree of stress and consequent adaptive requirements. (p. 151)

He found that the individual's success or failure in adapting to the new environment was strongly correlated with the similarity or dissimilarity of the pre-transition and post-transition environments, despite the individual's attitude toward or definition of the change.

Wapner compared pre-transition and post-transition environments ranging from nursery schools to nursing homes (1981). Each person lives in "multiple worlds" in the family, work, and community. Thus, positive, desired changes may have as great or even greater impact as negative ones because individuals may find it harder to recognize the need for support in such situations.

Wapner's "psychological distance map" (1981, p. 225) provided a graphic opportunity to compare the interactions in the old and new environments. By using such maps, we can look, for example, at families who move geographically and ascertain the degree to which they maintain prior contacts as well as the number of new contacts made. Thus, we have a better idea of the impact of the transition on relationships, routines, assumptions, and roles. A person who moves or enters a nursing home, who is able to maintain most of his or her former contacts, will experience the transition very differently from someone who loses all contacts.

Parkes (1971), however, believed that changes in the "life space" are important only insofar as they affect the individual's "assumptive world," which includes "everything we know or think we know. It includes our interpretation of the past and our expectations of the future, our plans and our prejudices. Any or all of these may need to change as a result of changes in the life space" (p. 103). The life space is changing constantly, but not all these changes call for a major restructuring of the assumptive world.

This conflicts with the views of theorists like Holmes and Rahe (1967), who originally showed the impact of multiple life events on physical health. To study this, they developed a Social Readjustment Rating Scale (1967) that assigns numerical values to different kinds of life events, with "death of a spouse" ranking at the top of the scale and such items as "vacation," "Christmas," and "minor violations of the law" at the bottom. The Holmes-Rahe scale ascertains the probable degree of stress connected with a given life event and its relationship to an individual's general state of mental and physical health. The cumulative numerical values of the life events that a person experiences during a given period of time—for example, a year—serve as an index of that person's general health. The person who has gone through a number of changes in a relatively short period of time is more vulnerable to illness.

But as Dohrenwend and associates pointed out, the Holmes-Rahe scale must be used with reservation (Dohrenwend, Krasnoff, Askenasy, & Dohrenwend, 1978). In the first place, the numerical values represent empirically derived averages and are subject to individual variation. Thus, a person who has suffered the loss of a loved one around Christmas time may for many years afterwards find the holiday season more stressful than other events given a higher value on the scale.

In the second place, the stressfulness of a particular event depends not so much on the event itself as on the balance between a person's liabilities and assets at the time the event occurs. The Peri Life Events Scale (Dohrenwend et al., 1978, p. 205) expands the Holmes-Rahe scale by including 102 items covering such categories as school, legal matters, finances, social activities, and health; it also differentiates between whether the event happened to the individual directly or to a significant other. Finally, the important point is that the birth of a baby, say, will have different meanings for the newly widowed or newly fired person than for a person in a relatively quiescent period.

To summarize impact: Assessment of a transition's impact on relationships, routines, assumptions, and roles is probably the most important consideration in understanding a given situation. For example, think of a retirement transition and its impact on such factors as self, family, friends, health, work or economics. As we assess the impact on each, we may find that in some cases retirement affects family more than self, or health more than economics.

Summary

To understand the meaning a transition has for a particular individual, we need to examine the type of transition (anticipated, unanticipated, or non-event), the context of the transition (relationship of person to transition, setting in which the transition occurs), and the impact of the transition on the individual's life (on relationships, routines, assumptions, roles). This point needs to be further underscored. Often people in the midst of one transition experience other transitions, which makes coping especially difficult. One man forced to take early retirement, explained that it was particularly difficult since that year his wife left him and his father had moved in because of a debilitating illness.

THE TRANSITION PROCESS

Although the onset of a transition may be linked to one identifiable event or non-event, transitions are really a process over time. Six months, a year, sometimes two years pass before one moves fully through a major transition. For example, if you interview a person before a move, during the move, six months after the move, and again two years later, you will get entirely different responses. Reactions continually change. The only way to understand people in transition is to study them at several points in time.

Transitions may provide both opportunities for psychological growth and dangers of psychological decline. For example, some of the elderly subjects who moved to nursing homes (Lieberman, 1975) "remained intact in the face of radical environmental change" (p. 156), "whereas about half suffered marked declines behaviorally, physically (including death), socially, or psychologically" (p. 142).

Interviews with men whose jobs had been eliminated (Schlossberg & Leibowitz, 1980), with couples who had recently undertaken geographical moves, with adult learners in undergraduate programs (Schlossberg, Lynch, & Chickering, 1989), and with clerical workers (Charner & Schlossberg, 1986) confirmed that the transition process often has both positive and negative aspects for the same individual.

In the job elimination study, one man saw his job loss as a "kick in the back" but at the same time recognized it as an "opportunity to get out of both my job and my marriage." Another man reported feeling "a little shaky but at the same time hopeful." In the geographical study, one woman talked about the miserable experience of moving: "I kept thinking, if only I were back home," but at the same time she described the move as an opportunity for her husband and herself to break away from their families, with whom they were "almost too close." The ambivalent nature surrounding many transitions explains the different stories a person tells a helper or friend at one point in time and two months or a year later.

Lipmen-Blumen (1976) described the transition process as moving from "pervasiveness" (an awareness that the transition permeates all of a person's attitudes and behaviors), to "boundedness" (the change is contained and integrated into the self). Thus, in the early stages, a person is totally conscious of being a new graduate, a new widower, a new mother. In the later stages, the person is aware of having graduated, having been widowed, having become a mother—but this awareness has become only one of the dimensions of living. Knowing this makes it easier for a counselor to help a client see a light at the end of the proverbial tunnel.

White turned his attention to the time dimension of adaptation. He stated that an individual's ability to adapt should not be judged on the basis of short-term observations: "Strategy is not created on the instant. It develops over time and is progressively modified in the course of time" (1976, p. 29). Similarly, Moos and Tsu (1976) identified two phases to the transition process: "An acute phase in which energy is directed at minimizing the impact of the stress, and a reorganization phase in which the new reality is faced and accepted. In the acute period feelings may be denied while attention is directed to practical matters . . . The reorganization phase involves the gradual return to normal function" (pp. 14–15). Hill (1965) believed that reaction to crisis takes a roller-coaster form: the crisis event occurs, the individual dips down into a period of disorganization, then gradually rises up again, and levels off into a period of reorganization.

There is also a wealth of literature dealing with human adaptation to specific types of transitions that presupposes a series of phases. For example, based on her work with terminal cancer patients, Kübler-Ross (1969) identified five stages experienced by people who realize they are dying:

1. Denial and isolation,
2. Anger and resentment,
3. Bargaining,
4. Preparatory depression over impending loss, and
5. Acceptance.

Similarly, bereavement over the loss of a loved one moves from "almost global denial or 'numbness,' . . . bitter pining and frustrated searching, . . . succeeded by depression and apathy . . . with a final phase of reorganization when new plans and assumptions about the world and self are built up" (Parkes, 1971, p. 106). Lindemann (1965), who has done extensive research on grief, maintained that if the person does not do the necessary "grief work"—passing through each of the stages in its turn—trouble can erupt later on.

Brammer and Abrego (1981) identified a seven-stage transition process model applicable to most transitions. At first the individual experiences temporary *immobilization*—either with despair or elation. The intensity depends on the impact of the transition. Then follows a period of *denial or minimization,* which serves a "stop-time function to provide the person some relief from suffering" (1981, p. 21). The next phase, *self-doubt,* can take many forms including depression, anxiety, anger, or sadness. Then comes a *letting go* when the person experiences the transition deeply.

Following this is the *testing-out* stage during which mood swings occur, accompanied by irritability and impatience. The next phase, *search for meaning,* becomes apparent when the individual begins to ask, "What did I learn from this experience?" The final phase, of internalization, is *integration*. Hopson wrote, "Integration not only involves renewal but also incorporates an acceptance that the transition is now complete. This means that it has become part of one's history. . . It will have an influence over future directions, but it is not imprisoning one in the past" (1981, p. 38). This outcome can take the form of acceptance, deterioration, or renewal. It is not possible to assess the final outcome until the person has experienced the range of phases or stages outlined. Thus, a helper interviewing a client in the self-doubt phase might consider that the person has opted for deterioration only to find six months later a new sense of hope.

William Bridges—Endings, Neutral Zones, Beginnings

Bridges discussed the transition process as having three phases: endings, neutral zones, and beginnings. Although we intuitively like to begin at the beginning—that is, the new job, the new baby, the new relationship—Bridges makes a convincing case that every beginning, every transition, starts with an ending. He wrote, " . . . endings are the first phase of transition. The second phase is a time of lostness and emptiness before 'life' resumes an intelligible pattern and direction, while the third phase is that of beginning anew" (1980, p. 17).

Endings. Bridges provided an example of endings when he described a woman dealing with a new baby. She was really confronting the ending of the family of two, moving into the relationship of three in a family. He wrote, "Considering that we have to deal with endings all our lives, most of us handle them very badly. This is in part because we misunderstand them . . . We take them too seriously by confusing them with finality—that's it, all over, never more, finished" (1980, p. 90).

Endings involve disengagement, disidentification, disenchantment, and disorientation (1980, p. 92). Not everyone experiencing an ending has to go through these in any prescribed sequence, however; nor does everyone have to go through all four aspects. Still, in one way or another, people do disengage by separating from the old roles and routines. Bridges offers the example of a woman's reactions to her husband's leaving her. She says, "My self-esteem, as a woman and as a person, was all tied up with his reactions to me. I didn't just lose a husband. I lost my way of evaluating myself. He was my mirror. Now I don't know how I look any more" (p. 95). After a period of mourning for her losses she began to see that there were some possible opportunities. "Connie's life transition was a turning point in her life . . . It had begun with an ending, and the ending had begun with a disengagement" (1980, p. 95). "Divorces, deaths, job changes, moves, illnesses, and many lesser events disengage us from the contexts which we have known ourselves. They break up the old cue-system . . . with disengagement, an inexorable process of change begins. Clarified, channeled, and supported, that change can lead toward development and renewal" (1980, pp. 95–96).

Related to disengagement is the need to disidentify with one's previous role. One man who had presided over an international agency was not reappointed. The same year he was pushed out of his job, his daughter died of cancer. This was the first time he did not have an assistant handling the mechanics of a trip abroad. At one point, the ticket agent said, "Well, who are you anyway?" The man said, "I know who I was. I don't know who I am." He had had one identity—a top executive and father. All that had changed. He did not know who he was.

As Bridges says, "No longer being . . . wife or a salesman, no longer being the old me or a young person is a source of panic. That is when it is important to remember the significance of disidentification and the need to loosen the bonds of who we think we are so that we can go through a transition toward a new identity" (1980, p. 97). Endings can also include periods of disenchantment and disorientation—periods during which, as Bridges describes it, we may become a "person floating free in a kind of limbo between two worlds" (1980, p. 98).

Neutral zones. Disenchantment and disorientation are preludes to the next phase, neutral zones. Bridges wrote: "We need not feel defensive about this apparently unproductive time-out at turning points in our lives, for the neutral zone is meant to be a moratorium from the conventional activity of our everyday existence" (1980, p. 114). For some who can afford it, it might be going to a spa. For others, it might be a weekend in the country; and for some it might be a leave of absence from the job or a massage. One woman, with a limited income, and no chance for a weekend away, requested a day with no responsibilities each Mother's Day. Whatever it is, it is a time to be—not to think of who you were or who you might become, but just a time to experience the "here and now" and to "smell the roses."

Bridges described this as a period of emptiness, almost like being suspended in time between the old life and the new life. During this period, a person is betwixt and between, having left old roles, relationships, routines, and assumptions but not yet in a new life with new roles, relationships, routines, and assumptions. In one way it is like being in a rudderless boat.

Beginnings. Beginnings come "when the endings and the time of fallow neutrality are finished" (Bridges, 1980, p. 134). These beginnings often take the form of external career changes. We read about doctors who become artists, housewives or househusbands who take up real estate. A 25-year-old man debating between social work or medicine, chose social work because he could not make the kind of commitment to the required lifestyle and rigor required of medical students. However, he feared that at 40 he would regret his decision. The counselor pointed out that what he did for the next 15 years did not have to determine his whole life. At 40 it is not too late to make a new beginning; in fact, new beginnings are possible all through life.

Bridges's work is an example of a theory-to-practice model. He conceptualized the transition process. He showed its relevance for individuals as they deal with their own transitions (1980), and he demonstrated its applicability to the corporate world in his book, *Surviving Corporate Transition* (1988). He showed how everyone—including business firms—go through endings, neutral zones, and beginnings. He provided many illustrations that help individuals understand transitions, and even relax in the face of change. The knowledge that every beginning begins with an ending; that endings break up habits, routines, and roles, helps explain why so many individuals hold on endlessly to bad relationships or stultifying jobs. Bridges specifically illustrated how managers can use this knowledge. For example, every change—whether a new boss or an introduction of technology—results in potential loss of attachments, turf, structure, future, meaning, and control (1988, p. 40). Employees must be allowed to grieve for what is lost.

A study of adult learners (Schlossberg, Lynch, & Chickering, 1989), found that graduation forced a reformulation of goals. As one set of goals is reached—finishing a degree—there is an inevitable letdown; for once again a sense of purpose must be reconstructed. The adult learners are giving up classes, advisers, and the goal of becoming, but have not yet moved to a new set of activities and self-definition. Change involves loss as well as new possibilities. Bridges summarized the entire transition process when he wrote, "Endings and beginnings, with emptiness and germination in between" (1988, p. 150).

Meryl Louis—Entering a Transition

Meryl Louis focused on what happens as people enter a new setting. People who move into a new situation, whether a new marriage, the Peace Corps, an educational environment, or even a new class, have some common agendas and needs. They must become familiar with the rules, regulations, norms, and expectations of the new system. In a theoretical discussion of employees moving into organizations, Louis (1980) proposed that employees should have clear expectations about what is in store, and be socialized into the explicit and implicit norms, roles, and culture of the organization. Louis suggested that the way to minimize employee turnover is to pay systematic attention to the beginning of a transition. In essence, Louis attributes turnover to unrealistic, inflated, or unmet expectations that are not addressed at the beginning of a transition.

Counselors, psychologists, social workers, ministers, and other helpers can help individuals learn the ropes and teach them about available resources and information-seeking strategies. The clergy and judges offer "words of wisdom" to those about to get married; managers and supervisors theoretically offer the same to new employees. We say theoretically because in a study conducted of new employees it was clear that most managers did *not* take the role of socializer seriously (Leibowitz, Schlossberg, & Shore, 1991, pp. 43–49). As a result of the study, Leibowitz, Schlossberg, and Shore developed materials for new employees and for managers to help both during this introductory period (1992).

Helen Rose Fuchs Ebaugh—The Process of Role Exit

Ebaugh, a sociologist, concentrated on endings, the process of leaving a role. She interviewed ex-doctors, dentists, police officers, air traffic controllers, teachers, military personnel, athletes, professors, convicts, prostitutes, transvestites, and nuns.

She found that exiting from a role is a unique process. "Role exit is a process of disengagement from a role that is central to one's self-identity and the reestablishment of an identity in a new role that takes into account one's ex-role. Role exit is a process that occurs over time" (1988, p. 23). The process begins with an individual having doubts, then looking for reactions that can be either positive or negative, and then seeking alternative roles (p. 84).

A student wrote a paper on mothers giving up custody of their children. She selected the topic after reading Ebaugh's book—mainly because she had such negative feelings about women who would voluntarily give up custody. Using the role exit framework, she looked at the process of women as they made the decision and the process of creating a new role—still mother but not with custody. It is a painful process. Incidentally, her views of this group changed dramatically after the study—she gained great respect for many, did not categorize them negatively, and became aware of the stigma we attach to certain ex-roles.

Ebaugh's studies were mainly of those individuals voluntarily exiting from their roles. Unstudied are the many forced into leaving a role they loved—the push to make people retire early, the announcement of a spouse or partner that he or she is in love with someone else and therefore is forcing the end of a relationship. In a pilot study of college presidents leaving the presidency, we found that the major difference was whether the person left voluntarily or saw the "handwriting on the wall" (McEwen, Komives, & Schlossberg, 1990). In another major difference related to gender, the men we interviewed were not as open in their responses, not as willing to talk about the pain of leaving one role and carving out a new role as the women were.

Ebaugh pointed out that many therapists "first encounter role exiters who are going through the vacuum stage of the process . . . this period is one of extreme anxiety and creates a sense of normlessness . . . Sometimes the greatest help a therapist can give an individual 'caught' in the vacuum stage is to help [the individual] . . . begin to identify as an ex and move on to the creation of new role" (1988, p. 209).

Self-help groups offer support to people seeking to connect with others "in the same boat," and thereby reduce loneliness and confusion. It takes time to leave a role, and establish new roles, new reference groups, new norms. The new life, though, is always built on the identity that went before. As one learns new roles, some remnants of the previous role always remain. For example, there is a tremendous difference between two elementary school teachers, one of whom had belonged to a religious order while the other had served as a police officer. They each have a "hang-over identity" from their previous roles.

Arnold van Gennep and Barbara Myerhoff—
The Rites of Passage

Arnold van Gennep, an anthropologist, identified a process common to all societies. "The life of an individual in any society is a series of passages from one age to another and from one occupation to another. . . . For every one of these events there are ceremonies whose essential purpose is to enable the individual to pass from one defined position to another" (1960, pp. 2–3). Rites of passage include events that:

1. separate the individual from the group, such as graduations;
2. incorporate the individual into a new role, such as marriage; or
3. acknowledge an in-between status, such as pregnancy, labeled as a period of "liminality."

Whether it is a rite to acknowledge separation, incorporation, or liminality, the rites have an "over-all goal to insure a change of condition or a passage from one magico-religious or secular group to another" (p. 11). Though written in 1960, these concepts apply today.

In the film *Rites of Renewal*, the late anthropologist, Barbara Myerhoff, discussed the role of rituals, ceremonies, and rites of passage in helping people mark "the transition of an individual from one phase of life . . . to another" (1984). In this film, Myeroff described the three stages of a ritual.

First, the individual is segregated. Observe any ceremony—graduation, retirement, wedding—and note the separation made obvious by the placement or dress of the persons in question.

Second, the individual moves into a state between the old role and the new role, liminality in Turner's terms and the Neutral Zone in Bridges's. The person is still a baby and not a baby; still a worker and not a worker. As Myerhoff stated in the film, "That middle stage, the marginal one, the liminal one, is an especially interesting one because that's where the person is neither one thing or another" (1984).

The final phase of the ritual is "reincorporating the person . . . back into society as a new creature with a new identity" (Myerhoff, 1985). For example, high school graduates entering college are not sure of their identities. The final phase of the transition occurs when they develop identities other than those connected to the high school roles and

MOVING IN

New Roles, Relationships,
Routines, Assumptions
(Schlossberg)

Learning the Ropes;
Socialization (Louis)

Hang-over Identity (Ebaugh)

MOVING OUT

Separation or Endings (Bridges)

Role Exit (Ebaugh)

Disengagement from Roles,
Relationships, Routines,
Assumptions

MOVING THROUGH: BETWIXT OR BETWEEN

Period of Liminality (Turner, Myerhoff)

Groping for new: Roles, Relationships, Routines, Assumptions

Neutral Zone: Period of Emptiness and Confusion (Bridges)

FIGURE 2.2 Integrative model of the transition process.

relationships they previously had. Rituals thus help people make sense out of the paradox inherent in many transitions—that there is no single truth, there are many truths; that individuals are part of the past, but also the future.

AN INTEGRATIVE MODEL OF THE TRANSITION PROCESS

Bridges presented an overview of the transition process that applies to both individuals and organizations. Louis focused on the entry process of moving into organizations, and Ebaugh delineated exiting from a role. Each of these theorists focuses on transition, but each comes to the topic with a different perspective. (See Figure 2.2.)

To restate: In any transition, the first stage can be conceptualized as either moving in or moving out. Using moving in as a starting point, people who move into a new situation, whether a new marriage, a new job or an educational environment, have some common agendas and needs. They need to become familiar with the rules, regulations, norms, and expectations of the new system. Institutions need to devote a great deal of time to orientation, a process designed to help individuals know what is expected of them.

As mentioned earlier, Louis (1980) proposed that new employees be given clear expectations about what is in store for them, and be socialized into the explicit and implicit norms, roles, and culture of the organization. Previous research focusing on "recruit turnover" and "organizational socialization" (p. 226) suggested to Louis that to minimize employee turnover, more systematic attention is necessary when employees enter an organization. We can extrapolate from Louis's work that entering any new system, whether a new marriage, a new educational experience, a new relationship, "Turnover" occurs because of unrealistic, inflated, or unmet expectations that are not addressed at the beginning of a transition.

Once in, adults confront such issues as how to balance their activities with other parts of their lives and how to feel supported and challenged during their new journey. Applying this to adult learners, we see that the *moving through* period begins once learners know the ropes. Because it can be a long transition, learners may need help sustaining their energy and commitment. In other areas of life, this in-between time can evoke new questions about the transition: "Did I do the right thing?" "Why am I bored?" "Can I commit to this transition?" Many jokes about the "seven-year itch" stem from this middle period when reevaluation takes place.

Moving out can be seen as ending one series of transitions and beginning to ask what comes next. Grieving can be used as a model to explain this phase in the process. People feel grief in many situations of loss other than those most commonly recognized as bereavement. When leaving familiar surroundings and people or ways of functioning and interacting to which one has become accustomed, one experiences disequilibrium. Changing jobs, moving, returning to school, all are transitions in which adults mourn the loss of former goals, friends, and structure.

Louis (1980) pointed out that organizations have not paid the same attention to helping employees move out as they have to helping them move in. In her view no one has really developed a detailed conceptualization of what is needed to help people leave, let go, and reinvest.

Another important point is that the larger the transition—either good or bad—the more it will pervade an individual's life. At first, one is a beginning student, new widow, or new parent. A period of disruption follows, in which old roles, relationships, assumptions, and routines

change and new ones evolve. Then finally, gradually, the sharp awareness of having graduated or having become a parent becomes only one
of the many dimensions of living—the transition has been integrated.

SUMMARY

The transition framework is based on the premises that:

- Adults continuously experience transitions.
- Adults' reactions to transitions depend on the type of transition,
  the context in which it occurs, and its impact on their lives.
- A transition has no endpoint; rather, a transition is a process
  over time that includes phases of assimilation and continuous
  appraisal as people move in, through, and out of it.

3

Factors That Influence Transitions

The transition framework presented in Chapter 2 and here in Chapter 3 is designed to depict the extraordinarily complex reality that accompanies and defines the human capacity to cope with change. Four major sets of factors (see Figure 3.1) influence the ability of the individual to cope during a transition:

1. The Situation variable—(What is happening? For example, the transition to retirement differs from the transition of having a first baby.)
2. The Self variable—(To whom is it happening? Each individual is different in terms of life issues and personality.)
3. The Support variable—(What help is available? Supports and available options vary for each individual.)
4. The Strategies variable—(How does the person cope? People navigate transitions in different ways.)

We call them the 4 S's.

THE 4 S SYSTEM: SOME CONSIDERATIONS

The 4 S System—Situation, Self, Support, and Strategies—describes the factors that make a difference in how one copes with change. These four sets of variables can be regarded as potential assets and/or liabilities. To understand how these assets and liabilities work, we need first to examine their interrelationship and how one goes about appraising them, but it is equally significant to examine options faced by different individuals and groups in our society.

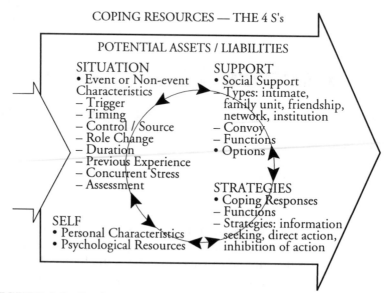

FIGURE 3.1 Coping resources—The 4 S's.

Balancing Assets and Liabilities

Coping effectiveness is best examined and explained by using a model that balances opposing forces. Individuals have both assets and liabilities, resources and deficits, as they experience transitions. Fiske and Chiriboga (1990) have identified individuals high on both resources and deficits; those high on one, low on the other; and those low on both. They argue that a model that incorporates both resources and deficits, rather than the degree-of-impairment model, is more meaningful because people have multiple strengths and limitations.

To clarify this mix of resources and deficits, we will look at two women diagnosed with multiple sclerosis. For both, the experience is painful, incapacitating, and psychologically distressing because of the uncertainty of the condition. One of the women has ample assets to balance this deficit in her physical well-being. She has a tenured position in a university, a highly supportive family, as well as friends and colleagues who rally around her, and a coping personality. The other woman is low on assets at this particular point in her life. She has recently had a double mastectomy, thus her physical stamina and her self-esteem are low, and she has just gone through a divorce, which suggests that part of her support system has crumbled. Moreover, this particular disability threatens her very economic survival by making it impossible for her to work as a carpenter, a job requiring great physical stamina. Moreover, her ability to cope has never been better than average. At this benchline, her liabilities far outweigh her assets, making life especially difficult.

The 4 S model then, rather than assessing a person's mental condition in terms of health or sickness, employs a ratio of assets to liabilities and allows for changes in the ratio as an individual's situation changes. This approach partially answers the question of why different individuals react differently to the same type of transition and why the same person reacts differently at different times. The difference may be that the assets–liabilities balance has changed; assets may outweigh liabilities, making adjustment relatively easy. Or, liabilities may now outweigh assets, so assimilation of the transition becomes correspondingly more difficult. It is important that psychologists and others in the helping professions delay diagnosis of someone as "ill" when, in fact, all that may be needed is a temporary shift in the balance of assets to liabilities.

Appraisal of Transitions

Lazarus and Folkman (1984) defined a transition as a transaction between individuals and their environment. The individual's appraisal of the transition is key. Does the individual see it as positive, negative, or benign? An individual's appraisal will clearly influence how that individual feels and copes with the transition event or non-event.

Lazarus and Folkman wrote:

> Although certain environmental demands and pressures produce stress in substantial numbers of people, individual and group differences in the degree and kind of reaction are always evident. People . . . differ in their sensitivity and vulnerability to certain types of events, as well as in their interpretations and reactions.
>
> Under comparable conditions, for example, one person responds with anger, another with depression, yet another with anxiety or guilt; and still others feel challenged rather than threatened. Likewise, one individual uses denial to cope with terminal illness whereas another anxiously ruminates about the problem or is depressed. One individual handles an insult by ignoring it and another grows angry . . . In order to understand

variations among individuals under comparable conditions, we must take into account the cognitive processes that intervene between the encounter and the reaction, and the factors that affect the nature of this mediation. If we do not consider these processes, we will be unable to understand human variation under comparable external conditions." (1984, pp. 22, 23)

Lazarus and Folkman suggested that individuals make two types of appraisals simultaneously. Primary appraisal refers to the perception of the transition itself—is it positive, negative, or irrelevant? If stressful, is it perceived as a challenge, a threat, or a loss? For example, ten parents experience having their youngest child begin college. For some it may signify the end of their parenting role; to others, it may mean freedom to follow their own interests; to still others, it may have no impact at all.

In addition, individuals engage in secondary appraisal during which they assess their resources for coping with the transition. These coping resources include the 4 S's—Situation, Self, Support, and Strategies. A woman might be facing job loss, a negative transition, but feel she has the resources to cope with it. Or she might be dealing with a positive transition like a promotion, but deem her resources for coping with it as low. One woman declined a wished-for job offer because her personal situation was negative—her son had just been diagnosed with cystic fibrosis, and her husband had left her. Her situation and supports were so low that she could not deal with any major transition—even a potentially positive one.

The results of the secondary appraisal influence the individual's selection of coping strategies. There is a feedback loop. For example, a person might appraise early retirement as a great opportunity but then may become anxious about taking advantage of it due to the assessment of the 4 S's. This might then force a reappraisal of the desirability of early retirement, and a decision not to take it. People make assessments and arrive at decisions like this all the time.

As we pointed out in Chapter 2, the transition process consists of reactions over a period of time. As reactions change, an individual's perspective can shift from feeling "this is forever" to one of "this too shall pass." It is useful for helpers to share this knowledge. Caine (1974) pointed out in writing about widowhood, "I am convinced that if I had known the facts of grief before I had to experience them, it would not have made my grief less intense . . . [but it] would have allowed me to hope" (1974, pp. 91–92). An individual's appraisal and reappraisal of a transition, and of his or her resources for coping, can be examined in light of the 4 S's.

A Multicultural View of Options

As we have already noted, individuals constantly assess their transitions and resources for coping. These resources, according to Sussman (1972), include the individual's options, which may be actual, perceived, utilized, or created. Sussman developed "an option-maintenance model" that stated that the central variable in determining whether people feel successful when coping with a transition resides in the number of options that people feel they can exercise. Sussman further contends that options are directly related to self-esteem. Chronic job loss, feeling forced to stay in a low-level job or an unsatisfactory marriage can erode an individual's confidence and self-esteem.

Sussman discussed two levels of options: structural and psychological. Structural options are related to the availability of options. When unemployment is structural, more people are affected and the individual alone can do less about it. Opening up the opportunity structure requires political action, such as legislative changes in the retirement age, thus changing the options for older people. Psychological options are related to the individual's skill in perceiving and utilizing alternatives (Sussman, 1972, pp. 28–73).

The history of oppressed groups in this country—African Americans, other ethnic minorities, women, the old—reflects a shift from a time when many individuals accepted that there were no options for their group, to a time when the group organized to fight to change the opportunity structure. The ability to create new options is not restricted to political activists. Career development experts run workshops designed specifically to help people take control of their lives, break out of their boxes, identify what they want, and create their own jobs and options.

Thus, options can be both objective (at one time there were few professional jobs for African Americans) and subjective ("because I am African American I will not apply to medical school"). A fine line exists between actual options and the perception of actual options. Further, political action groups may assist in the creation of options for some groups, for example, women wanting to be astronauts. Thus, any discussion of options is highly complex, and involves the interaction of the actual world with the individual's perceptions and actions.

At a recent workshop on transitions, counseling psychologist Donelda Cooke was asked to critique the 4 S model from a multicultural perspective. According to Cooke, a multicultural perspective is not one of just numbers or labels. Reporting cases or vignettes which reflect diversity of color, ethnicity, gender, or age is only a first step.

Cook's overriding message concerned the necessity of carefully examining the assumptions and world view of others, the ways that different people make meaning in the world. As she said:

> It is important to ask how the model applies to the low-income African American mothers from an inner-city Baltimore community I interviewed for a research project, the caucasian female client I saw in counseling who had cerebral palsy and was a victim of rape, the student who struggled with her sexual identity because her traditional Italian family would never accept that the one girl in the family was a lesbian, the 19-year-old caucasian male student who was confined to a wheelchair three years ago and experiences insensitivities and discriminatory practices on a daily basis. (1994)

Cooke urged that sociopolitical and cultural values be the context in which others are understood:

> By looking at various groups' experiences regarding domination, oppression, and co-existence, you can begin to understand the amount of control individuals have over the circumstances in their lives, or the limited choices they may have in their assets, liabilities, and resources. While the theory leaves room to explore the sense of control one has over one's transitions, unless sociopolitical constraints are boldly articulated, readers from privileged classes can too easily overlook them. (1994)

Everyone uses coping strategies, everyone has some kind of support system, everyone has a personal way of being in the world, and everyone has a unique situation. Yet there is an overriding concern. Some individuals' Situation, Self, Supports, and Strategies are qualitatively so restricted that one cannot consider the 4 S's alone. As Cooke said, one's resources for coping—the 4 S's—are determined by the outside world. If people's concerns relate to feeding their families, dealing with ill children without health insurance, their resources are qualitatively different than those of middle-class professionals.

THE 4 S SYSTEM: A DETAILED VIEW

Situation

Every individual's situation varies according to the following factors:

- Trigger (What set off the transition?)
- Timing (How does the transition relate to one's social clock?)
- Control (What aspects of the transition can one control?)
- Role change (Does the transition involve role change?)
- Duration (Is the transition seen as permanent or temporary?)
- Previous experience with a similar transition (How has the individual met similar transitions?)
- Concurrent stress (What and how great are the stresses facing the individual now, if any?)
- Assessment (Does the individual view the situation positively, negatively, or as benign?)

Trigger. A transition, as we have defined it, can be anticipated or unanticipated, an event or a non-event, as long as it alters one's life. Triggers can be external, like a decade birthday, and have internal consequences, like an awareness that time is running out. Triggers stimulate individuals to look at themselves and their lives in a new way. For example, a change in health—a heart attack or cancer—can act as a trigger for rethinking work and relationships. Job changes, especially job losses, trigger reevaluation. For one man, the trigger was being in bed for five months with a slipped disk, coupled with the death from cancer of one of his closest friends: "If I can get sick, if John can die, then life is not forever." For another, being at a wedding of a friend's child can trigger the realization that one's adult children are not married and one might never be an in-law or a grandparent.

A transition can also be triggered by something that happens to someone close to the individual: a husband's retirement may trigger a fear of aging in his wife; a wife's mastectomy may trigger fears of death in her husband. Other triggers can be class reunions, movies, books.

Aslanian and Brickell (1980) differentiated transitions from triggers: A *transition* is a "change in status . . . that makes learning necessary. The adult needs to become competent at something that he or she could not do before in order to succeed in the new status" (1980, pp. 38–39). A *trigger,* however, is a specific life event that precipitates "the decision to learn at that point in time" (p. 39). The trigger is not necessarily directly related to the transition—as in the example of an unemployed woman, suddenly widowed, who enrolls in a medical technology course in order to become qualified for a job. The transition is her change of status from nonworker to worker; the triggering event is her husband's death, in itself, a major transition.

Timing. As noted, most adults have built-in social clocks that are their barometers to judge whether they are "on time" or "off time" with respect to family, career, and self issues. To be "off time," whether early or late, can make individuals feel uncomfortable. Certain transitions, for example, getting married, having children, going to college, taking a job, and retiring, used to be linked in people's minds to a certain age. Today, these rigid time tables are loosening as people's lives follow irregular paths. Despite the more fluid life span, many still use age to define how they are doing.

Transition events or non-events are also experienced as happening at "good" or "bad" times. For example, an adolescent in senior high school will resist a family geographical move as being at a bad time. A newlywed couple may define a move away from parents and in-laws as happening at a good time. The couple's parents, who have recently become in-laws, however, may see it as a bad time. A major illness at a time of job loss would be both "bad" and "off time." Thus, events—both anticipated and unanticipated—can be at better or worse times, making it easier or more difficult for individuals to go through the transition process.

Control. The source of some transitions is internal, a deliberate decision on the part of the individual, whereas the source of others is completely external, and the transition is forced upon the individual by other people or by circumstances. The worker who retires because of ill health or a plant closing probably finds retirement more difficult and troubling than the worker who retires voluntarily. Similarly, couples often experience considerable negative stress in connection with residential moves when the move is forced upon them by the job requirements of one of them. The issue here is how an individual perceives control over his/her own life.

Judith Rodin, the psychologist who studied the relevance of control in determining one's mental health, has paid particular attention to aging and control. She wrote: "Across the life-span, every significant developmental transition provides new challenges for perceived and actual control ... Through middle adulthood and into old age, new demands and issues impact on one's sense of control ... Therefore, one's overall level of self-efficacy may remain stable, although the domains in which one feels competent are likely to change and become less numerous" (1990, pp. 11–12).

Even if the transition is beyond the individual's control, the response to it can be within the individual's control. The two sources of control—internal and external—interact. Counselors can help adults explore the degree to which the trigger or transition is in or out of their control and the degree to which they can control their reactions to it.

Role change. Many, but not all, transitions involve role change. We have already noted that role changes are an important aspect in determining the impact of a transition. Fiske and Chiriboga (1990) distinguished between role gains (such as getting married, becoming a parent, taking a job, getting a job promotion) and role losses (such as getting divorced, retiring, being widowed). Regardless of whether a transition involves a role gain or loss, some degree of stress accompanies it.

For instance, LeMasters (1957) found that the period after the birth of the first child often constitutes a mental health crisis for the mother; along with her feelings of joy and satisfaction, she may be physically exhausted, anxious about her responsibilities, frustrated over her loss of freedom, resentful of her husband for not sharing more of the duties, and—on top of it all—guilty about her negative feelings. Similarly, though an individual may look forward with pleasurable anticipation to retiring from employment or seeing the last child launched into the world, the actual event may carry with it feelings of pain. Again, any role change—whether primarily positive or negative—involves some degree of stress.

Role is the "behavioral enacting of the patterned expectations attributed to a position" (Merton, 1957, p. 368). "Role theory in sociology centers on others' expectations as to the behavior of the individual who occupies a given position. These expectations sustain order and consistency in human interaction. These expectations are essentially normative prescriptions for behavior" (Zaleznik & Jardim, 1967, p. 210). The more an individual engages in "anticipatory socialization"—that is, orientation toward the values and norms of the new role—the sooner the individual will be comfortable (Merton, 1957, p. 265). When there are no role models available for the new role, the individual remains marginal for a longer period, as did the first women executives in American business.

Thus, a given role change can be more or less difficult (and have greater or lesser impact) depending on whether the new role is a loss or a gain, positive or negative, or has explicit norms and expectations for the new incumbent. As Pearlin and Lieberman conclude, "It is not the tearing away from old roles that matters to well-being, but what is discovered in the context of the new roles" (1979, p. 239).

Duration. The expected duration of the transition affects the ease or difficulty of assimilating the transition. A change that is regarded as permanent will be perceived differently from one that is viewed as temporary. A wife may be willing to tolerate the inconvenience involved in moving to a new location so her husband can attend graduate school if she believes that the move is temporary and that they will return to their former home when he has received his degree. A transition that is painful and unpleasant may be more easily borne if the individual is assured that it is of limited duration; for example, when someone enters the hospital for surgery knowing that the discomfort is temporary. Conversely, if the change is desired, then the certainty that it represents a more or less permanent state may be reassuring.

Uncertainty about duration, however, is connected with perhaps the greatest degree of stress and negative effect. Chodoff (1976), talking about the psychological stresses of being in a German concentration camp, said, "A healthy personality [can] defend itself against a peril, which, though grave, is predictable and is at least potentially limited in time, but the absolute uncertainty of [the concentration camp inmate's] condition was a barrier to the erection of adequate psychological measures" (pp. 337–338). To have an illness whose cause and prognosis is uncertain may be more stressful and unsettling for an individual than to know for sure that he or she has a terminal disease.

Previous experience with a similar transition. It is generally assumed that the individual who has successfully weathered a particular kind of transition in the past will probably be successful at assimilating another transition of a similar nature. Conversely, the person who has been defeated by a situation may become more vulnerable and less able to cope in the future. Past experiences to some extent determine the person's mental set, and if that past experience was unfavorable, then the mental set may be something of a self-confirming prophecy. Of course, given possible changes in the balance of assets and liabilities (discussed earlier), the correlation between successful assimilation in the past and at a later point in time is by no means perfect.

Some types of loss seem to have long-lasting negative effects. For example, Fiske and Chiriboga (1990) found that of the one-quarter of their sample who had suffered an early childhood loss through death or divorce, one-half belonged to the "overwhelmed" category; that is, they were preoccupied with stress. Undoubtedly, some experiences are so harrowing that many people are left permanently damaged.

Concurrent stress. Often transitions in one area stimulate other stresses and transitions. Consider the transition faced by a middle-aged couple whose first daughter is marrying. Can we rate that transition? We would say no. Understanding the transition requires examining the impact on the middle-aged couple's life. If the daughter lives across the country and will remain there, the marriage will not have a significant impact on the daily or weekly life of the parents. Some changes will, of course, occur. If, however, the daughter who has lived away returns to the parents' city to marry, has one small stepchild and little money, comes home three times a week to do laundry, and asks the parents to babysit, then it is a transition of much greater impact.

Assessment. An individual's view of who or what is responsible for the transition affects how that individual appraises the transition (and himself or herself and the environment). Does he/she see the divorce as attributable to the other's deficiencies, to his or her own deficiencies, to societal problems, or to idiosyncratic causes? The individual's attributions about self and situation provide a theoretical basis for many studies explaining behavior, some of which were summarized by Kelley and Michela (1980).

Situation review. Each transition event or non-event is different. The same individual can get divorced, become a grandparent, lose a job, inherit a million dollars, or not have a baby. Each of these transitions will be different in terms of the following:

> What triggered it?
> Was it at a good time in the individual's life?
> Did the individual initiate the transition or did it happen to him/her?

Did the individual experience a role change?

Is the transition permanent or temporary?

Has the individual had previous experience with similar transitions, and if so, were they helpful or harmful?

Is the individual experiencing stress in other areas of life?

Does the individual assess the transition as positive, negative, or benign?

The Self

We stated earlier that every individual has both assets and liabilities— resources and deficits. In addition to the Situation itself, we now look at what the individual brings to the transition. We all hear clients who state, "I'm a pessimist and always see the glass as half empty," or "I'm usually up for change but this one has really knocked me out." It is complex to get a handle on the Self, but we have identified some characteristics that are particularly relevant for individuals as they cope with change.

- Personal and demographic characteristics
  Socioeconomic status
  Gender
  Age and stage of life
  State of health
  Ethnicity
- Psychological resources
  Ego development
  Outlook—optimism and self-efficacy
  Commitment and values

Personal and demographic characteristics. An individual's
personal and demographic characteristics—socioeconomic status, gender, age and stage of life, and state of health—bear directly on how he/ she perceives and assesses life. Research that combines societal and individual perspectives illustrates the importance and value of an integrated approach to the study of transitions. Such research clarifies the differences we refer to when we say that research results "vary as a function of age, sex, and social class." People who inhabit different parts of the social system live, in many ways, in very different contexts, have different resources, and are affected differently by different events.

Sociologists Leonard Pearlin and Morton Lieberman interviewed 2300 adults, both white and nonwhite, ages 20 to 60 in 1972. In 1976–77 they again interviewed these adults, looking particularly for "the persistent problems of everyday life" as well as the life-course transitions and crises through which they had passed in the intervening four-year period. The researchers identified the stresses and hardships the group had experienced as well as ways they coped with them.

Pearlin and Lieberman divided life strains into those that are unexpected (non-normative—like a serious illness), those that are expected (normative—like getting married, becoming a parent), and those which they call "persistent role problems" (like an unaccepting spouse or children's failure to act responsibly). They then examined the effects of these life strains (or transitions) on anxiety and depression, at the same time identifying the ways people from different walks of life experienced these different life strains. Pearlin and Lieberman reported that, by and large, "The events, transitions, and persistent role problems are not scattered helter-skelter throughout the population, but tend to be more or less prevalent among groups having distinguishing social characteristics"—that is, the life strains seemed to depend on age, sex, and socioeconomic status (1979, p. 230).

The importance of socioeconomic status is underlined in Rubin's study of the empty nest (1981). Women from advantaged situations can anticipate that their children will go away to college; therefore, children's departure from the home is expected, and those women engage in anticipatory socialization. Women from working-class homes, for whom money is often a problem and children's attendance at an out-of-town college is uncertain, experience a more difficult transition in the event of their children's departure. Rubin stresses the fact that the empty nest is not a problem for most women. What makes it a problem is when it is unplanned or when feelings about it are ambivalent (Rubin, 1981).

The effects of an individual's racial and ethnic background on his/her ability to navigate transitions are probably mediated through other factors such as value orientation and cultural norms. They should not, however, be underestimated. We hope the next decade will see an increase in studies of many populations so that insights will be gained into the differing adult experiences.

The relationship between gender and the transition process is complex. Many observers have suggested that because men are socialized to hide emotion and deny problems (whereas women are given greater freedom to express their feelings), men present a more favorable picture with respect to mental health. Despite appearances, however, women's greater capacity for intimacy and mutuality may make it easier for them to assimilate certain transitions; the example of widowhood has already been cited. Moreover, evidence suggests that women "can apparently integrate many and diverse emotional experiences. Men seem more distressed by ups and downs of emotional life; they apparently thrive either on a preponderance of positive emotional experiences or a relative lack of any kind [of experience]" (Fiske & Chiriboga, 1990, p. 97).

Wherever we look, we see gender as a critical determiner of work and family issues. Deborah Tannen investigated the different ways men and women communicate. Because boys and girls grow up in different cultures, they speak and listen from different vantage points. Tannen wrote, "If women speak and hear a language of connection and intimacy, while men speak and hear a language of status and independence, then communication between men and women can be like cross-cultural communication, prey to a clash of conversational styles. Instead of different dialects, it has been said they speak different genderlects" (1990, p. 42).

Her research corroborated others', showing that men like to problem-solve and women like to discuss and develop ideas. "When men and women talk to each other, the problem is that each expects a different kind of response" (1990, p. 61). Tannen's message is even more forceful when she describes the power differences between men and women as seen through their communication. This power differential is reflected over and over in different wages, different job titles, different opportunities. These differences in power and communication styles reflect the different world views of men and women, and these views in turn have an impact on how transitions are viewed.

Although there have been significant strides in reducing sex-role stereotyping, there is still a great deal of difference that results from gender. Therefore, helpers need to explore with individuals how such differences may affect their response to their transition.

Again, the wealth of data about the relation between *age* and ability to assimilate transitions precludes all but a cursory discussion here. One point that makes analysis difficult is that most experts agree that chronological age is relatively unimportant compared to *psychological age* ("the capacity to respond to societal pressures and the tasks required of an individual"), social age ("the extent to which an individual participates in roles assigned by society"), and functional age ("the ability to function or perform as expected of people in one's age bracket, which in turn, depends on social, biological and personality considerations") (Spierer, 1977, p. 10).

Another complication is that the process of aging itself constitutes a series of events that require adaptation on the part of the individual. That is, the biological and physiological changes that occur over the life-span may themselves be regarded as transitions.

As mentioned, life stage may be a more useful concept than chronological age in examining transitions. Fiske and Chiriboga (1990) identified numerous stage differences with respect to the sources and nature of stress, the number of significant life events, and the ratio of positive to negative experiences. The younger subjects (high school seniors and newlyweds) reported more "stressor events" during the last ten years of their lives than older subjects (middle-aged and preretirement couples). As was pointed out previously, in the later stages of life more subtle factors cause changes in self-perception and satisfaction—the realization that one has not achieved as much as one had planned or the shift in time perspective so that one thinks in terms of years left to live rather than years since birth.

Middle age is a period of contrasting stereotypes. One is that middle agers are the command generation, powerful, in charge of themselves and others; another is the unhappy man or woman, bored at work and with love, in the midst of a face lift or an affair. So what is the truth about midlife?

If only we could define midlife by chronological age, we at least would have the parameters. However, there is no agreement about when it begins and when it ends. Some scholars define it as between 40 and 60, others as starting at 35 with no end, and others who specify it as the fifth decade. Neugarten (1979) suggested it is when we begin to think of time left to live rather than time since birth. Women are labeled middle aged and old before men, and those from higher socioeconomic groups begin midlife later and it lasts longer than for those from working-class and low-income groups. Chronological definitions of midlife are so variable that age, per se, is no indicator.

If only there were a midlife crisis, we could plan for it, handle it, and move on. However, the midlife crisis seems to be an artifact of the media. Pearlin and Lieberman found that despite fears that life will get harder as we age, younger people experience a clustering of work/family transitions in a relatively short period. They experience more disruptions in employment, more activity in both the formation and dissolution of relationships, and more persistent problems that accompany raising young children.

There is a wider timetable for the events and non-events during middle and old age. For example, one can lose both parents by 40, yet many in their 60s still have a parent living. This lengthened time period enables anticipation and preparation for the inevitable ups and downs connected with aging.

To test out the midlife crisis, psychologists Paul Costa and Robert McCrae (1980) administered a midlife crisis scale to a number of men of all ages. They hypothesized that those in midlife, whatever that is, would mark more problems than others. They discovered no clustering of crises by age. Ronald Kessler, a researcher for The MacArthur Foundation's research program on Successful Midlife Development (MIDMAC), and his colleagues found that only 10 to 12 percent of those surveyed reported a midlife crisis. (Kessler, Foster, Webster, & House, 1992).

As with age and aging, the individual's state of health not only affects his or her ability to assimilate a transition, but also may itself be a source of stress. Ill health in itself, of course, constitutes a transition. In some cases, a person may recover quickly from an acute illness and be left relatively unaffected, with little change in self-perception. In other cases, an illness—though brief—may remind a person of his or her own mortality and thus have lasting psychological effects. In still other cases, an illness may be chronic, leading to a gradual decline in physical resources and energy level and thus profoundly affecting the individual's coping ability. Moreover, health has a subjective as well as an objective aspect. For instance, some people are health pessimists, others are health optimists.

Both demographics and personal characteristics are important as filters and mediate whether or not an individual's life will be altered in ways basic to the particular person. As an individual's social class, sex, age, life stage, and health all bear on his/her options—perceived and real—these variables need to be explored.

Psychological resources. Psychological resources are the "personality characteristics that people draw upon to help them withstand threats" (Pearlin & Schooler, 1978, p. 5). This includes ego development, optimism, self-efficacy, and commitments and values.

People approach the same transition from different frames of reference. For example, if there were 100 45-year-old women enrolled in the same educational program, they would react according to their frame of reference and their level of maturity. Loevinger (1976) used the term "ego development" to describe this process and identified several levels of maturity. At a low level, the conformist will think in stereotypes, conform to the rules, and follow instructions without question. At a higher level, autonomous individuals are more critical and better able to tolerate ambiguity.

Knowing the level of ego development of a client can be useful to counselors in many situations. Consider such diverse transitions as navigating a divorce or a layoff. If you can identify the level at which this person operates, you may better tailor your interventions. In this schema, self-protective people are motivated to satisfy immediate needs; conformists are motivated to impress significant others and gain social acceptance; conscientious people are motivated to achieve skills and competence; and autonomous people seek to deepen understanding of themselves and others as well as to develop increasing capacity to tolerate ambiguity, uncertainty, and be responsible for their own destiny.

Another way to understand clients is by knowing whether they see life as half full or half empty. Thus, an individual's *outlook*, itself a result of the complex interplay of many factors, colors the way change is viewed. Optimism and self-efficacy are two critical aspects of one's outlook.

Psychologist Martin Seligman's (1990) work has focused on different ways people react, especially to negative, uncontrollable, or bad events. Those who feel they have control over their lives, or who feel optimistic about their own power to control at least some portions of their lives, tend to experience less depression and achieve more at school or work; they are even in better health.

One study showed that men's optimism following bypass surgery positively correlated "with a faster rate of recovery during hospitalization, a faster rate of return to normal activities after discharge, and higher quality of life at six months after the surgery" (Scheier, Matthews, Owens, Magovern, Lefebre, Abbott, & Carver, 1989, p. 1034) The importance of this study is that data were collected at three points in time— before surgery, right after surgery, and six months later. This fits in with what we know about transitions—they are a process over time rather than a point in time.

Seligman (1990) suggested that the individual's "explanatory style"—the way a person thinks about an event or transition—can explain how some people weather transitions without becoming depressed or giving up. As many transitions are neither "bad" nor "good" but a mixture, a person's "explanatory style" becomes the critical key to coping. A person with a positive explanatory style is an optimist, while one with a negative style is basically a pessimist.

For example, we can ask a client, Steve, who has lost his job, to explain what happened. Did he blame himself and say he lost the job because he was inadequate? Did he conclude that he would always be inadequate at work? People who blame themselves for everything that happens and then generalize to think they always "foul things up" have a good chance of being depressed and passive. On the other hand, if Steve saw that he clearly had some role in the job decision and that, in general, he handled complex situations well, he has a good chance of coping effectively with this transition.

Seligman also suggested that people's explanatory style can predict their success on a job. In a study of insurance sales people, those representatives with a "positive explanatory style" were twice as likely as those with a "negative style" to be still on the job after a year. Following up on this study, a special force of a hundred representatives who had failed the insurance industry test but who had a "positive explanatory style" were hired. They were much more successful than the pessimists who had passed the test.

A related concept, and one that predicts how one will negotiate transitions is self-efficacy. "Bandura has argued that, among the different mechanisms of personal agency, none is more pervasive than people's beliefs in their capabilities to exercise control over their own motivations and behaviors and over environmental demands. Self-efficacy depends on the individual's belief that he or she can cause an intended event to occur and can organize and carry out the courses of behavior necessary to deal with various situations" (Rodin, 1990, p. 2).

Related to self-efficacy is the notion of perceived control. "The illusion of control is . . . the inverse of . . . learned helplessness . . . Although learned helplessness is the erroneous belief that one has no control to affect the outcome of a given event when contingency does in fact exist between response and outcome, the illusion of control involves the erroneous belief that one can produce a positive outcome when such a contingency does not exist" (Rodin, 1990, pp. 4–5).

Shelley Taylor, a psychologist, wrote: "My task . . . is to persuade the reader that normal human thought and perception is marked not by accuracy but by positive self-enhancing illusions about the self, the world, and the future . . . these illusions [are] . . . adaptive, promoting . . . good mental health" (1989, p. 7). Taylor described different, but related, types of positive illusions: "self-enhancement, . . . personal control, involving the perception that one can bring about primarily positive but not negative outcomes, and unrealistic optimism, namely perceptions that the future holds an unrealistically bountiful array of opportunities" (p. 6).

Taylor's book argues for the importance of perceived illusions and control. She demonstrates that a cancer patient's belief in a particular treatment and/or doctor can influence how the patient copes with the disease. When recovery does occur, it is attributed to a person's belief system. We do not know how many people with positive illusions die, but the very fact of having positive illusions, of being optimistic, serves as a resource even in the case of impending death. Of course, self-efficacy makes a difference, as does optimism and one's style of processing the world. However, it can be a disadvantage to assume that a client with an upbeat attitude and a sense of personal power can control the entire transition. The transition model is intended to show the interrelatedness of Situation, Self, Support, and Strategies. So yes, self-efficacy and optimism are crucial, but they are not the entire story.

For instance, the style one uses to process the world is important. Some rely on intuition, doing what feels right to them. Others use their senses to gather data on the world, and then process this data in a logical, systematic way, arriving at reasoned decisions. People differentiate themselves along these lines, and many counselors spend time helping their clients recognize that their styles might be different from that of their partner, boss, or friends. Acknowledging these differences can be helpful in building collaboration rather than conflict. The Myers Briggs Type Instrument (1980) is one way of identifying one's style.

Fiske studied men and women's changing commitments over the life-span (1980). An individual's major commitment—whether it lies in his/her relationships (interpersonal), in working for others (altruism), in self-improvement (competence/mastery), or in survival (self-protection)—determines his/her vulnerability.

The father of a 26-year old boy who committed suicide explained how differently he and his wife reacted. He said it was easier for him because he could bury himself in work—commitment to mastery—whereas his wife, whose lifelong commitment had been to relationships, especially in the family, was unable, even after five years, to reinvest in life. Clearly individuals' reactions to and assimilation of transitions are greatly influenced by their commitments—which, of course, change over time, thereby changing those individuals' areas of vulnerability.

An individual's basic values and beliefs are also a factor in his/her ability to assimilate transitions. On the basis of subjects' responses to the question, "What is the main purpose in life?" Fiske and Chiriboga (1990) developed a seven-category value typology:

1. achievement and work (economic competence, rewards, success, social status);
2. good personal relations (love and affection, happy marriage, friends);
3. philosophical and religious (including concern with the meaning of existence and an adherence to an ethical code);
4. social service (helping others, community service . . .);
5. ease and contentment (simple comforts, security, relaxation);
6. seeking enjoyment (recreation, exciting experiences . . .); and
7. personal growth (self-improvement, being creative). (p. 216)

A value system that contributes to assimilation at one life stage may be dysfunctional at another. People at different stages tend to emphasize different values.

The specific content of a person's religious beliefs, and the cultural norms associated with particular religions, should also be considered. For example, a woman from a Catholic background facing divorce may find her distress exacerbated by the church's strictures against divorce. A man from a Protestant background who has grown up with a strong commitment to the work ethic may find forced unemployment especially hard to take, quite apart from the financial strain it entails.

Beyond the comforts of religion, strong commitment to an ideology or cause may be a necessity in some situations. Thus, those draft dodgers who moved to Canada, not to escape from some difficult personal situation or to seek adventure, but for ideological reasons—because they believed the Vietnam War to be immoral, or regarded themselves as political refugees from an oppressive system—were more likely to adapt to the new situation (Levine, 1976). Concentration camp victims who saw themselves as surviving for some greater purpose were able to mobilize their coping resources more effectively (Dimsdale, 1976).

People face transitions, problems, and joys with characteristic psychological patterns and resources. These vary according to ego development, outlook, commitments, and values.

Review of the self. Every person brings different assets to a transition. The following are some ways to assess clients.

- Are they able to deal with the world in an autonomous way? Can they tolerate ambiguity?
- Are they optimists? Do they see the glass as half-full or half-empty?
- Do they blame themselves for what happens?
- Do they feel in control of their responses to the transition?
- Do they believe that their efforts will affect the outcome of a particular course of action?

Support

The importance of social support is often said to be the key to handling stress. Support, however, needs to be defined operationally because it comes in many sizes and shapes, and can be for better or for worse.

Types of Support. The types of support people receive are classified according to their sources: intimate relationships, family units, networks of friends, and the institutions and/or communities of which the people are a part.

With respect to the first of these four types, Lowenthal and Weiss (1976) maintained that "intimate relationships—involving trust, support, understanding and the sharing of confidences" (p. 12)—are an important resource during stressful transitions. There are gender differences. Some suggest that the death of a spouse may be more traumatic for men than for women, in part because men may have more difficulty forming intimate relationships. Men's difficulty in forming close ties with other people may also contribute to their shorter life expectancy.

As further indication of the power of intimate relationships, Lowenthal and Weiss suggested that "former intimate relationships, disrupted by death, distance, or interpersonal conflict, may continue to be a resource in terms of crisis, chronic and acute, throughout the life course . . . Knowing through past experience that one is capable of having an intimate relationship, romantic or otherwise, may prove nearly as important a resource in difficult life situations as actually having an intimate at the time of crisis: a former relationship is reinforcing, and at the same time sustains hope for a future one" (1976, p. 147).

The family unit has long been a subject for study by sociologists and others, many of whom have attempted to define those qualities of the family that contribute to its ability to adapt to a crisis or to ease the process of adaptation for one of its members. For example, the already mentioned study of draft dodgers and deserters who fled to Canada during the Vietnam era (Levine, 1976) indicated that those who received parental support for their move adapted better to the new situation than did those whose parents disapproved of their action.

An individual's network of friends is also an important social support system. One of the most stressful side effects of divorce is the loss of friendships that were based on couple relationships. Loss of the network of friends may also result from a residential move or from the death of a spouse, thus exacerbating the difficulties of those transitions. Conversely, the presence of friends can cushion sudden shock.

The fourth type of support involves those organizations individuals can turn to for help, such as religious institutions, political groups, social welfare or community support groups, and other more-or-less formal agencies. As discussed in Part III of this book, the need for such agencies has become more widely recognized. There has been a proliferation of programs—which may take the form of seminars, lectures, workshops, or simply discussion groups—aimed at people experiencing particular transitions: midcareer change, divorce, retirement, a return to school.

Functions of Support. According to Caplan, support systems function mainly to help "the individual mobilize . . . psychological resources and master . . . emotional burdens; they share . . . tasks . . . they provide . . . extra supplies of money, materials, tools, skills, and cognitive guidance to improve . . . handling of . . . situations" (1976, pp. 5–6). Developing this even further, Kahn and Antonucci (1980) identified the functions of social support as an incorporation of one or more of the following key elements: affect, affirmation, and aid. Affect refers to expressions of liking, admiration, respect, or love; affirmation refers to expressions of agreement or acknowledgement of the appropriateness or rightness of some act or statement of another person; aid (or assistance) includes the exchange of things, money, information, time, and entitlements (pp. 267–268).

In addition to the functions of affect, affirmation, and aid, we include another—honest feedback. This refers to re-actions offered that might be negative as well as positive. For example, if a parent is complaining about a teenager's behavior and telling how the teenager is going to be punished, a counselor might suggest the coping strategy of selective ignoring; or if the parents always selectively ignore, a counselor might suggest providing more structure.

Measurement of Social Support. Robert Kahn (1975) introduced the concept of the "convoy" of social support, "the idea that each person moves through the life cycle surrounded by a set of significant others related to him [or her] either by the giving or receiving of social support" (p. 1). Two notable features of this concept are, first, that it implies movement and change, and second, that it emphasizes "the giving as well as the receiving of social support . . . " (p. 1)

Kahn used several methods to measure social support, based on some operational definitions. "Convoy is a person-centered network; each convoy is a personal network of social support, defined around a focal person whose activities and well-being we wish to understand . . . The network stops with that set of other persons with whom the focal person has direct relationship of support—receiving or giving . . . The convoy structure is the delivery system" for social support (p. 278). An individual's convoy includes those who are stable over time and not role dependent, those somewhat role related and likely to change over time, and those "tied directly to role relationships, and most vulnerable to role changes" (p. 273).

Figure 3.2 (see p. 71) illustrates a convoy with the focal person in the center. The first circle around the person represents his or her stable supports, irrespective of roles; the second circle represents the group that is somewhat role dependent; the outside circle represents those supports most likely to change. Techniques for using the convoy are discussed later in the book.

Kahn recommended a procedure to measure support, based on the convoy model. The adult in transition identifies people close to him/her and places them in such categories as family, co-workers, other organizational members, neighbors, professionals, and friends. The adult then rates each person listed in terms of the social support offered. Three measures are thus obtained: one for affect, one for affirmation, one for aid (pp. 279–280).

Support Summary

In summary: To take stock of their clients' supports counselors can ask:

- Is this client getting what he/she needs for this transition in terms of affect? Affirmation? Aid?
- Does the client have a range of types of support—spouse or partner, other close family or friends, co-workers/colleagues/neighbors, organizations, strangers, and institutions?
- Has the client's support system or "convoy of social support" been interrupted by this transition?
- Does the client feel the support system for this transition is a low or a high resource?

Strategies

"By coping we refer to the things people do to avoid being harmed by life strains" (Pearlin & Schooler, 1978, p. 1). "We will define coping as the overt and covert behaviors individuals use to prevent, alleviate, or respond to stressful situations . . . Coping can occur before, during, or after a stressful or challenging situation" (George & Siegler, 1981, p. 37). "In my view, stress itself as a concept pales in significance . . . compared with coping . . . Stress is ubiquitous, an inevitable feature of normal living . . . What makes the difference in adaptational outcome is coping" (Lazarus, 1980, p. 52).

Pearlin and associates identified major life strains and the coping strategies people use to deal with them. Coping "represents . . . concrete efforts to deal with the life strains they encounter in their different roles"; that is, those things an individual does in his or her own behalf (Pearlin & Schooler, 1978, p. 5).

The researchers distinguished three types of coping:

1. "Responses that modify the situation" (such as negotiation in marriage, discipline in parenting, optimistic action in occupation, and seeking advice in marriage and parenting);
2. "Responses that . . . control the meaning of the problem" (such as responses that neutralize, positive comparisons, selective ignoring, substitution of rewards); and
3. Responses that help to manage stress after it has occurred (such as "denial, passive acceptance, withdrawal, magical thinking, hopefulness, avoidance of worry, relaxation"). Specific mechanisms include "emotional discharge versus controlled reflectiveness, . . . passive forbearance versus self-assertion, . . .

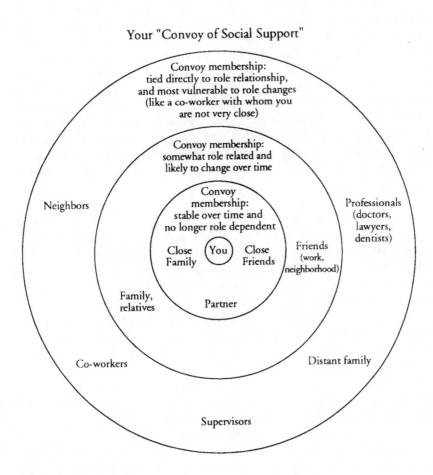

Your "Convoy of Social Support"

Convoy membership:
tied directly to role relationship,
and most vulnerable to role changes
(like a co-worker with whom you
are not very close)

Convoy membership:
somewhat role related and
likely to change over time

Convoy
membership:
stable over time and
no longer role dependent

Neighbors

Professionals
(doctors,
lawyers,
dentists)

Close
Family

You

Close
Friends

Friends
(work,
neighborhood)

Family,
relatives

Partner

Co-workers

Distant family

Supervisors

FIGURE 3.2 "Convoy of social support" (*Source:* Based on work from "Convoys over live course: Attachment, roles, and social support," by R.L. Kahn and T.C. Antonucci, in *Life-Span Development and Behavior,* edited by P.B. Baltes and O.C. Brim, Jr. New York: Academic Press, © 1980, p. 273. Reprinted with permission.)

potency versus helpless resignation, . . . optimistic faith" (1978, pp. 6–7)

Coping strategies are related to people's "psychological resources of self-esteem and mastery" (p. 5). With chronic unemployment, damage to the ego can limit the individual's flexibility in selecting coping strategies. In discussing chronic unemployment, a physician commented on her unemployed husband's shattered ego. Despite the fact that they tried to manage the stress, redefine the situation, and change the situation, there were some lasting and damaging effects on their marriage. Another family—the wife a nurse, the husband an unemployed air traffic controller—reported feeling at the end of their rope. They did not know how to change the situation, redefine the problem, or manage their stress. Counseling could help them develop strategies in one or all of these areas.

Of course, the question crops up as to which coping strategies are best in different situations. Pearlin reports there are many options for people to use in every area of their lives, and that certain strategies do reduce stress in certain role areas, but he also reports that individual coping has the greatest chance of being efficacious with interpersonal problems rather than work-related problems. He further cautions against assuming that coping efforts will work in all settings. The need is to see coping in a broader context. In some cases, collective coping, that is, helping people share in a problem they cannot undo individually, is essential. Structural unemployment is just such a case, for it needs to be addressed collectively and politically. Some individuals, however, are clearly going to cope more effectively than others, and the person with a repertoire of responses—at least five or six—for each role area will most likely handle the strains of life more effectively.

The coping strategies identified in the Pearlin study "constitute but a portion of the full range of responses people undoubtedly call upon in dealing with life-exigencies" (Pearlin & Schooler, 1978, p. 5); nevertheless, they indicate a systematic way to think about strategies. The following outline is adapted from the study; questions or descriptors illustrate each strategy or coping response. The items for the responses are taken from Appendix 4 in "The Structure of Coping" by L. I. Pearlin and C. Schooler, *Journal of Health and Social Behavior,* Volume 19, 1978. (Reprinted with permission.)

1. Responses that modify the situation and are "aimed at altering the source of strain" (p. 20).

- Negotiation. "How often do you try to find a fair compromise, . . . sit down and talk things out?"
- Optimistic action. "When you have difficulties in your work situation, how often do you take some action to get rid of them, or to find a solution?"
- Self-reliance vs. advice-seeking. "In the past year . . . have you asked for the advice of friends . . . relative . . . doctor . . . or other professional?"
- Exercise of potency vs. helpless resignation. "How often do you decide there's really nothing you can do to change things?"

2. Responses that control the meaning of the problem in order to cognitively neutralize the threat (p. 6).
   - Positive comparisons. "A device . . . [to enable] a temporal frame of reference, . . . captured in such idioms as count your blessings."
   - Selective ignoring. A "positive attribute . . . within a troublesome situation. When you have difficulties in your work situation, how often do you tell yourself that they are unimportant [and] try to pay attention only to your duties and overlook them?"
   - Substitution of rewards. "Hierarchical ordering of life priorities . . . to keep the most strainful experiences within the least valued areas of life. If I have troubles at work, I value other areas of life more and downplay the importance of work."

3. Responses that help the individual manage stress after it has occurred to help "accommodate to existing stress without being overwhelmed by it" (p. 7).
   - Emotional discharge. "Expressive ventilation of feelings: How often do you yell or shout to let off steam?"
   - Self-assertion. "When you have differences with your spouse, how often do you fight it out?"
   - Passive forbearance. "When you have differences with your spouse, how often do you keep out of his or her way?"

Pearlin relates the selection of coping strategies to the individual's psychological resources, which we discussed earlier.

Coping, in sum, is certainly not a unidimensional behavior. It functions at a number of levels and is attained by a plethora of behaviors, cognitions, and perceptions. It is useful . . . that coping responses be distinguished from what we have identified as psychological resources for coping, those personality characteristics that minimize threat to self . . . we cannot completely understand coping without looking beyond the personality attributes of individuals to the specific responses to problems in different social roles. (pp. 7–8)

Pearlin and his associates identified a number of coping strategies. None contains magic; rather, effective coping means flexible utilization of a range of strategies as each situation demands.

Like Pearlin, Lazarus and Folkman (1984) see the coping strategies a person employs as more relevant than the event, hassle, or strain, and the person's appraisal of the situation as more central than the event. As we described earlier, the key is the way the person sees the strain, stressor, event—whether it is perceived as harmful, benign, or challenging.

Concurrent with appraising and reappraising events, resources, and results, an individual engages in coping behavior. Lazarus classifies coping in two major ways: instrumental or problem-focused behavior that aims to change the situation, and palliative or emotion-focused behavior that aims to help minimize emotional distress.

Whether individuals want to change their situation or reduce their distress, they can choose from among four coping modes: information seeking, direct action, inhibition of action, and intrapsychic behavior. The first three seem self-explanatory; the last one (intrapsychic) refers to the mind sets individuals employ to resolve problems that arise. These mind sets, which include denial, wishful thinking, and distortion, enable people to carry on. Lazarus finds that "effective copers use both direct action and palliative coping modes" (1980, p. 54). Similarly, Pearlin identified "selective ignoring" as an adaptive strategy.

Lazarus emphasized the fact that selection of a coping strategy depends on whether or not the situation can be changed. If it can be, then problem-focused instrumental strategies will be used; if not, then emotion-focused, palliative will be employed.

An important point for helpers to remember is that effective copers are flexible and utilize a number of methods. Ability to cope is not a trait, but a dynamic process constantly in flux throughout the continuing process of appraisal. For example, Cohen looked at ways people coped with surgery. She reviewed studies based on a theoretical framework suggesting that people's appraisal of a situation determined subsequent emotion and behaviors (1980, p. 376). She studied 59 hernia, gall bladder, and thyroid patients the night before surgery and rated them on a continuum from avoidance (avoid information and knowledge about surgery and outcome) to vigilance (seek out information about surgery). Then she measured recovery on a number of dimensions. Contrary to expectation, neither age nor life change score was a factor in recovery, but the coping strategy of denial was. Those who knew the most had more "complications and a longer hospital stay" (p. 377). In this kind of situation, too much knowledge can lead to panic. Furthermore, trying to be in charge in a situation the individual is unable to control can lead to frustration. Although, in general, most of us will work to help people take control, in some situations this strategy is counterproductive.

How effective such strategies are overall is a complex question. Some theorists and counselors focus on outcomes. Did the client get accepted into an apprentice training program? By focusing only on outcome, however, we may overlook a client's coping effectiveness. A client may employ many strategies flexibly but still not be able to achieve the stated goals. Just as being assertive doesn't guarantee "winning," using flexible coping strategies doesn't always guarantee the desired outcome.

Summary of coping responses. The preceding section has described the way several researchers have conceptualized and studied coping. According to Pearlin, most individuals—when faced with a transition—try to control the situation (for example, by publishing a great deal to ensure promotion), control the meaning of the situation (by seeing promotion as irrelevant), or control the stress (by jogging to release tension caused by promotion worries). Lazarus identified two major coping orientations—changing the situation (instrumental) or relaxing oneself (palliative) and suggests four possible modes of coping: direct action, inhibition of action, information seeking, and intrapsychic.

The following questions can be used to assess ways of coping among your clients:

- Does the client use a range of strategies?   Yes   No
- Does the client sometimes take action to change
  the transition?   Yes   No
- Does the client sometimes try to change
  the meaning of the transition?   Yes   No

- Does the client try to take stress in stride?   Yes   No
- Does the client know when to do nothing?   Yes   No
- Does the client feel that he/she can flexibly choose different strategies depending on the challenge at hand?   Yes   No
- Taking all of the above into account, does the client rate his/her Strategies as:
  A high resource   Yes   No
  A low resource   Yes   No
  A mixed bag   Yes   No
  Okay   Yes   No

ASSETS AND LIABILITIES: ANOTHER LOOK

An individual's ability to cope with transitions depends on the changing interaction and balance of his/her assets and liabilities. Thus, to study or understand an individual's balance, we need to ask such questions as these:

- What are the variables characterizing the particular situation in terms of timing, assessment, duration?
- What are the personal and demographic characteristics of the individual at the time of the transition—the Self?
- Is the client sick or well?
- What is the client's level of ego development, personality, and outlook?
- What coping strategies does he/she use?
- What types of support does the client have?
- What are his/her actual and perceived options?

These variables could also be scored as to whether the individual sees them as assets or liabilities.

Often clients ask, "Should I initiate a change? Should I go back to school? Should I get a divorce? Should I move?" Or they may wonder, "How can I weather the transition imposed upon me?" To answer these questions, one rates the client's 4 S's—the variables characterizing the Situation, the Self, the Supports and the Strategies. From these ratings, a balance score can be derived that will indicate whether or not the client has many or few resources. Further, the client can determine where his/her liabilities lie (Personnel Decisions, Inc., 1994).

Now that the framework, which conceptualizes the way an individual copes with transitions is in place, we move to a discussion of transitions from the clients' points of view. We will hear their views of the balance of their liabilities and assets. Then in Part III of the book we consider how that balance suggests to helpers the areas in which they can be most effective in providing motivation, support, and resources in order to help adults who experience disabling problems at love, work, or play.

Part II
WHAT ARE WE LIKELY TO HEAR?

INTRODUCTION

In this section we move to a discussion of what counselors are likely to hear as they deal with adult clients anticipating or experiencing transitions. As you read this section, we hope you will visualize the clients whose stories we tell you. More than that, however, we hope that these stories will be a trigger for you, encouraging you to think about adults you know—friends, family, and co-workers, as well as clients—who are by choice or necessity in the process of reshaping their lives.

Assume that you are the unseen audience, watching, listening, and interpreting what goes on in the counselor's office. It may help to imagine that you are observing through one-way glass, as in a practicum lab. Many of these stories are ones we have heard directly from clients, students, friends calling somewhat desperately, even seat mates on airplanes. Whatever the source, the stories are often poignant as they illuminate the struggles and challenges of adults navigating transitions. They are designed to help you understand transitions from the client's point of view.

This section is divided into three chapters that focus on different areas of life in which we experience transitions—internally, in relationships with family and other intimates, and in our work lives. Clearly the classifications used here are somewhat arbitrary. For most people there will be considerable overlap among the categories. Almost always a transition in one area of a person's life has an impact on other areas of that person's life, as well as on the lives of the person's "significant others."

Chapter 4 focuses on transitions that are mainly intrapersonal in nature. While decisions made by the individual may ultimately have a dramatic effect on others, the basis for the transition is an internal one. Recurring issues here deal with questions of identity, autonomy, and making meaning of one's life.

Chapter 5 deals with close interpersonal relationships, often but not always within families. Transitions may take the form of events or non-events as people couple or uncouple, have children or decide not to, become grandparents or realize they will not. Here, too, adults face changes in relationships with lovers, siblings, close friends and aging parents, as well as the fear of losing people close to them. Recurring issues in this chapter focus on intimacy, mattering, and belonging.

Chapter 6 surveys the place of work in our lives and the many transitions that occur in this arena. Adults constantly re-examine where they want their careers to go and where they want to invest their energies. Counselors see people looking for their first jobs—some as teenagers, others as mature adults; they also deal with people wanting to change careers, "fix" their present jobs, or leave the paid work force. Recurring issues here deal with work salience (the centrality of work in people's lives), resilience (career adaptability), mastery (self-efficacy), and balance.

In each of these chapters, we include several case studies and a discussion of the types of transitions that may bring adults to a counselor. Using the transition model explicated in Part I, we listen for what clients tell us about their resources for coping with these transitions, that is their 4 S's: their Situation, Self, Supports, and Strategies.

4

Individual Transitions

Listen. Jack Williams, a man in his late thirties is telling you the following:

I woke up one morning a few months ago, looked in the mirror to shave, and saw my father. I don't mean that I hallucinated. I knew it was me, but I looked just like him—colorless, tired, bored. It scared me half to death. I don't want my life to be anything like his. He's retired now and bored to tears, but even when he was working, he always seemed bored. I don't remember his ever being excited about anything. It's like he went, and still goes, through the motions of living without enjoying it. I can't face a lifetime like his.

I've been married for 18 years. My wife and I have two darling kids, a girl 15 and a boy 13. They have their whole lives ahead of them, and I find I'm kind of envious. There is so much they can do, experience, try. My daughter now has a chance for a basketball scholarship. I'm excited for her, but again, I'm jealous. My job is OK. I am the manager for Roberts' furniture store in our small town about an hour and a half outside of the city. It's a job I do well, and I enjoy the contact with everybody I see all day. But all I can think about is if this is all it's going to be for the rest of my life? Is it enough for me?

When I was a teenager I had such dreams. I was the star pitcher on the baseball team in high school, in the same town where I now live. I expected to get a college scholarship. But then I injured my arm, and it didn't happen. There wasn't money to send me to school, and to tell you the truth, I wasn't that interested in more education. I worked a couple of years at the furniture store where I continue to work, married my high school sweetheart, and settled down. I've done well at the store, moving from stock boy to manager in the last 20 years. I've been involved in the community, done all the "right" things. I've coached little league, gone to Rotary luncheons, been an active member of our church, even taught Sunday school for a few years. My wife's and my families live in town. We've been lucky that everyone is still healthy. We spend most Sundays with either my parents or hers. It sounds like the good life doesn't it? So why am I so unhappy?

I've had fantasies about having an affair. It might bring some excitement into my life. But I wouldn't even know how to go about it, and anyway it wouldn't be right. But if I don't do something, I think I'll just wither away. I've always been the "good kid." My older brother was wild when he was a teenager, but I was always solid Jack—the one you could count on. I still am. I shovel my parents' and in-laws' snow in the winter; I'm a volunteer fireman; I always call if I'm going to be late for dinner—though even that much change of routine rarely happens. Good old solid, boring Jack.

I thought if I waited a bit, this feeling would pass. But it hasn't. Sometimes I don't even know who I am. I'm Roberts' store manager, Susan's husband, Cindy and young Jack's father, the Williams's son, the Paines's son-in-law; you get the idea. If none of those people existed, would I? I think I've just drifted to where I am, and I don't have any sense of the future except bleakness. What will it all matter in 100 years?

I've tried to talk to my wife about some of this. (Except the idea of the affair of course.) She says everyone goes through these times of doubt and it will pass. But it hasn't. And I'm finding it harder and harder to get up in the morning. I can't face that face of my father's in the mirror.

Jack Williams's poignant story describes his confrontation with several event and non-event transitions that often occur in midlife. His children are getting close to graduation from high school, and he is anticipating their leaving home. He is asking himself, "Is this all there is?" The peace and joy he expected to find in his middle years have not happened. Clearly, it is a rare individual who lives in a vacuum; relationships and work are almost always an important part of life. But in this chapter, we will use Jack's story to clarify transitions—events and non-events—that pertain primarily to the individual.

We will focus on what counselors *hear* from their adult clients about intrapersonal transitions, interweaving Jack's story with illustrative literature. We will show how individuals experience their transitions in a unique manner, depending on their particular Situation, the aspects of Self that come into play, the Supports they have available, and the Strategies currently being employed.

SITUATION

What makes Jack's situation similar to and different from other people's transitions? Here we will first discuss the triggers to internal transitions, some of which may come from internal awarenesses and some of which may be stimulated by external events. We will then turn our attention to the timing of these transitions. Are they off time or on time? Do they come at a time of relative peace in the person's life, or at a time of turmoil? Next we will talk about the duration of the transition, and finally we will address the source of control—or perceived control. As we discuss these general questions, remember that as people's answers differ, their experiences are unique.

Triggers

Jack went to a counselor to talk about his malaise, his discomfort with his life. He is experiencing a transition in how he views himself—indeed, it seems that he is looking at himself in a conscious way for perhaps the first time in his adult life. What triggered this transition? On the surface, seeing his father's face in the mirror is the primary trigger. And he sees his aging father leading a sterile life—one that he wants to avoid. But what caused the experience? Jack seems to be confronting a change in perspective from seeing life as time spent to seeing life as time left. He worries, wondering, "Is now forever?" He fears that his future will continue in the present pattern and does not like what he sees. It was all right as long as he could imagine a different future. Suddenly that seemed unlikely, and he became terrified.

Isenhart (1983) compared the midlife transition to river rafting. She stated that:

(a) The current of the river is like adult development; it can be anticipated but never completely controlled.
(b) Submerged rocks below the surface of the river are like stressful periods in the transition that often present themselves first as smooth non-events.
(c) The circular currents of water reflect the sense of limitless time when no progress appears possible.

Jack seems to be stuck in this time of circular water, and his perspective of the future has changed.

Such change in perspective can be brought on by an external event, such as being called "sir" or ma'am" for the first time; it can also be caused by a sudden awareness of the changing physical self, such as a twinge in the knees, needing bifocals, or that first gray hair. For people whose self-esteem is closely tied to their appearance, the awareness of aging may be very painful. For people whose work roles require a youthful appearance, for example, models, this transition may be an agonizing one. In American culture, women are probably hit harder than men. Our society is more accepting of aging actors than actresses. Gray sideburns make a man look distinguished, but graying hair makes a woman look less desirable.

For some women, the onset of menopause is the trigger that begins their internal transition. Raphael (1994), a therapist who runs self-discovery groups for mature women, described her own experience, bemoaning some aspects of aging, but ending on a positive note:

> Beginning menopause also signals getting older, and, like it or not, our physical appearance is a large part of how we view ourselves. Distasteful as we may find the leers and come-ons that youthful beauty attracts, becoming invisible is no better bargain. I had no trouble getting older until it showed. In my early fifties, I would brag about my age, confident of hearing, "but you don't look it." The absence of that response can still feel chilling. I don't like being addressed as "Ma'am" and I don't like reminding grown people of their grandmothers. But it is all part of the process. One cannot sort through the various accumulated labels, judgments, and programs of one's lifetime without looking inside. And this kind of self-examination is actually facilitated by the kind of invisibility that accompanies midlife in our culture. Menopause really is a Change of Life. It is about becoming your own person. I am healthier, happier, and more energetic now than at any previous time in my life. (p. 10)

Clients describe many triggers to awareness of transitions. Among them we have heard an impending high school reunion, becoming eligible to join the American Association of Retired Persons or to take advantage of senior discounts, being ineligible for a management training program or the junior league, being offered a seat on the bus or a face cream for mature skin. The death of one's last parent creates an awareness for many of now being "the older generation."

Whether internally or externally triggered, sudden or gradual, the realization of aging can be disturbing. In Jack's case, the trigger included his awareness of his children's growing up and the lives he sees them having *ahead* of them. Different cultures may have differing systems for recognizing aging. Some East African tribal societies organize their population into age groups. "Men in their prime may resist initiating a new cohort of young warriors. The entry of a new cohort automatically advances those above it by one grade and so places the senior men into the respected—but terminal—grade of elder" (Plath, 1980, p. 117).

Furthermore, awareness of time left often includes for the first time a personalization of death. As William Saroyan is rumored to have said on his death bed, "I knew everyone had to die sometime, but I always thought I'd be the exception." Decade birthdays often stimulate this kind of awareness. Card shops sell a variety of paraphernalia with the theme, "Over the hill," and even though this is meant to be humorous, it implies that one is on the downside of the hill—with death at the bottom of the slope. Consider this line from a middle-aged character in the play *Change of Life* (Dubin, 1994):[1] "People always said, 'You have your whole life ahead of you.' Well, my life isn't ahead of me anymore." Even the daily comic strips show an awareness of this phenomenon. The following conversation took place in *For Better or For Worse* (Johnston, 1994):[2]

> "You know, Connie . . . I thought I'd never get old. Other people got old . . . but not me."
> "Yeah."
> "Then suddenly you realize that it is happening. I *am* following my parents, as my parents followed their parents. The laws of nature apply to *me* too! . . . It's scary."
> "Yeah . . . we're on the great conveyer belt of life, . . . and from this point you can look up and see the end."

For some, the realization of the finiteness of life can lead to a determination to live life fully, to appreciate existence, to, in the words of the cliché, pick more daisies. For others, the awareness can lead to depression or panic, occasioned by a sense of urgency to "do it now!" As will be discussed in Part III, the challenge for counselors is to help reframe this awareness into appropriate goal setting.

Jack's transition is a complex one. It includes the events of his children getting ready to leave the nest, his own aging, and what he perceives as diminishing opportunities for himself. His recognition that he

---

[1] *Change of Life*, unpublished play by K. Dubin, 1994. Quoted material used with permission of the author.

[2] *For Better or For Worse* by Lynn Johnson, © 1994 Universal Press Syndicate, used with permission.

has advanced as far as he is probably going to at work and that he really never will achieve his dreams of sports stardom are non-events also affecting his life at this point. (Even though he may have grieved in the past for his injury and the lost scholarship, his current recognition is different in that it encompasses the future.) Jack seems, in Hudson's (1991) words, to have "run out of dreams and . . . [to] lack the ability to envision new ones" (p. xii) . . . [He feels] vulnerable instead of visionary, trapped instead of empowered" (p. 13).

Timing

In Jack's case, the transition is created largely by the time in his life in which it is happening. He is established in his career, in his community, and in his family. He is close to the statistical midpoint of life. He sees his children heading off to partake of opportunities he feels he missed.

Jack is also at a time when he has some freedom to be introspective. His children are "on track," his place in his marriage, his work, and his community are secure. One might speculate that it is because of this secure base that he feels safe enough to risk looking at his life in this way. Maslow's (1954) hierarchy would indicate that basic needs for physiological and psychological safety precede the need for belongingness and self-esteem, and later, the search for self-actualization. The internal transition of meaning-making seems to be such a search, indicating that this sort of midlife transition is a phenomenon of the comfortable. It seems unlikely that the homeless or others desperately struggling to survive have time or energy to ask meaning-making questions. There is, however, little research on the psychological aspects of that population.

Age is an important, but not the sole, determinant of a typical adult's midlife awareness. Internal or external triggers may precipitate this awareness at a variety of ages and invite the existential question, "Is this all there is?" And age may also have an effect on how an individual reacts to a transition event. A classic example comes from a study of men aged 37 to 67 who were hospitalized following heart attacks (Rosen & Bibring, 1968). Whereas the younger men were generally cheerful and the 60-year-olds fatherly and easygoing, the 50-year-olds were hostile, withdrawn, depressed, and difficult as patients. The authors interpret these age differences as follows: Those under 50 simply denied the seriousness of their condition; those in their 60s accepted it as an on-time event; but those in their 50s experienced "open conflict from the active orientation of youth . . . A heart attack theoretically accentuates the very issues with which the [middle-aged man] has been actively struggling" (p. 207), that is, with his anxiety about aging and his reluctance about shifting from an active to a passive role.

Different cultures may attach different meanings to certain ages. "Old" is changing its definition as today's generation ages with greater health and longevity than previous generations. Gloria Steinem's classic statement, on being told she looked young for 40, "This is how 40 looks!" reflects this. Yet, in American culture there is also the paradox of the worship of youth. As mentioned, for women, this is particularly poignant. Fashion magazines rarely portray older women in either editorial or advertising photographs. Television advertisers consistently use young models to sell their wares. Some good news on that front was reported in the *Beauty News* section of the February, 1994 *Mirabella*, a fashion magazine for women. "Clinique removes the word *younger looking* from all its ads and replaces it with *better looking*. At the same time, the company plasters New York City with black and white posters that read, 'Beauty isn't about looking young.' "

In Finland, one's 50th birthday is noted and celebrated. Indeed, in a small community one must have a party and invite everyone, or one must leave town and put a notice in the newspaper. Niemela (1987) studied Finnish women aged 49–55 and found that:

> The 50th birthday had shaken up these women, starting a process of rethinking and reevaluating their total lives. If middle-aged women no longer reflect the cultural image of the ideal woman as a young, attractive sex object, what can they be? My study showed that they start thinking about what they really are; get more in contact with their real feelings and thoughts, needs, and wishes. The older women of the study expressed more independence. They felt they were more in the center of their own lives, more responsible for themselves . . . "Instead of material goods, I have started evaluating other things. I have started valuing health and small joys." (p. 5)

Further in the same piece, Niemela speculated about why an artificial event such as a birthday can lead to such profound changes in a woman's life, in particular, how it becomes an impetus to individuation. She stated, "It is not the age per se, but the woman's awareness of being 50, which starts the developmental processes. The 52–55-year-old women had worked through life matters which the 49–51-year-olds had only started to confront" (p. 5).

Counselors need to be alert for client comments that demonstrate concern about aging, fear of future limitations, or more positively, excitement about future possibilities. They need to be alert for artificial barriers to change that may be revealed by statements such as, "You can't teach an old dog new tricks." Clients who feel hopeless about their abilities to manage a transition may say things like, "It's too late for me to change; I'm too old." Sometimes a humorous interchange like the following may help break that cycle:

Client: I can't learn a new trade, it would take me five years and I'll be 55 by then.

Counselor: How old will you be in five years if you don't learn the new trade?

Client: Fifty-five . . . Oh . . .

The insight represented by that "Oh" can be the beginning of a new view of life's possibilities.

Pearson and Petitpas (1990) examined the unpredictability of athletes' careers, which often make their transitions "off time." They cited Mihovilovic's (1968) finding that 95% of professional soccer players leave the sport against their will, usually by not making the team or by being injured. As we saw with Jack, this loss may stay with a person for many years. According to Pearson and Petitpas, when " . . . a person's identity and activity increasingly center on athletics" (p. 7), the transition becomes even harder to manage. The "macho" tradition that makes it difficult for athletes to ask for or accept support complicates the issue. Counselors may see athletes who come in for help with career planning or for marital counseling and who also, or perhaps primarily, need to deal with a transition regarding their athletic life.

Similarly, older actresses no longer able to secure ingenue roles, or actors forced to change from leading man to character actor, must, because of an external trigger, change internal assumptions as they change roles. The performer who tries to retain a youthful appearance by cosmetic surgery and excessive make-up has become a commonplace butt of comedians' put-downs, but the real limitations in possible roles created by aging are no joke to the performer.

Duration

The duration of an individual transition is not always obvious. The time it takes for the new self to be accepted and integrated varies widely from individual to individual. The menopause process, for example, can last ten years. Some questions that may help a client gain a better understanding of the duration of a transition include: Is it perceived as permanent, temporary, or unknown? Does the individual assess it as positive, negative, or mixed? Is it of great importance to the individual? For example, waiting a year to take one last class to complete a degree may be agonizing to Person A and a minor nuisance to Person B.

In one study, 50 clerical workers were questioned about ways they coped with transitions. One woman selected remarriage as the transition of most recent impact. When asked whether she saw the remarriage as permanent or temporary, she thought a moment and said it was too hard to answer. She would like it to be permanent, but, as she was on her fourth husband, she would probably have to say temporary (Charner & Schlossberg, 1986).

Health crises are examples of internal events with varying durations. A person may be temporarily immobilized by back surgery or permanently disabled due to a spinal injury. Someone may have to restrict activities due to a bout of pneumonia, another may have to lead a permanently quiet life due to a heart condition.

Even health events with temporary durations, however, can trigger a more lasting transition. If a health crisis leads to a redefinition of self, a sense of vulnerability or frailty, it may affect future goals and plans or lead to a different life style. Of course, some health events may be of unknown duration, for example, knee surgery or cancer treatment. Counselors will hear some people with orthopaedic problems complain that the athletic side of their lives is over; they will hear others investigate what kinds of braces to wear as they resume their sport or look into which sports they can play with their new handicap. Some tennis players, as their knees and backs give out, make the move from playing singles on a hard court to playing doubles on a clay court; others, with the same level of deficit, quit the game entirely.

Although some cancer treatments are so devastating that one can barely manage one's daily life, others allow more freedom. However, helpers hear adults in similar circumstances describe their health transitions in widely different ways. The duration, uncertain, is the same for all; the interpretation is again quite different. Some of the reasons for these different interpretations will be treated below in the discussions on hope and selective denial.

The duration of non-events is even more difficult to assess. As one woman, bemoaning what she saw as a static life, said, "I thought this was to be the 'change of life,' but nothing has changed!" Perhaps the duration of non-events is more appropriately considered as the length of time it takes people to accept as permanent a condition they thought was temporary. When concern about the non-event ceases to take center stage, the transition can be thought of as having been integrated into one's life.

Source of Control

The source of Jack's transition is internal, although fed by external factors. Having a sense of control is often critical to success in managing transitions. Many self-related transitions have an internal genesis, and therefore an internal locus of control. Some, however, are a combination of internal and external. Health problems are a good example. If your asthma is aggravated by smoking, you have some control over the course of the disease. If you have a bad back, it may be improved by appropriate exercise. Careful management can allow a person to control diseases like diabetes or high blood pressure. Many believe that our minds have great influence over the state of our health in general (e.g., Pearsall, 1987; Siegel, 1986). Counselors may hear adults bemoan the fact that they have lost control to the medical establishment. Many determine to influence their treatment; others find letting go of control can lessen the stress of the situation.

Two women developed emphysema and needed to adapt to a future with limited mobility. One sat in her chair and rarely moved. She saw the illness as not only permanent but one over which she had no control. Another used portable oxygen, acquired a good backpack to carry it, and took walks with her family. Even if the walks were slow, she was able to be outdoors and participate in activities she had enjoyed previously. For both of these women the limitations imposed by the disease were similar, but the two women took different amounts of control, and therefore the amount of change created by the event differed.

A difficult decision for many gays, lesbians, or bisexuals is whether or when to "come out" to family, friends, or work colleagues. Although individuals control this decision, they cannot control others' reactions to it. Sometimes a partner forces a revelation; sometimes a person is "found out" by being seen in a gay environment, or by contracting AIDS or having a "roommate" contract AIDS. Some people make an active decision to let those close to them know about their sexual orientation but not to tell the world in general. Regardless of the etiology, the transition from secret to public is an important one to the individual and those close to that individual. A mystery novel by Alison Gordon (1990) dramatized the pain and loss of privacy when teammates and press respond with great hostility to a baseball star's "coming out." The shock of his teammates and the sports world that an athlete could be gay provides a dramatic illustration of the misconceptions of many about homosexuality.

SELF

Here, as we focus on the Self issues related to internal transitions, we will look at issues of identity, autonomy, meaning-making, and self-efficacy. These are added to the personal, demographic, and psychological characteristics of the individual presented in Chapter 3.

Identity

It is tempting to assume that most self-transition issues relate to identity. The answer to "Who am I?" changes as life situations change. For Jack Williams, the old answers no longer satisfy. For a person with a chronic illness, "I" has changed. Perhaps even more importantly, people often ask, "Who will I be?" With help, they may find answers that differ from those in the past. Many young adults believe that they will find out who they are one of these days. They see older people seemingly knowing this, and make an assumption that this kind of wisdom comes with age. They retain the childhood wish of someday being and feeling "grown up," with its attendant assumption of self-knowledge. Perhaps one of the triggers to a midlife self transition is the recognition that this "grown-upness" may never happen, that it is a myth. Perhaps at the same time comes a recognition of ultimate aloneness—the so-called existential awareness we mentioned earlier.

Older people, on the other hand, may be asking themselves, "Who was I?" Counselors hear older clients reviewing their lives, looking at the past as a way of assessing the present. Erikson (1950) discussed the developmental crisis of old age as being one of integrity versus despair.

Integrity is found by assessing one's life as having been meaningful. But-ler (1963) theorized that an internal life review was a universal occur-rence. Counselors often hear older clients asking such questions as, "Was I successful as a parent, spouse, worker, citizen, friend?" and "All in all, has it been a good life?" They may also be making summary statements such as, "Given where I started, I've done OK," or "Nothing I've done has worked out. I guess you could say my life has been a failure." Coun-selors need to be alert for these types of statements so they can foster appropriate follow-up exploration.

For some, issues of identity are non-events. If my dreams of being a spouse and parent, or grandparent, chair of the board, or chief stew-ard, do not happen, my identity changes. Although Erikson (1950) talked of identity formation as a task of young adulthood, midlife adults often recapitulate this issue. Counselors may hear people simultaneously grieving for the loss of a planned identity and questioning how they can reshape their dreams (Schlossberg & Robinson, 1993). If my desire to be a parent, as it often does, comes out of my need to be nurturing to the next generation, I may talk about volunteering in a childcare cen-ter, being a "Big Brother" or "Big Sister," spending more time with my nieces and nephews, or becoming a foster grandparent.

Sometimes people use humor to help in their struggle to accept the non-event. Tom Lehrer, mathematician, satirist, pianist, folk singer, once said, "It's a sobering thought to think that when Mozart was my age, he had been dead for 10 years" (Personal communication, June, 1972). Judith Viorst's (1976) poem, "Facing the Facts," listed all the things she would probably never do, such as cure the cold, paint a Picasso, or advise presidents, and ends with, "I must still face the fact that they'll never be able to say, 'and she did it so young' "(p. 53).

One's past experience is clearly a central component of identity and often determines how a person approaches a current transition. Counselors may hear, if they ask the right questions, stories of previous challenges faced by their client. When these stories describe a track record of successful coping, clients are usually more prepared to take risks and confront their current transition with verve. When these sto-ries are largely descriptive of negative outcomes, clients may be afraid to trust their own instincts and will ask for solutions from the counse-lor. Counselors can help people recall positive coping experiences and look for the skills they used in making them positive.

Autonomy

The dictionary defines *autonomy* as independence or self-directed freedom (Webster, 1980). A great deal of research substantiates that life satisfaction depends on one's perception of autonomy. Whether you believe the autonomy is real or an illusion may not matter. People who feel in control of their lives tend to describe their lives as happier. We must remember, however, Gilligan's (1982) work on women's development. She stated, "Illuminating life as a web rather than a succession of relationships, women portray autonomy rather than attachment as the illusory and dangerous quest" (p. 48). She posed autonomy as an aim in conflict with compassion and connection, a narrower definition than that which we are using. We would suggest that personal autonomy can include the choice, but not the compulsion, to be compassionate and connect. We take the androgynous position that intimacy and autonomy are both desirable if men and women are to lead satisfying adult lives.

Kincade (1987) suggested that individuals develop along the following lines: (a) The young child is *dependent* for all its needs on a nurturing parent. With growth, comes a period of (b) *counter-dependence,* a time of rebellion where individuation and autonomy take place, followed by (c) a period of *independence,* where the individual leads or attempts to lead a completely separate life. Many individuals stop developing at this point, but Kincade suggests that fully mature individuals move to (d) *interdependence,* where there is a recognition of the connections and mutuality suggested by Gilligan (1982). It is the authors' position that this interdependence includes a true autonomy. One cannot fully participate in an interdependent relationship without being at first an independent, autonomous person. Adults who believe that they are able to function independently can willingly join with another in true mutuality. Adults who believe that they need another to survive, will not be able to be a true full partner in a relationship—the risks are too great.

Levinson (1986) supported this position. He stated:

> One developmental task of this [midlife] transition is to begin a new step in individuation. To the extent that this occurs, we can become more compassionate, more reflective and judicious, less tyrannized by inner conflicts and external demands, and more genuinely loving of ourselves and others. (p. 5)

Fouad and Fahje (1989) studied the psychological effects of infertility on women. Although others, for example, Shapiro (1982), studied the impact of infertility on couples, this study focused on the women themselves, identifying variables that fit well with our discussion of locus of control, self-esteem, depression, and social support. Using the Coopersmith Self-Esteem Inventory (Peterson & Austin, 1985), the Beck Depression Inventory (Beck, Ward, Mendelsohn, Mock, & Erbaugh, 1961), the Social Support Inventory (Brown & Heath, 1984), and Rotter's Internal-External Scale (Rotter, 1966), they found:

(a) depressed women needed more support and were less satisfied with the support they received;

(b) women with higher self-esteem had a better match between the support they wanted and the support they received, but women with higher self-esteem needed less support;

(c) self-esteem and internal locus of control were positively correlated; and

(d) more depressed women felt less in control of their lives.

These women lacked autonomy. They felt that they had lost control because of their inability to control their childbearing and the invasive medical procedures associated with infertility, and they felt dehumanized by the procedures. The interaction among many variables stands out as we consider the lives of these women. Counselors need to listen carefully to their clients' descriptions of complex scenarios as they help individuals assess their resources and liabilities in terms of the Self, the Situation, the Supports available, and the Strategies employed.

Clients will also talk about fears related to loss of autonomy or expectations of increases in autonomy. People may be afraid that changes in relationships, such as marriage or childbearing, or changes in work, such as joining a large corporation, may have a deleterious effect on their autonomy. They may see other transitions, for example, getting divorced or having children leave home, becoming self-employed or retiring, or an increased sense of interiority, as leading to more autonomy. And to further complicate matters, some people may *fear* increased autonomy. (We never promised you this would be simple!)

Meaning-Making

An important element of many midlife transitions is the need to make meaning—of the transition and of life itself. Certainly Jack is questioning his values and his purpose—in life. And surely his hope and optimism are shaky. Transitions often shake spiritual sureties as well. All we know about Jack's spiritual life is that he is active in his church, but we might suspect that he is questioning that church as he is everything else in his life. Counselors frequently hear middle-aged clients moving away from organized religion, particularly if they have been involved "for the children" who are now grown up. But they also often hear a commitment or recommitment to spirituality, defined more broadly than when the adult was younger. It now often includes hope and optimism, purpose in life, love, and moral values.

Finding one's life mission often relates to spirituality. This can relate to finding work that is meaningful in a deeper sense, but many people seek their life mission in other arenas of life. For example, one woman's search for meaning stemmed from a divorce. She took a six-month leave from her job and spent time on an island near Singapore where she worked with a United Nations team providing mental health services to Southeast Asian refugees. While there she met two young Vietnamese refugees. After her return to the United States, she became their sponsor here, and in the process changed her views about what was important in her life. This example illustrates the intertwining of internal and external triggers that invited one adult to search for life's meaning in a new way. Her divorce, together with her children's becoming adults and leaving home, provided both the spur and the possibility of a creative, new way to look for "more" out of her life.

There is, of course, no "right" way to find meaning. Another woman quit a good professional job to spend a year in South America doing things she had always wanted to like swimming with dolphins and exploring more fully her own inner life. These "quests" are a way that some, whose life circumstances and financial means allow, seek to find meaning in midlife. Quests have a long tradition in many cultures. Sometimes relegated solely to the young, many cultures encouraged the middle-aged or old among them to seek meaning in exploration, for example, American Indian vision quests. Many Catholics see a visit to a shrine, such as Lourdes in France, Guadaloupe in Mexico, as fulfilling a lifetime dream. A Moslem's trip to Mecca is considered an important component of spiritual health.

Weenolsen (1986) conducted a study to investigate empirically some of the ideas contained in existential philosophy, fiction, and psychology. Using the concept of transcendence, she described her paradigm as follows:

The central thesis of the loss and transcendence paradigm is that we are in a continuous process of creating our lives and our selves. Our lives are the external aspects of our identity; our selves are the inner aspects. This creation of lives and selves . . . [includes] loss and transcendence. Loss is defined very broadly: it is any event, thought, or feeling that destroys some aspect of one's life and/or one's self (the one cannot be affected without the other). This can be the loss of a loved one, a job, a material possession; it can be a loss of will, freedom, control, plans, expectations, hopes, ideals, or illusions. It can be a loss that is chosen or imposed, originating within the individual or without. Transcendence is the overcoming of loss and the re-creation of the life-self. There is no human activity, major or minor, that does not represent a loss and a transcendence of some kind to the individual experiencing it. (p. 2)

Weenolsen interviewed 48 women aged 25–67, asking open-ended questions related to the meaning of life. Although she found that 38 of the 48 women in her study believed that life has meaning, there was a distinction between those oriented to loss and those oriented to transcendence. In telling their stories, "The loss-oriented answered in terms of what they did not have, whereas the transcendence-oriented replied in terms of losses overcome" (p. 6).

Most women found meaning through conducting a life review. Although usually discussed as a later-life phenomenon (c.f., Butler, 1963), Weenolsen (1986) found that 71% of her middle-aged interviewees reported frequent or occasional life reviews, and only one individual reported that she never engaged in such an activity. Clearly then, counselors can encourage life-review activities for clients at all ages. This strategy can be encouraged or expanded upon as clients face new challenges.

Weenolsen found four primary ways whereby people find meaning: (a) being preordained and coming from God; (b) part of a process of personal and spiritual growth; (c) a specific individual purpose such as being productive or helping others; and (d) a more general personal purpose such as being loving or sharing joy. The women who believed that God has a divine plan for them believed they would find life's meaning in that plan. The majority of subjects, however, believed that meaning could be created.

Counselors will want to listen for statements that reveal where a person is in this process and how a particular client makes meaning. They can then plan interventions to help individuals find meaning as they manage their transitions.

An interesting example of using the life review process to find life meaning is found in *Inscape: A Search for Meaning* (Young, 1983). This memoir "records the backward look over a personal journey, a search to discover in the changing circumstances of my life, over a period of eight decades, my own meaning" (p. 1). Young commented near the end of the book that " . . . the voyage of discovery consists in seeing with new eyes all that has woven the tapestry of one's life" (p. 98). Not everyone will write a book, but many can benefit from the introspective process used by Young.

Self-Efficacy

Counselors hear self-descriptions that run the gamut from confident to inadequate. Bandura (1982) coined the term *self-efficacy* to describe the belief that one can make a difference in one's own life and have an impact on one's environment. Self-efficacy enables a person to tackle a new problem with an optimistic expectation that it will be solvable.

Consider Sylvia, a 55-year-old divorced teacher who had been offered an early retirement package from her school district. She sought counseling help to decide whether or not to accept the offer. In describing her dilemma, she discussed her fears that in retirement she will be bored, that she will have no social life, which currently is made up mostly of school-related events, and that she will "wither away." She also talked about opportunities for visiting her children and grandchildren who live in distant states and for spending more time on her crafts and hobbies. She explained that she has made many bad decisions in her life, has no confidence in her ability to make this one, and is feeling panicky over its irrevocacy. Clearly her appraisal of the situation includes both present threat and fear of future harm, as well as possible challenge. This mixed bag, common to stressful situations, is coupled with low self-efficacy estimates.

Counselors can intervene in each of these arenas—evaluating the harm and threat, reinforcing the challenge, and changing the client's beliefs in her self-efficacy by helping her explore past successes and current resources. As counselors get to know about the balance of Sylvia's assets to deficits, they need to consider not only the situation she faces and the areas of her self that impinge on that situation, but also where else she can obtain assistance to face her current challenges.

SUPPORT

When individuals hear the word "support," they usually think of other people. Counselors, with judicious questioning, can find out the shape, size, and range of a person's support system—who is in it and what function each person plays in the system. During times of transition, we often hear of great disruptions to a support system. An important first step to planning ways to enhance a system is to learn about its present status. Although we will discuss methods for improving support systems with individuals in Chapter 7 and with groups in Chapter 8, in this discussion we will describe what counselors may hear as clients describe their "people" supports. As with all of the discussions in this section of the book, our purpose here is to heighten your awareness of issues brought to counseling by people in transition. It is our hope that this heightened awareness will enable you to listen more productively as you help your clients explore their lives.

Types of Support

Waters and Samson (1993) used Pearson's (1990) research to provide a list of typical support needs. They included: (a) acceptance, (b) self-esteem, (c) love and physical intimacy, (d) personal and work connections, (e) peers (people like one in a particular arena, such as other parents of adolescents), (f) stimulation and challenge, (g) role models, (h) guidance (mentors or sponsors), and (i) comfort and assistance.

Let us look at one of the needs listed above, "role models." In Jack's case, the potential for his father to be such a role model is lost. Positive role models can be important components of support, but Jack's father is a negative role model—helpful only in clarifying for Jack what he doesn't want to become. Jack's counselor will want to help him think about who else may have been or could be role models for him. The counselor and Jack may also want to think together about whether there are any positive aspects of his father that he could use as a pattern for his own adult life.

As you elicit the stories of your clients in transition, listen for such support issues as: having very few people filling many functions, having areas with little or no support, and statements such as, "I don't need support" or "Grown men don't depend on others." Often you can help people to feel more comfortable accepting support if you remind them of the times that they have supported others and encourage them to think of times in the future when they will again be able to be givers. It may also help to remind them of the pleasure they get in giving to others. When they do not let others assist them, they deprive the people they care about of the opportunity to be givers.

For instance, a man attending a party saw a list of emergency numbers next to a friend's telephone and asked, with some dismay, why he wasn't on the list. The unstated messages of: "I thought you knew you could count on me in an emergency" and "I want to be able to help you out when you need it" were expressive of his desire to give. Many clients do not recognize the supportive function played by people in their lives. Sometimes a delightful serendipitous outcome of exploring support systems is that clients share this awareness with those closest to them who are generally very flattered and pleased.

People often receive support from groups designed specifically to provide supportive functions. A plethora of such groups have arisen, both self-help and professionally led, to provide a forum for adults with specific problems. These include support groups for people who have lost breasts or colons, groups for people newly divorced or widowed, and groups for new parents or those who have decided not to have children. These groups, which will be discussed more fully in Chapters 8 and 9, offer information and support, and, with luck, help individuals both to acquire and to perceive more control over their situation.

Spirituality

For many, faith in a higher power is an important component of the support they get from "others." Although we discussed spirituality under meaning-making previously, we write about spirituality here because therapists as well as religious leaders recognize the comfort in a belief system that includes an all-powerful or all-forgiving God. People draw on this support in a variety of ways, many extremely individualistic. Many people find it in an organized religious setting—church, mosque, synagogue, or temple. The support comes from the beliefs of the religion, from the clergy or other religious leaders, and from the people who come together to worship.

Others find spirituality outside of organized religion. Clients often describe communion with the natural world or with special people as being of a spiritual nature. They may talk about their sense of connection to the universe as they look at a summer sky, admire bare tree branches in the snow, or gaze at the majesty of mountains. Or they may talk about love of children and grandchildren, or of a life partner, or they may describe the spiritual joy they feel in listening to great music or watching a beautiful dance.

For counselors, it is important to listen for the ways clients find spirituality and how they use it supportively. The challenge, perhaps, is to be open to hearing about forms of spirituality quite different from one's own. This may be an area where cultures are indeed diverse— and where our own biases make it hard to recognize other's supports.

STRATEGIES

Part III is dedicated to counseling interventions—things we can do to help our clients develop strategies that will help them move forward in their lives. The goal of this part is to identify what you may hear from clients about strategies they currently employ. We have found that it is usually easier for clients to do more of what they already know than to learn new things. Thus, finding out in some detail what successful strategies clients already use is a productive aim of counseling.

Reframing

Folkman, Chesney, McKusick Ironson, Johnson, and Coates (1991), refer to a process of reappraisal, reframing, as central to the coping process. In their model, this is a continuous process that can move in either a positive or negative direction. Clearly, we hope that the reframing will be in a positive direction, but the important point is for counselors to listen for either type of statement. One woman we know, in despair over a painful divorce, talked about her pride in being able to care so deeply. In doing so, she reframed at least some of her pain into hope for a future deep relationship. Another woman described her graying hair as a "free frosting."

Two men were forced into early retirement by companies that were "right-sizing." One saw it as an opportunity to spend more time with his family and in pursuing several hobbies. Another, a negative reframer, over-generalized and saw it as a total condemnation of his worth. He felt that if he was not valuable enough to the company to keep, then he was valuable to no one. He gave up his volunteer activities, quit his golf league, and retreated to his den where he watched television and generally exhibited symptoms of depression. He was not able to separate the cause of his lay-off—economics, and not a comment on his work performance—from his total worth as a person.

Bandler and Grinder (1975) discussed this process from the perspective of linguistics as well as psychology. They described three processes through which we narrow the real world into our perceptive world. They are: (a) generalization, in which we apply learning from one situation or experience to others we deem similar, (b) distortion, in which we change what we think, see, and feel about the world to match our internal perceptions, and (c) deletion, in which we selectively screen out parts of our perception, again often to match some internal sense. Counselors need to listen to their clients' uses of each of these processes to determine if the use is self-enhancing or self-destructive.

Let us look in more detail at the case of the depressed laid-off man described above. He extended his negative feelings about his work abilities to include his feelings about all of his abilities—*over-generalization.* It is likely that he *distorted* what he heard from the personnel office. Perhaps he was told that they had to let a certain number of people go and chose everyone earning above a certain amount. Or perhaps he was told that his department was being absorbed by another, and that all the managers in his section had to be let go. But our hypothetical man probably already had a fairly low self-esteem, perhaps based on a lifetime of negative thinking, so he *distorted* what he heard to match his internal perception of his value. Perhaps they even told him they were sorry to lose a good worker, and that they would be glad to give him excellent references. Because he did not, deep down, believe that he was worthy, he "didn't hear" or *deleted* the positive message. Whenever any of these processes become evident to a counselor, the stage is set for reframing.

The classic example of positive reframing is the reference to the Chinese pictograph for crisis, said to be a combination of the brushstrokes for threat and opportunity. The Western version might be represented by the adage that, "Every cloud has a silver lining." A negative example might be the so-called Murphy's law, "If anything can go wrong, it will." Counselors can listen to a client's abilities to reframe positively so they can reinforce, modify, or teach this coping strategy.

Selective Denial

The technique of selective denial is closely allied to reframing. Counselors can listen for the ways that people "forget" parts of their situations.

A 60-year-old man had surgery for cancer. Although the odds for re-covery were about fifty-fifty, he believed that his cancer was all gone. He took the recommended chemotherapy and followed other medical recommendations, although he believed they were unnecessary. His se-lective denial allowed him to enjoy life during this unpleasant time, and, if we believe researchers like Siegel (1986), increased his chances of com-plete recovery. The difference between healthy and unhealthy denial in this situation is that an unhealthy denier might refuse treatments. People can deny facts, as in the above example, deny the meaning of a situation, deny that the situation applies to them, or deny that the situ-ation is pervasive or will be long-lasting.

A client moved across the country by herself to a place where she knew nobody. She stated that she didn't consider herself alone or lonely. She enjoyed her own company, she said, and knew that eventually she would meet people and form new friendships. This denial of the pos-sible ill-effects of her move might get her in trouble if she did not then reach out to others in her new community. But at the moment, it gave her the energy to focus on settling into her apartment and finding a job.

People who deny that their own aging means slowing down, even if it means so for others, may be the same people we see competing in the "over 80" field in a marathon, triathlon, or swim meet. Selective de-nial for these athletes creates a true change in the reality. Unhealthy deniers might continue to compete when it is causing permanent harm to their knees or even their hearts.

Denying the pervasiveness or long-lastingness of the situation is the last type of selective denial. Counselors will hear people making such pronouncements as: "It was only my job, not my life." "This will feel like home in a few weeks." "I may look old on the outside, but inside I'm still a lad of 21." Counselors should be alert to the coping strategies re-lated to selective denial currently being used by their clients. They can then support the ones that are functional and help to redirect those that are less so.

Hope and Optimism

Hope has been described as "the passion for the possible." According to the dictionary it is "desire accompanied by expectation of or belief in fulfillment" (Webster's, 1980, p. 546). According to the same dictio-nary, optimism is "an inclination to put the most favorable construction upon actions and events or to anticipate the best possible outcome" (p. 799). Hope only exists when there is also doubt—otherwise it is expectation. Take the case of Marie, who had two adult children. She expected her children would marry, and she would become a grandparent. However, one daughter became emotionally unstable and was in and out of hospitals; the other daughter married but postponed having children. As the possibility emerged that she might not have grandchildren, her hope increased. In other words, when she fully expected to be a grandmother, there was no need for hope. As the possibility became ambiguous, hope became her "powerful ally." After her daughter announced that she and her husband had decided never to have children, hope went out the window. She became despondent; she gave herself time to grieve over the loss of what might have been. Finally, she modified her dream by becoming a foster grandparent.

According to Hof (1993), hope is an important, and often overlooked aspect of the therapy process. Reviewing the literature in family/couple counseling from 1975–1992, he found only two mentions of hope. He said, "One of the first tasks of the therapist is to uncover hope, to help create hope, or to instill hope" (p. 223). Counselors often find that people in transition can be divided among those with hope, those without, and some, who he calls Paul or Paula Pollyanna, who may even have so much that they fail to appropriately avoid danger. Some people come to counseling as a last hope!

What is it about hope that is so important in a transition? Again, we see the intertwining of experience and emotional state. The naturally hopeful can lose this world view during times of crisis, but can regain it afterwards. The naturally gloomy may struggle even harder to cope with difficult times. We recall an experienced school counselor who found himself stultified in a job he did easily and had done for a long time. He returned to school for an advanced degree solely to energize himself in his profession. He described the experience with enthusiasm, both for his own learning and renewal, and for the renewed empathy he had for his students' academic tribulations. This man clearly believed he had the ability to change his life through his own efforts—an optimist. We recall another man, also bored with his work in education, who counted the days to retirement for several years, and withdrew more and more into a cocoon. He felt helpless to change his situation and believed that he had to suffer in silence—a pessimist.

Crow (1987) discussed the possible loss of optimism for women in midlife:

At midlife this optimism may be gone; time is no longer the great escape. Feeling trapped at midlife can be described as "lifestyle claustrophobia." It is an overwhelming feeling of being caught in a set of circumstances, or personal life box, from which there is no escape. The world is closing in and circumstances seem to be set in stone. It is too late to change things now. (p. 413)

In her study of 146 female educators, who averaged 48 years old, Crow found that two-thirds experienced, or were currently experiencing, a midlife crisis. She described these women as follows: "She no longer believes she is capable of living with the prices she pays for earlier decisions or behavior. The box gets tighter, the escapes are fewer and less feasible, and the feeling of entrapment more overpowering" (p. 413). Crow implied that women return to optimism after experiencing a successful change.

In his book *Learned Optimism*, Seligman (1990) described several components of optimism/pessimism. Counselors can listen for the following aspects of their clients' explanatory style—their habitual way of explaining both bad and good events. Explanatory style has three dimensions:

1. *Permanence.* Do you believe causes are permanent or transitory? Optimists believe causes of good things are permanent, bad things transitory; pessimists believe just the opposite—that causes of bad things are permanent, good things transitory. Counselors need to be alert for such words as "always" and "never" and the context in which they are used.

2. *Pervasiveness.* "The optimist believes that bad events have specific causes, while good events will enhance everything he does; the pessimist believes that bad events have universal causes and that good events are caused by specific factors" (pp. 47–48). Pervasiveness can determine whether people who experience a painful transition will allow that event to spill into all areas of their lives, or whether they will contain the event in its own "box." Counselors need to listen for "catastrophizing" statements as they listen for the pervasiveness dimension. The same process holds for positive transitions. Counselors need to listen for whether people will allow the event to permeate their entire sense of self. Transitions relating to the self are particularly subject to pervasiveness *because* of their internality. It is hard to see "angst" or joy as anything but pervasive. A person

who declares, "I really seem to have a new sense of who I am
and what matters to me" is unlikely to keep that feeling in a
small box.

3. *Personalization.* The third dimension of explanatory style, personalization, refers to whether one takes responsibility for one's
own successes and failures or attributes them to others. Optimists take responsibility for their successes and blame others
for their failures. A middle-aged optimistic man with healthy
teeth said he had worked hard all of his life to keep them that
way—flossing, brushing, getting regular check-ups, etc. The
pessimistic man with similar dental health said it was because
his parents and then his employer made him go to the dentist
regularly, and that his dentist was a genius. The middle-aged
optimist with bad teeth absolved himself from responsibility saying that it was because his employer hadn't provided dental insurance and his parents hadn't taken him to the dentist as a
child. The middle-aged pessimist, also with poor dental health,
said it was his own fault for not paying attention to oral hygiene
and being lazy about visiting his dentist. This dimension of explanatory style is closely related to locus of control.

Researchers Suzanne Kobasa and Salvatore Maddi with others have
been studying what they call "hardiness" for several years. They questioned the oft-quoted connection between stress and illness and found
that hardy people handled stress better and were healthier than the non-
hardy during stressful transitions. In an article written with Stephen
Kahn (Kobasa, Maddi, & Kahn, 1982), they defined *hardiness* to include
commitment, control, and challenge. These are defined as follows:

> The commitment disposition is expressed as a tendency to involve one-
> self in (rather than experience alienation from) whatever one is doing
> or encounters . . . The control disposition is expressed as a a tendency to
> feel and act as if one is influential (rather than helpless) in the face of
> the varied contingencies of life. . . . The challenge disposition is expressed
> as the belief that change rather than stability is normal in life and that
> the anticipation of changes are interesting incentives to growth rather
> than threats to security. (pp. 169–170)

The hardiness model provides counselors with additional clues to
their clients' state of mind. One person may describe awareness of life's
finiteness as a time to fulfill dreams, experience more, set new goals,

or make more careful choices about how time is spent. This person may come to seek help in implementing these plans or in managing other's reactions to his/her new lifestyle choices. A person at the other end of the commitment continuum may describe group self-hatred, saying things like, "I don't want to spend time with all those old people." Still another person may cling to the past by dressing in the clothing of his or her youth, reading nothing written after a certain date, or refusing to acknowledge changes in the world and its customs.

Listening for the control dimension may help counselors be alert to such statements as, "I've handled other tough situations, I'm sure with a little help I'll be able to handle this one, too"; or "There's nothing anyone can do. I guess I just have to suffer." Kobasa, Maddi, and Kahn (1982) stated that control "does not imply the naive expectation of complete determination of events and outcomes, but rather implies the perception of oneself as having a definite influence through the exercise of imagination, knowledge, skill, and choice" (p. 169). In addition to managing transitions better, people who perceive that they have more control over their lives experience fewer of the deleterious effects of stress.

Popular culture describes the challenge disposition with adages such as, "If life gives you lemons, make lemonade"; or, "When you get to the end of your rope, make a knot and hang on." Kobasa, Maddi, and Kahn (1982) stated:

> Challenge mitigates the stressfulness of life events on the perceptual side by coloring events as stimulating rather than threatening, specifically because they are changes requiring readjustment. In coping behaviors, challenge will lead to attempts to transform oneself and thereby grow rather than conserve and protect what one can of the former existence." (p. 170)

We are reminded of the man who saw turning 60 as an opportunity to increase his chances of winning tennis tournaments as he would then be one of the youngest in his new age group. A similar positive view is expressed in a poem found in a book with the delightful title of *When I Am An Old Woman, I Shall Wear Purple.* In the poem from which the title is drawn, "Warning" (Joseph, 1987), a woman describes how her age gives her the freedom to be nonconforming.

Counselors will hear statements from clients in transition that give clues to their optimistic or pessimistic outlook on life. Perhaps one of the most important interventions we can apply is to help a person establish or reestablish hope.

5

Relationship Transitions

The first client you are observing today is Martha Smith. All you know about Mrs. Smith from the intake interviewer is that she is 48 years old, married with two children, and employed by an insurance company. She is smartly dressed in a gray suit with a bright print blouse and contemporary jewelry. As soon as you introduce yourself and explain a little bit about how you work, Mrs. Smith, who says most people call her Marty, launches into the following story.

I'm not sure just why I'm here today. When I think about my life, it seems like I should be really happy. And in many ways I am. My husband is a wonderful man. When we met about five years ago he was a widower and I had been divorced for three years. I was a little gun shy about remarrying, but he is such a kind, generous man and was so eager to get married that I agreed. I think it was a good decision, but we're in different places. He's ten years older than I am and thinking about taking an early retirement. And he wants me to slow down at work too so we can have more time to spend together. After being in a very cool marriage for several years, then alone, it feels awfully good to have somebody who really wants to be with me. Having someone really love me is very special, but it's not the only thing in my life.

I was out of the work force for a number of years while the children were young. My first husband wasn't around a whole lot even when we were still married. So in some ways I was both mother and father to the children. They are both out of the house now. My son had some trouble "finding himself"—isn't that the phrase that young people use—but he's now at the community college and living with two friends in an apartment. He still comes back all the time to do his laundry and get some home-cooked meals. And we do help him a little financially.

My daughter is married, has two little children, and lives in another part of the state. She calls almost every week and asks if I can come for the weekend. I'm glad that she wants me, and I do love to spend time with my grandchildren, but my husband wants me to be here with him and his widowed mother who lives near us and needs a lot of help. She counts on me to do her shopping and take her to the doctor and the beauty parlor. She's a really nice lady, but I don't know why she calls me all the time instead of her other daughter-in-law who has been in the family for 20 years. She hasn't said anything directly, but I think she'd like to move in with us. She has commented on how we must rattle around in the house since the children have left.

My husband's two children are both married and live nearby. They drop in with the children at least twice a week. They're nice kids, but they do make a mess. I know I should be flattered that they want to spend time with their stepmother. And I am. But they do tire me out. So you see why I say I should be happy. I've always wanted to be needed and I am. But sometimes I feel like an octopus, with everybody pulling on one of my tentacles.

Even at work, I'm very involved. I started as a clerical worker, and I've received several promotions. When I first went back to work, before I met my present husband, the social life I developed with the other people at work was very important to me. Some of them are really nice and included me in many of their activities. I'm also the oldest woman in my group, and the others sort of count on me to arrange the birthday celebrations, Christmas party, and other social events. Lots of them also come to me to talk about personal problems.

My boss has offered to send me to Dallas for a two-week training program, which he says will make me eligible for a substantial promotion. I'm really excited about the prospect, but when I told my husband he looked startled. He tried to say how nice for me, but I could tell he didn't like the idea. Now isn't it silly that with all this good stuff going on in my life, I feel so unsettled?

Given what we know about adult development, it really isn't "silly" for Marty to feel unsettled. She has experienced a number of transitions in recent years—being divorced, remarried, becoming a stepmother and a grandmother, and launching a new career. The transition she is currently grappling with is whether to take training and go for advancement at work, given her complex family situation. If she were our client, we could help her make that decision, using the transition model to help her analyze her resources and deficits in each of the 4 S's.

In terms of the Situation, Marty's transition decision has to be made in the context of multiple demands on her time. Given the many stresses in her life, it may not be the best time for her to make a major change in her work role. At the same time, she may see it as a "now or never" offer. With respect to Self, we could help her explore her values concerning work and family. On the surface, she seems to be healthy, economically secure, and in a positive marriage.

Marty's Support system, including her husband, blended family, friends and co-workers, seems to be both an asset and a burden. We don't know much yet about her Strategies, other than that she managed to cope with a poor marriage, a divorce, a remarriage, and a return to the work force and seems to make friends easily.

Marty's story suggests a number of recurring issues that clients bring to a counselor's office. She is experiencing a new sense of intimacy or attachment which she apparently treasures; she certainly belongs in her new and old families, and in her work place; and she "matters" to many people. In fact, the presenting problem may be that she matters too much.

In this chapter, we first discuss various types of relationship transitions—of which Marty's is only one example—that bring adults to counseling. We then review the major recurring issues mentioned above: intimacy, belonging, and mattering. In the final section, we consider ways to utilize the transition model to help us evaluate Marty's case and those of other adults facing relationship transitions.

Throughout this chapter it is important to remember Howard's (1978) statement, "The trouble we take to arrange ourselves in some semblance of families is one of the most imperishable habits of the human race" (p. 15). Although definitions of what constitutes a family change over time and differ from one culture to another, family units are the basic units of society.

While listening to clients' stories, counselors also should remember that many people, particularly women, think of their lives in terms of relationships and key family events. Hagestad (1986) stated: "We place ourselves on the axis of chronological time by orienting ourselves to key transitions: when we graduate, marry, have children. In such temporal construction and reconstruction, family members play key parts: 'It was the year Pete started school, so it must have been . . . ' In the work of creating an autobiography we need the help of family consociates" (p. 691). Plath (1980) also talked of the key role of consociates, those with whom we have close contacts over long periods of time.

TYPES OF TRANSITIONS

One of the most common reasons for adults to seek counseling is that they are contemplating, experiencing, or having trouble adapting to transitions involving family or other close relationships. Often clients lend support to Bridges's (1980) view that transitions begin with endings, as we are more apt to hear about relationships that are "going sour," needing to be redefined, or already over, than about new loves.

As counselors, we may be asked to help our clients sort out their feelings about the unpredictability of family relationships today. Families come in many different shapes and sizes; there is no longer a "typical" family. Many young girls, some married, many not, have babies during their teenage years while other women delay childbearing until their late 30s or 40s. Therefore, first-time grandparents can be 40 or 70. An increasing number of adults, mostly but not always women, are responsible for parent care. But, once again, there is no specified age at which this occurs, no designated length of time that pinpoints how long parent care is necessary.

Today multigenerational families are common, and the term "sandwich generation" has crept into the popular vocabulary. The term refers to people in midlife who are caught between the needs of children and aging parents. As people live longer, and the number of generations increases, the metaphor becomes a "club sandwich." For the first time in history, the average married couple has more parents than children (Hagestad, 1986). This development represents the potential for many years of closeness and many changes in relationships. Following is a discussion of some of the more common transitions involving close interpersonal relationships.

Partnering Relationships

For many adults, having one committed relationship is a primary life goal. This relationship, if obtained, may be marked by satisfaction and/ or conflict requiring continuous renegotiation. One insightful man commented, "I've had one wife but several marriages" (Personal communication, 1991). Talking of people in their 50s, Bergquist, Greenberg, and Klaum asserted that:

> The relationship that is most likely to be sustained in this period of reinventing ourselves is perhaps, surprisingly, with our spouse or significant

other. While our children have often left home by the time we reach fifty and our friendships have changed and become fewer, our partner is often still there to support us and be our companion. This central, intimate, relationship can be a major source of generativity... When couples fail to develop a new intimacy in these years the problem is usually that they find they no longer have any common interests. They discover new time together in their fifties but have nothing to share in that time. (1993, pp. 80–82)

For some individuals who seek counseling, a basic concern is "Will I ever find the kind of partner I want?" and more significantly, "What will happen to me if I don't?" As adults contemplate marriage or other committed relationships, they may ask transition-related questions such as, "How will my life change?" or "He wants me to move across the country, but how do I know if I can manage without all the supports I have here?" "We both have good jobs, but in different cities. Can we manage a commuter relationship?"

Different value systems can create serious problems around the decision to marry. A woman recently said, "I think we should live together for a while before we marry, but he says his family will disown him if we do." Her desire for a trial period reflects her concern about not wanting to make a decision without being really sure, while his reluctance may stem from family or religious scruples about living together "out of wedlock."

Gay and lesbian couples may experience even more value conflicts, both their own and those imposed by an often disapproving society. One man in considerable anguish recently said, "My partner wants me to take him to our company Christmas party. He accused me of being ashamed of him and of our relationship. Of course I'm not, but the truth is I don't know how my co-workers would react. I'm not sure they know I'm gay."

For gay men and lesbians, as for heterosexuals, the presence of a committed partner can be a source of satisfaction and a buffer against stress. When the relationship is longstanding, partners can draw on a reservoir of shared experiences and patterns of relating to each other. However, problems may arise when one member of a gay or lesbian couple is hospitalized or needs long-term care because that partner may not be perceived as "family" by the bureaucracy or the family of origin. In such situations both the ill person and the partner may be denied opportunities to support each other, to enjoy continued intimacy, or, in cases of terminal illness, even to say good-bye. An additional problem for gay and lesbian couples is the scarcity of societal rituals for some-one whose same-sex partner leaves or dies. Yet the pain and loneliness is every bit as intense as in heterosexual relationships. Furthermore, in-dividuals from the gay culture may be leery of counseling with "straight" mental health professionals.

Divorce

In many counselors' offices, coping with divorce is the most frequently discussed transition. Despite the fact that approximately 50% of mar-riages currently end in divorce (U.S. Department of Commerce, 1993), it can be among the most painful of life's experiences. Whether your client is the instigator of the divorce or the partner being rejected, he or she is likely to describe a sense of failure. For some the pain of re-jection is uppermost in their minds, for others the guilt as to what they are doing to other people is paramount. What they tell you may also depend on where they are in terms of stages of the divorce transition.

One particularly difficult stage, characterized by lack of clarity, has been termed a "limbo loss" by Colgrove, Bloomfield, and McWilliams (1991). During this stage, counselors may hear statements such as "I do all right alone, and better together, but I do very poorly when semi-to-gether" (p. 5). A similar angst is expressed in one of the writers' po-ems:

> Limbo losses often feel like this . . .
> this slow erosion from below
>   —or within—
> it's me falling down around my life
>   because you're still in that life
>   —but not really
> And you're out of that life
>   —but not quite. (p. 4)[1]

One woman in her late 40s recently told a counselor, "My marriage doesn't do it for me anymore, but I don't know if I have the guts to leave. What will happen to me? to him? to the children? to our dream

---

[1] From *How to Survive the Loss of a Love,* by Melba Colgrove, PhD, Harold H. Bloomfield, MD, and Peter McWilliams, © 1991, published by Prelude Press, 8159 Santa Monica Boulevard, Los Angeles, CA, 90046, 1-800-LIFE-101. Used with permission.

of being grandparents together?" Another woman said between her tears, "I think my husband is having an affair. Shall I confront him or just hope it will play itself out? Is this his midlife crisis?" Both these women are grappling with a major decision as to whether to initiate a divorce, thus embarking on a major transition. They probably need help in examining their resources for coping, regardless of the decision they make.

Alcoholism or other substance abuse is often involved when one or both partners are considering divorce. Counselors may hear heart-wrenching stories from people who are uncertain as to whether to believe their partner's statements that "they really are going to stop." Women married to alcoholic or substance-abusing husbands are more likely to "stick by" their husbands than are men married to alcoholic women (Covington, 1994). However, one of the reasons why alcoholic women often get into treatment late in the course of their disease is that their families have engaged in an elaborate cover-up to avoid embarrassment. Peluso and Peluso stated that "For every woman drug addict hiding in a closet, there are usually several family members leaning against the door" (1988, p.7).

Widowhood

Much has been written about the major life transition of widowhood. Books for the bereaved person such as *Living with an Empty Chair* (Temes, 1984), and *How to Survive the Loss of a Love* (Colgrove, Bloomfield, & McWilliams, 1991), as well as books for professionals (e.g., Kalish, 1985; Lopata, 1987; Worden, 1991), discuss the devastation and mix of intense feelings that may be experienced, and of the fear of many people that they hurt so much they must be going crazy.

Counselors hear statements such as, "I don't think I can live without him," or "We always thought I'd die first." This is not an unusual reaction on the part of widowers as demographics and conventional wisdom agree that wives usually outlive their husbands. Early studies by Neugarten (1968) indicated that a major difference between the sexes is that women are more likely to rehearse for widowhood. This is probably related both to differences in life expectancies and to the greater emphasis women put on connectedness in their thinking about and planning their lives (Belenky et al., 1986; Gilligan, 1982).

The value of such rehearsing may depend on the kind of rehearsing that is done. Although behavioral rehearsal (e.g., planning and making decisions, beginning to assume control of family finances, and making new friends) was helpful in the adjustment to widowhood, cognitive rehearsal, defined as the "work of worrying," was associated with increased emotional disruption (Remondet, Hansson, Rule, & Winfrey, 1987). Counselors can help widows and widowers think about which rehearsal techniques will help them most.

Clients whose spouses are suffering from a long-term serious disability are clearly grieving, but may be unclear about "how to do it." One woman whose husband had a serious stroke and was unable to talk said, "I know I'm grieving but I'm not sure for what." There are no clear rituals, such as funerals, to assist people in this limbo status, so counselors may want to help clients develop their own. Lustbader (1994) told a moving story of a woman whose husband's personality and behavior had been altered by a major illness. The woman explained to her counselor that "I had to divorce him in my mind and marry him again on new terms."

Counselors may also hear poignant statements such as "We did everything together," or "Why did I leave the running of the house to my wife/husband. I have no idea how to . . . " "How-tos" can refer to handling everything from finances to household chores and social arrangements. A principal role of counselors in working with widowed persons, and people whose spouses are severely disabled, is to assure them of the normality of their intense, and often vacillating, feelings. Referrals to support groups as well as to attorneys, financial planners, and other advisors may also be helpful.

Some widowed persons complain that they are being ignored, or they hesitantly express resentment that everybody else seems to be just going along with their lives. At the approach of one holiday season, a widow asked with much pathos, "Will I ever be happy again?" When confronted with such questions, counselors may be able to help widowed persons see that while they will never be their "old selves" again, they can become reasonably comfortable "new selves."

Alternatively, other widows may express feelings such as "I'm tired of people feeling sorry for me. I guess I should be grateful, but I can't stand it when people talk to me as if my life must be over." A widowed friend recently explained, "Sure I miss Joe, but I really do have a full life now, with many friends and interests."

Differences among widowed persons may reflect not only their personal styles, but also the social context in which they live. Comparative studies of widows in different communities in the United States and

Canada revealed "tremendous variation in life frameworks, social roles and relations, support systems, life-styles, and self concepts" (Lopata, 1987, p. 273). A major role of counselors may be to listen carefully for information about those aspects of a widowed person's life. Such attention may provide clues, for example, as to whether the person's primary need is for self-esteem building, help in finding or utilizing informal supports, or referral to formal community resources.

Members of some social groups in this country may be effectively deprived of services because they do not understand their availability and/or do not think it appropriate to ask for such assistance. In this situation, as in many others, counselors working with individuals from a different cultural group than theirs may need to refer the client to a counselor more familiar with that group, or else seek consultation.

Remarriage

For some widowed persons, particularly those who have spent many years in caregiving, the idea of remarriage holds no appeal. For others it may be a primary goal or emerge as a surprising opportunity.

Counselors may hear comments ranging from, "I hate the thought of living the rest of my life alone, but how can a woman my age ever find another husband?" to "My wife has only been dead three months, but I really want to get married again. What will people say? What will the children think?" Divorced persons often talk about being "gun shy," or fearful of making "another mistake."

Gender differences with respect to remarriage are significant. For many men, particularly those whose business responsibilities involve entertaining, or whose ability or willingness to perform household tasks is limited, the thought of being without a wife may be too difficult to contemplate. Given the high ratio of widows to widowers among most social groups in this country, such men may be able to find another wife with relative ease. Women seeking remarriage may need to take more dramatic steps. One woman we know who was widowed in her 40s thought about where she had the best chance of finding a second husband and decided to take flying lessons. She was indeed the only woman in her piloting class, and her quests for a pilot's license and a husband were both successful!

Many widowed persons have no desire for remarriage. Lopata (1987) found that some widows engage in what she labelled "husband sanctification." When deceased husbands are idealized to this extent, no real person can measure up. If counselors hear such themes, they have to decide whether gentle confrontation would be helpful.

Whether their clients are divorced or widowed, counselors may hear a variety of questions—logistical, emotional, and financial—relating to remarriage. For example, "How will we deal with all those children and grandchildren? How will we decide where to spend vacations and holidays?" "Do we live in his house, my house, or start all over?" "How do we deal with the "exes"? Sometimes emotional and economic issues may be interwoven. "He says he loves me, but I'm worried he is really just interested in my money." "I'm not sure I love him, but he could certainly support me and make the rest of my life more comfortable." or "Will she think I don't trust her if I ask for a prenuptial agreement?" In many such discussions counselors can help concerned clients explore their values, their resources, and their deficits. Discussions of life meaning may also come into play with respect to transitions involving a very different relationship, that of parenting.

Parenting Issues

Parenting, like many other intimate relationships, can be a source of utter delight and/or unbelievable frustration. Counselors will talk to clients dealing with a host of issues, such as whether or not to have children, how custody should be arranged, or what child-rearing techniques are most effective. Parents of older children may have questions about how to encourage children to leave home or whether to allow them to return. Sometimes parents wonder how to deal with their disappointment over non-events, such as when children don't do what the parents expected.

All such decisions are complicated by the fact that many people, and many dimensions of a person's life, are affected. Consider the dilemma of a woman on the fast track at work who says, "My husband really wants to start a family, but I know I'd have to be the one to stay home when the baby is sick. I'm not sure I'm willing to sacrifice my career."

Counselors may hear considerable talk about the ticking of the biological clock. Some couples, particularly those with professional careers, may postpone childbearing, but there comes a time when partners must face such questions as: "Do I really want to have children, and if I do, how will it change my life?" "If I don't, am I letting my parents down? I know they are eager to become grandparents." "If I decide now not to have children, will I be sorry later?" Sometimes the difficulty of the decision is masked with humor, "If we have a baby and then change our minds, can we return it to the store within five years?" The decision as to whether or not to have children may be one of the few irrevocable decisions many people ever make.

For some groups, the decision about parenting may be especially difficult. Counselors working with gay or lesbian clients may hear statements such as, "Just because I'm gay doesn't mean I wouldn't make a good parent. I'm thinking about fathering a child for my lesbian friend who wants to be a mother." or "My partner and I really want to raise a child together. We're trying to decide if one of us should be artificially inseminated or whether we should look for a baby to adopt. Apart from the logistics of how to do it, we wonder if it would be fair to the child. What would its friends think?"

If an individual or a couple decides to have or adopt a baby, it is only the first of many transitions they will face. Kimmel (1990) summarized a number of studies on the impact of becoming parents and found such a step to be a profound transition leading to changes in individuals' views of themselves as well as the couple's relationship.

The myriad of child-rearing issues that arise for married couples, single parents, divorced couples, and extended families are beyond the scope of this book. Such issues as finding appropriate day-care, selecting schools, permitting dating, or fostering healthy sibling relationships, however, are often the subjects adults in transition most want to discuss. Adult counselors are likely to hear about the triumphs and travails experienced by their clients in their role as parents, and, life not being tidy, such experiences undoubtedly affect other aspects of their clients' lives.

Grandparenting Issues

For most people, becoming a grandparent is an exciting and heartwarming experience. For others, however, it may be an unwanted confrontation with their own aging or a mark of their children's "problems." Becoming a grandparent serves as a reminder of the continuity of the generations and provides an opportunity, to varying extents, to again help shape a young life. Conversely, the realization that one will not become a grandparent may be a prime example of a ripple non-event (Schlossberg & Robinson, 1993). When an adult child informs his or her parents about a decision not to—or an inability to—have children, this can lead to unfulfilled expectations that alter the roles, relationships, and assumptions of the older person. A very disappointed "nongrandparent" may need to discuss his/her sadness about the non-event.

Reactions to becoming a grandparent may depend in part upon the ages and life situations of the newborn's parents, as well as the life situation of the grandparent. Hagestad and Burton (1986) found that black women who became grandmothers "on time" were much more positive about their role than those who became grandparents "off time." Many who felt they became grandmothers too early said that the new role interfered with their own parenting, work, education, friendships, and romantic involvements. Some actively rejected the role, bringing consequences to several generations.

Responsibility for raising grandchildren may be thrust upon some grandparents because the children's parents became disabled. This phenomenon has captured the interest of the popular press and become the focus for a limited number of support groups. *Family Circle* magazine frequently profiles "women who make a difference." One such profile (R. Waters, 1994), quoted a woman who captured the situation thus, "I felt guilty when some of my kids got on drugs. But now I'm gonna save my grandson." In recognition of the growth of the situation, the American Association of Retired Persons (AARP) has set up model programs and prepared resources for grandparents raising their grandchildren (AARP, 1993a). In 1995 the National Council on Aging and the Center of Human Services Development at the University of Maryland, College Park, held a mini-White House conference on "Grandparents Raising Grandchildren."

Paradoxically, as more people become grandparents, the role becomes less clear. Today's grandparents range in age from 30 to over 100, their grandchildren may be newborn or themselves retired. Some grandparents live with or very close to their grandchildren, others may be across the country or the world. Cherlin and Furstenberg (1992) identified three styles of grandparenting: companionate, remote, and involved. Companionate grandparents are affectionate, but somewhat passive in their behavior. They clearly see the child's parents as "in charge." Remote grandparents are geographically distant and thus have difficulty establishing intimate relationships. Involved grandparents, in their terminology, are those who engage in active parenting. This style tends to emerge at times of crisis or transition, such as after the child's parents divorce. If the children's mother is forced to devote more time and energy to earning a living, the grandparent may take over more of the child rearing responsibilities.

Not infrequently grandparents may be asked by divorced children, usually daughters, if they may move back home. So-called "boomerang" children, with or without children of their own, clearly represent a lifestyle transition for all generations involved, and this may trigger a request for counseling.

Another issue that brings grandparents to counseling is concern about losing contact with grandchildren. When parents divorce, grandparents on the noncustodial side, typically the father's parents, may find it difficult to maintain close relations with their grandchildren. After hearing rumblings about a separation or divorce in the family, a grandparent may tell a counselor, "I'm devastated for them and from a selfish point of view I'm terrified I'll lose contact with my grandchildren." Myers and Perrin (1993) noted, "To the extent that grandparents are denied access to grandchildren as a result of divorce, they may experience difficulty in resolving their own developmental issues, feel a sense of dissatisfaction with their lives, or feel that some part of themselves is missing or incomplete" (p. 64).

Counselors may help grandparents concerned about losing contact with their grandchildren by suggesting legal assistance, support groups, or appropriate reading material. In recognition of legal battles that may arise, grandparent-rights provisions are written into some divorce settlements. Some self-help groups provide information and support for people who fear or experience a major interruption in their relationship with the grandchildren. A poignant article by Lindeman (1987) entitled "Nana, I can't visit you" dealt with the plight of grandparents and grandchildren who are cut off from each other.

Counselors may hear of mixed feelings and values conflicts from people who become grandparents under nontraditional circumstances. One of our clients almost furtively showed pictures of a grandchild she yearned to hold, but felt reluctant to visit because the child's parents were not married. On the other hand, there are grandparents who have a close relationship with the child of their gay son and a cordial relationship with the child's mother, who lives with her lesbian partner. In many families grandchildren, as well as their parents, may be highly involved in elder care, an important relationship issue to which we now turn.

Eldercare

For many midlife adults, the realization that they are, or may soon be, responsible for caring for their parents can constitute a major life transition. Often the realization is triggered by the parent's sudden illness, which typically comes as a shock, even though to use Brody's now classic phrase, parent care has become a "normative family stress" (1985). The ubiquity of the problem can be understood by listening to informal conversations of people in midlife, and reading the popular press and business publications, as well as by hearing concerns voiced by clients. There is even a special magazine, *Answers*, which describes itself as "the only national consumer magazine devoted to the questions, issues, and concerns that arise when caring for an elderly parent or relative."

A special report in the magazine, *Money* (Hedberg, 1989) began with the following alert: "Face this fact: If you have a parent alive today, you likely have a crisis waiting for you somewhere down the road. Sooner or later that parent will need help. The problem . . . may be financial, medical, or emotional. Often it will be all three at once. And inevitably you will be central to the solution. However you choose to lend your support . . . the effect upon your own life will undoubtedly be seismic" (p.136). The warnings may be overstated, but they do point to a concern apt to be heard in many counseling sessions. Some adults who talk about feeling that they have changed roles with their parents may be helped by Silverstone's (1994) terminology. She described the change not as role reversal, but as moving from being dependent on parents to being dependable for them.

Becoming responsible for one's parents can radically change individuals' roles, responsibilities, and assumptions about themselves. Although most of us "know" that America is graying and that many older adults need some kind of assistance, it is very different when the older adult is "ours." In dealing with issues of eldercare, counselors are likely to hear a range of feelings including: love and concern for the parent, grief over the anticipated death of a parent, guilt over not being able to do enough, resentment over the interruptions in their own plans, confusion about where they need to invest their energies, or despair at realizing the situation may be out of their control.

Expectations about caregiving may be strongly influenced by the cultural background of both informal and formal caregivers. The training director of a large nursing home in an urban area talked of the difficulties that staff and family members have in understanding each other's values. The staff, who are primarily African American or foreign born, come from a culture that expects family members to take in "their" frail older adults. Therefore they assume that the families of the residents "don't really care" or else they would have their relatives at home. Many of the family members, most of whom are middle class and white, think they are making a good choice to give their relatives the best possible care and opportunities for socialization.

In studying parent care, Brody (1990) found that the vast majority of caregivers to the old are women—primarily wives and daughters—and that daughters provide even more long-term care than spouses.

> The first, most powerful, and over-arching theme, one that appears and reappears for virtually all daughters and daughters-in-law, is their fundamental acceptance that parent care is a woman's role . . . and that they are responsible for more than performing the instrumental, personal-care and nursing tasks that are needed. The women also feel responsible for the emotional well-being of the older people. Indeed they often feel responsible for the happiness of everyone in their families. (p. 79)

Marty, our client, seemed to support this view. She expressed surprise, not that her mother-in-law didn't call her sons, but that she didn't call her other daughter-in-law.

In collecting data on the strains experienced by caregivers, Brody interviewed 1500 women, 300 of their husbands, and 150 of their siblings. She noted that the women's problems were exacerbated by the persistent myth that adult children don't take care of their elderly parents the way they used to in the "good old days." "It is ironic that many of the parent-caring women themselves believe that myth . . . even though they do much more parent care than their counterparts in the past" (1990, p. 6). Counselors who hear clients berating themselves for not doing enough may find it helpful to confront this misconception.

Although most caregivers are women, Silverstone (1994) cautioned that we not ignore the problems of male caregivers. Husbands and other male relatives may find themselves "odd man out" in terms of the provision of services.

Although children, particularly daughters, assume major responsibilities for eldercare, not all older adults have children. Special strains may come from caring for a frail relative who is not one's parent. Nieces and nephews, for example, may care for a childless relative largely out of loyalty to their deceased parents. While older women in this country greatly outnumber older men, this is not true for all ethnic groups. Because many Chinese and Filipino men came to this country and either left wives at home or never married, there are large numbers of childless older men among these groups who have special needs and problems (Markides & Mindel, 1987). In helping clients with issues of eldercare, counselors may need to supplement their usual counseling techniques by providing case management services or making appropriate referrals.

Clients involved in caregiving may also be concerned about the impact on the rest of the family. Cutler (1985) talked about the spread of distress within a family, and particularly the effect on grandchildren when an older family member has dementia. "The relationship between grandparents and grandchildren is often a close and special one, and when 'Grandpa' begins to be short-tempered and inappropriate, it can be devastating for the grandchildren" (p. 53). When a grandparent becomes incapacitated or dies, midlife adults may need to cope with their own grief as well as be a support to their children.

Death of a Parent

In terms of grief, counselors may find midlife adults surprised and confused by the extent of their reactions to the death of a parent. "Why am I so devastated when we knew it was coming?" is a common question counselors may hear. In a study of the impact of parent death, Douglas (1990) found that most of her sample reported that the death of a parent changed their outlook on life. They confronted their own mortality, at the same time they grappled with feelings of being alone and orphaned. Respondents also noted that the death of a parent was often a trigger for personal growth as it inspired them to look more closely at their own lives and appreciate the relationships they had.

For many midlife adults the death of the second parent may trigger much stronger feelings than the death of the first. Upon the death of the first parent, concern and attention are typically focused on the surviving spouse. But when the second parent dies, adult children may become increasingly aware of, and free to pay attention to, their own loss and orphaned status. Some orphaned adults may find their new responsibilities as the older generation daunting; others may view it as an opportunity to matter in a new way. In either case, they are likely to become the primary communication channels in the family, letting others know who needs help or who is to be congratulated.

The death of a parent may drastically alter sibling relationships. In some families siblings become closer, realizing they can no longer communicate through the parent. In others, where the family has stayed together only because of the parent, siblings may drift apart. Counselors are more likely to hear about the latter situation. Discussions with friends who have experienced similar losses may be particularly helpful.

Friendships

Though the well-known saying is, "that's what friends are for," counselors may hear a wide variety of concerns regarding friends. Some adults who have experienced a major life transition worry about putting too much of a burden on their friends, others are disappointed in lack of support from friends. Some yearn for more and deeper friendships, others worry that the pressures of work and family prevent them from nurturing friendships, fearing that this neglect can have long-term as well as short-term negative effects.

In listening to clients' concerns about friendships, counselors need to be aware of gender differences that may affect the type and depth of friendships. Both research and conventional wisdom suggest that women do more self-disclosing and have more intimate relationships with same-sex friends than men. Rubin (1986) distinguished between male bonding, which arises from shared experiences and common physical or intellectual exploits, and male intimacy, which involves open expressions of thoughts and feelings. Male clients who do not understand this distinction may be surprised at their feelings of isolation, despite the presence of friends with whom they share interests.

In their study of patterns of friendship among male graduate students over 35, Busse and Birk (1993) found that competitiveness was inversely related to self-disclosure. In addition, men who engaged in more self-disclosure perceived their friendships as being closer than those who disclosed relatively little. The authors suggest that counselors may help their male clients by making them aware of gender stereotypes.

Friends are important to us throughout our lives. The crucial role of peers in the lives of adolescents is both a developmental task and the bane of many parents' existence. To adults, friends are often the people with whom they can "be themselves." In his definition, Peter

(1978) said, "You can always tell a real friend: when you've made a fool of yourself, he doesn't feel you've done a permanent job" (p. 206). Going beyond the humor, our friends are often the people who help us keep our lives in balance and our sense of perspective in place.

Many transitions including geographic moves, job changes or retirement, divorce or widowhood can lead to drastic changes in friendship patterns. As people look at the balance between their resources and deficits, friends may move from one column to the other as they become harder to access. In interviews with people in their 50s, Bergquist, Greenberg, and Klaum (1993) found that many people treasured long-term friendships and believed there was not sufficient time to develop new deep relationships.

Quite a different view of late-life friendships is presented by Kidder (1993), who studied residents of a large long-term care facility. He talked enthusiastically of Lou and Joe, two men who had been assigned as roommates and become great friends. "The crucial thing about Lou and Joe is that they remain very good friends, better friends every time I visit. They present an antidote to despair, which is connectedness, and for me, I learned it is only the connectedness of the human tribe that can hold despair at bay" (p. 55).

Different groups of the population may have different friendship patterns. Lipman (1986) cited several studies that show that both older gay men and older lesbians have more friends than do heterosexuals of similar age. Such strong friendships may supplant or supplement traditional kinship support.

Other studies suggest that friendships and partners meet different emotional needs. After studying couples who moved and individuals in Parents Without Partners, Weiss (1976) concluded that both people with partners, who have a limited network of friends, and people with large support networks but no intimate partner, can be lonely. People seem to need to be part of a social network in order not to experience social isolation; people need intimacy to avoid experiencing emotional isolation. When counselors hear about either kind of void, they need to listen carefully for what clients are saying—perhaps unconsciously—about themselves. Such statements may be a signal that it is time to explore one of the recurring themes of adulthood.

RECURRING ISSUES

Marty, the client whose story started this chapter, expressed a number of concerns about herself and her values. She is involved in a new relationship, enmeshed in a blended family, and active in a work group. These relationships probably meet her needs for intimacy and belonging. She may well be over-committed and matter too much. Each of the major issues embedded in her story—intimacy, belonging, and mattering—is discussed below.

Intimacy

Intimacy is a major concern during the adult years. We may be intimate with a spouse, lover, parent, child, or friend as the term covers a wide range of close human relationships. The Random House Dictionary (1987) defined intimacy as "a close, familiar and usually affectionate or loving personal relationship with another person or group." Different people may describe intimacy differently, but the concept commonly involves relationships marked by strong caring, mutual support, openness, and a sense of being able to "be oneself" with another. Most people find a sense of intimacy an essential part of a complete life.

Concerns about intimacy—how to get it, keep it, or replace it—are issues frequently brought to counselors. We may see people who "glow" because of a new intimate relationship that adds warmth and color to their lives. Or we may see people whose lives look full, but who experience a void because they do not have a special person or persons with whom they feel really close. Many different kinds of transitions can trigger issues of intimacy. For example, loss of a relationship through death, divorce, a move, or a change in commitment, can cause adults a great deal of anguish. So can the realization that one is missing an important piece of a full life.

Adults experiencing similar transitions are likely to see very different options for themselves. An open discussion with three 60-year-old widows illustrated this. One said, "I don't care about men. It's finding a man or woman with whom I can be close. I figure I have more chances with women." The other two disagreed, saying they care about men. One said, "The demographics are against me. I'm miserable because I know I won't ever have another close relationship again." The other said, "I know I'll meet men—even if I have to run an ad in the local paper." Regardless of where they saw their options, all were discussing the pain of losing an intimate and were questioning how likely they were to be able to "reinvest" or replace their source of intimacy. Others may express doubt about whether a search for a replacement is worth the effort saying, "I don't ever want to hurt that much again."

According to Erikson's stage theory, achieving intimacy (versus isolation) is a developmental task of young adulthood (Erikson, Erikson, & Kevenic, 1986). Experience suggests, however, that concerns about intimacy, like the other conflicts identified by Erikson, can surface or resurface at any stage of life. Hudson (1991) summed it up by stating, "In today's world, intimacy is a series of bonds and attachments, not merely a significant other" (pp. 11–12). The importance of close interpersonal relationships can hardly be exaggerated. To many people, the character of their relationships is what determines their level of happiness and/or life satisfaction. Close relationships have been found to be a significant buffer against the negative effects of stressful situations (Berkman & Syme, 1979; Pearson, 1990). Parkes (1982) observed that people without significant attachment or intimacy are often considered at risk, while those who have such significant relations are better able to cope with transitions. Moreover, intimacy and attachment are often what add zest to a person's life.

There seem to be significant gender differences in the ability to form intimate relationships. In their longitudinal study of adults, Fiske and Chiriboga (1990) reported, "One of our research-based observations is that losing a spouse is often more traumatic for men than for women because men are less likely to have really close relationships with anyone but their wives . . . men name their spouses as confidants far more often than women do" (p. 255). Thus when a man's wife dies, he often loses his best friend along with the person who was responsible for his social life.

Despite increased attention to "men's issues" and the formation of men's support groups, (e.g., Bly, 1990; Doerr, 1993; Rubin, 1986), male friendships are often based on common interests and activities. However Bergquist, Greenberg, and Klaum reported:

> By the time they reach midlife . . . men find themselves increasingly concerned about connectedness rather than differentiation . . . as they move into their fifties, men often try to establish a community . . . They want to feel as if they belong and begin paying attention to their voices from other rooms that speak about increased sociability . . . or the importance of intimacy and interpersonal commitment. (1993, pp. 58–59)

Women's investment in establishing close relationships is documented in the research of Gilligan (1982), who observed that women define themselves in a context of human relationships. Such relationships are clearly involved in a sense of belonging, another major theme of adulthood.

Belonging

By the time we met Marty at the beginning of this chapter, she belonged in many places; that is, she was a part of a number of groups, home, family, work, in-laws, etc. She had apparently worked hard after her divorce to make sure she belonged to her work group. For many counselees, however, lack of belonging can be a major problem. Consider the following statements which a counselor is apt to hear.

"I've joined a new church, but I don't really feel like I belong. It sure is different from the church in our old neighborhood."

"Joe and I belonged to a couples group that met once a month for dinner. We rotated from one house to another. After he died, I didn't know whether to stay with the group or not. A couple of people asked me to, but I wasn't sure they really meant it. Maybe they thought they had to. I went once and felt like a fifth wheel. I'm really more at ease when I'm with other widows or even just the wives. There is another dinner coming up next week and I just can't decide."

"I just moved out of my girlfriend's house where I lived for five years. I really thought we'd get married some day, but it just didn't work out. Now I feel lonely and rudderless."

"The holidays are coming up and I don't know what to do. I wish I could get in bed and stay there for about a month. Before my son and his wife got divorced they used to come to my house for almost all the holidays and I loved it. Now my son is married to someone else. My stepdaughter is nice but she has her own family. She asked me if I wanted to come for Thanksgiving but I don't feel like I really FIT."

The clients above seem to be questioning where they belong. Their transitions have placed them in an unclear situation between belonging and marginality or, stated differently, between being central or peripheral to a particular group. Every time individuals move from one role to another or experience a transition, they risk becoming marginal. The larger the difference between the old and the new roles and the less knowledge people have about the new role, the more marginal they may feel. Counselors who can discuss this phenomenon with their clients may help them better understand their concerns about not feeling "part of it." Counselors can also help clients realize that this sense of marginality may be only temporary.

Societal changes also can affect an individual's sense of belonging. Increasing mobility and increasing divorce rates have meant that in many families, parents and children live far apart. The sense of not belonging experienced by many adults whose children have moved away is reflected in the title of an organization formed by an innovative religious organization. Members of the "Orphaned Parents Group" get together to discuss their concerns and provide support for each other, and to hold group holiday celebrations so people have somewhere they belong.

While the "orphaned parents" are meeting in one city, their children may be feeling equally lonely in another part of the country, where they, too, may be working to build friendship groups or "families of choice" with whom they can share holidays. Such groups may include courtesy "aunts and uncles," close family friends who are given honorary titles that may make them feel more a part of the family.

Societal changes can have a particularly negative effect on older adults. Difficulties may stem from a combination of internal and external factors. In a study of loneliness and adjustment to old age, Hansson, Jones, Carpenter, and Remondet (1986) found that loneliness was related to both poor psychological adjustment and to dissatisfaction with family and social relationships. They noted that loneliness can stem from "an underlying lack of skill in living, perhaps including social skills, planning, and control over actions and internal thoughts . . . or loneliness may interfere with effective interpersonal functioning resulting in unpleasant and self-degrading emotional experiences" (p. 51). If counselors hear concerns about loneliness, they may want to help clients explore the basis for the loneliness and consider ways to find places where they belong or matter.

Mattering

Mattering, the need to be appreciated, noticed, and acknowledged, is a concern of people at all stages of life and can strongly influence behavior. Rosenberg and McCullough (1981) found that nondelinquent boys differed from delinquent boys in that the former felt they mattered to parents and teachers. Depressed people who think they matter to family and friends are less likely to commit suicide. A rationale for pet or horticultural therapy is that having responsiblity for care of a pet or a plant helps people know they still matter.

To be sure, our client Marty may have mattered to too many people, but the opposite is more often the concern of those in transition. The rejected lover may think, "If my former partner no longer cares about me, I may not matter to anyone." What has been called the empty nest syndrome is an example of a loss of mattering. Some people—men and women alike—feel they are no longer important after their children leave home. Others view the emptying of the nest as a transition to a potentially exciting new stage of life. If adult children return home and refill the nest, it may be another example of mattering too much.

Mattering is clearly an issue outside of families as well as inside them. Employees who talk about constant put-downs and lack of appreciation at work, as well as people who complain that their teachers don't listen to them, may feel they don't matter. Schlossberg, Lynch, and Chickering (1989) gave examples of how adult learners might be helped to feel they matter to the school, basing their discussion on five dimensions of mattering identified by Rosenberg and McCullough: attention, importance, dependence, ego-extension, and appreciation (1981). For example, adult learners are more likely to feel accepted if they have a place to put their things, and receive mail and messages. Adult learners may feel important if there is evidence someone cares about what they want, and notices if they miss a class.

These same dimensions of mattering can be crucial to an adult facing a relationship transition. For example, a person who has lost a partner may experience lack of attention, feel unimportant, and think, "Nobody depends on me, is proud of my accomplishments, or appreciates what I do."

ASSESSING RESOURCES— LOOKING AT THE 4 S'S

When counselors hear concerns about interpersonal issues, it should alert them to use the transition model to help clients analyze their resources for coping with the change in their lives. Each client brings to a transition a unique combination of Situation, Self, Supports and Strategies. In discussing interpersonal transitions, clients typically talk first about the situations in which they find themselves. Counselors can then ask them to consider more carefully what they are saying about themselves. It is also important to hear what clients say about their support system and learn something of the strategies they have used in the past.

Situations

Let's take another look at Marty's situation. Marty and her husband seem to be in the throes of what has been termed the "dromedary/camel phenomenon," or the out-of-sync career commitment curve (Goodman & Waters, 1985), a not uncommon problem experienced by couples in late midlife. Men who have invested themselves highly in their careers for many years come to a decision that they want to turn to other interests and spend more time with the family. Their career commitment curve, which has "one hump," like a dromedary, has peaked and is on the way down. At the same time, their wives, whose interest may have peaked earlier and then dropped down during their child-rearing years (whether or not they were working), rises again as child-rearing responsibilities diminish. Like a camel, their career commitment curve has "two humps."

An article in the *New York Times* (Lewin, 1993), referring to several studies on the impact of retirement, reported, "In many cases, husbands and wives find themselves troublingly out of sync as they approach retirement age. Husbands who have worked for 40 years may be eager to leave their job pressures behind, while wives who entered the work force late find those same pressures exhilarating." Retirement often precipitates a renegotiation of marital roles, a situation that may bring one or both members of the couple to a counselor.

In terms of the facets to be considered when examining one's situation, the trigger for Marty to seek counseling may have been her need to decide about the training opportunity. Timing is an issue because she and her husband are in different phases of their careers. If Marty takes the training and receives a promotion, it may well lead to a role change, which may affect her relationships with her co-workers as well as her view of the importance of work in her life. The duration of the transition issue is not clear. Her bosses' suggestion to send her for training is an external stimulus, but the decision about the training is hers, so it represents an internal locus of control. A counselor can help Marty assess these situational factors and decide which aspects of the possible change she sees as positive, as negative, or as benign. The counselor can also help her explore her internal resources for coping with change.

Self

Many clients find it difficult to talk about—or even identify—their internal resources. These resources include the degrees to which they are optimistic or pessimistic in outlook, able to tolerate ambiguity, or inclined to act autonomously. Helping clients know themselves and clarify their values and their assumptions about themselves is a key part of self-assessment.

Fox and Halbrook examined the changes in how low-income women saw themselves after they ended a relationship with a male partner. The women, who were between the ages of 33 and 42 and had two or more children, went through a "three-phased process . . . 1) an early phase designated by original assumptions and "happily ever after" dreams; 2) a period of disintegration of original assumptions resulting in "shattered dreams"; and 3) a final phase when [the] women were actively involved in reconstructing new, meaningful assumptions" (1994, p. 152).

It is interesting to note that although these interviews were conducted in the early 1990s, after several decades of the current women's movement, women in the first phase consistently subordinated their interests to those of their husbands'. They also subscribed to strong beliefs about what women should do, say, and feel to maintain their marriage relationships. When they reached phase two, "shattered dreams," the women tended to blame themselves, often labelling themselves as failures because their marriages did not last. One woman whose husband abused her talked of her responsibility for his anger, explaining, "I guess I couldn't please him." As they moved to the third phase and began to reconstruct assumptions about themselves, they had to confront their own identity with the profound question, "If I am not who I thought I was, then who am I?"

Counseling interventions helped these women. The authors observed that after considerable work, "independence developed confidence; many discovered resilience and other assets which helped them cope. Their self-esteem began to expand, and they felt stronger, more in control" (1995, p. 17).

Unlike the women in the above study, Marty came for counseling in order to make a choice, not deal with a fait accompli. A counselor could help Marty examine her work and family values, her sense of autonomy, and her self-efficacy. The counselor could also direct her attention to her support system, and help her look at ways to utilize it more advantageously.

Support

As we listen to adults in transition talk about their relationships, support is often an integral part of the discussion. Indeed, providing emotional and instrumental support may be considered at least a partial measure of what constitutes a close relationship. However, such relationships can change over time. One older woman, whose close friends and relatives were suffering from many disabilities, told us in a weary tone, "My support group is no longer supportive. I still love them, but they're a drain now." In some ways Marty's support system has become a drain or a liability as well as an asset. A counselor who hears this concern may be able to help Marty understand the changing nature of her support system, and consider strategies for redressing the balance between nourishers and drainers.

Social support can be a major buffer enabling adults to cope with stressful situations. It can be provided by intimate relationships, family members, networks of friends, or by institutions. A paradox of support systems is that at the very time they may be most needed, during major transitions such as divorce, widowhood, or a long-distance move, they may be most in jeopardy.

When helping adults cope with transitions, it is important to listen to their ideas of who and what serve as supports for them. Counselors may hear concerns not only about the presence or absence of supportive people, but also about the way friends and family provide support. After finishing a trying course of radiation treatments, a colleague who had breast cancer wrote about what she most needed from her friends.

During a recent bout with cancer, I went through all the stages of grief. In the process, I relearned the importance of receiving helpful help, and that unhelpful help can actually hurt . . . Help came from many sources, and I feel lucky to have such a good support system. When special friends would call and tell me I sounded stronger, so they knew I was making progress, I would feel encouraged . . . [but I also received unhelpful help] from well-meaning friends of long standing. One told me about radiation sickness horror stories . . . I asked my family to keep her posted about my progress, so I didn't have to talk to her . . . Yet another friend seemed to have difficulty accepting my cancer, describing it as "my health challenge" while announcing that we would only speak of pleasant things. Fortunately I had enough power at the time to tell her that I needed to be with friends who would accept my need to be honest about the fact that I have cancer. While I had yet to find it pleasant, I did need to talk about it. She is still my friend but she does tip-toe up to me. (White, 1992, pp. 7–8)

Few clients are as clear and articulate about what they want from friends as this woman, but as helpers we can encourage clients to identify and express their needs. This is important as people in the same situation may vary considerably in their needs. Another co-worker with breast cancer, for instance, wanted very different support from her friends. She chose to talk about her cancer with only a limited number of people and wanted her friends to keep her involved in social activities to the extent her strength permitted.

In his introduction to Pearson's book, *Counseling and Social Support,* George Gazda expressed the hope that the book will refocus counselors on "the importance of utilizing natural and social support groups in the counseling process" (1990, p. 9). Such an orientation should sensitize counselors to listen more attentively to what clients have to say about the kind and amount of support they get from their close relationships. It may also assist them in determining whether problems with a support system stem from problems with the client or with the external sources of support. For example, a person going through a divorce may find that his/her friends feel they have to choose sides. If they choose the former spouse, the client may feel additional rejection and lack of support.

Pearson's analysis of sources of support was built upon earlier work by Caplan (1974), Kahn (1975), and Kahn and Antonucci (1980). Their schemas may help counselors listen more effectively to the stories clients tell. In Caplan's view members of an individual's support system function at different levels. They help the person mobilize psychological resources to cope with difficult situations, share tasks, and provide money, materials, tools, or skills that may be needed. Some clients may be able to express what kinds of support they most need.

Kahn suggested that the "adequacy and stability of social support is a determinant of objective and subjective well-being, of performance in the major social roles, and of success in managing changes in those roles" (1975, p. 3). As partial evidence for this proposition, he cited the findings of several investigations. For instance, in a 12-year study that compared the predominantly Italian American residents of Roseto, Pennsylvania, with residents of four surrounding communities, death from myocardial infarction was found to be much less frequent among the Roseto citizens despite bad dietary habits. This difference was attributed to their close-knit families, mutually supportive and gregarious behavior, respect for the elderly, and use of family conclaves for the resolution of problems (p. 4).

As mentioned earlier, Kahn and Antonucci (1980) suggested that we think of support systems in terms of convoys. They picture individuals moving through their life cycles surrounded by other people on whom they rely for support and to whom they provide support. As depicted in Figure 3.2 in Chapter 3, they envision a person as the center of a ring of concentric circles. This method of visualizing support enables us to see the impact of a transition upon an individual's support system. For example, geographical moves can negatively affect the relationship of husband and wife. Those wives who do not want to move, but who agree for the sake of the family, may experience deep resentment and anger. This may change their relationship from one of being close to becoming "intimate enemies." If a retired couple moves from an area with many supports to a place with no supports, the transition can be very difficult. If, however, an individual moves to an area with more support than in the one left, the transition will be much easier. Thus an important element in listening to clients talk about their transitions is to consider the effect upon their convoy. This may help you to identify strengths and weaknesses in the client's support system.

Major transitions can affect not only receiving support but giving it. Pearson noted that "most long-standing support relationships are reciprocal in nature. Therefore, one of the issues a person may confront on the death or disability of a loved one is what to "do" with the love, affection, companionship, and material assistance that had previously been expended on the lost one" (1990, p. 31).

Losing the ability to give can also stem from one's own disability. One woman who lost a leg to complications of diabetes became depressed over her inability to take care of other people as she had done all of her life. After listening to the woman and talking with various volunteer centers, her counselor was able to help her find a telephone job. A local hospital gave her names of newly discharged patients who lived alone. Calling these patients at regular intervals to make sure they were alright was helpful both to them and to her sense of being a supportive person.

Another perceptive woman, temporarily immobilized by a hip problem, said, "I think I've always gotten support, and felt good about myself, by being a support. Now that I'm having to stay off my feet for several months, I'm finding it really hard to ask for help." It helped her to learn the meaning of the term "cosmic accounting" (S. Uhle, personal communication, 1988), which refers to the need for people to be in relative balance in terms of the amount of help they give and receive. She realized that her reluctance to ask for help deprived members of her support system of the opportunity to assist her. As a result, she began to work on a new strategy to deal with her, she hopes, temporary transition to the state of invalid.

Strategies

It is important for counselors to help people identify the strategies they have used for coping with past relationships. Counselors can ask clients how they made friends or dealt with past family tensions. By listening carefully to the answers, both counselor and client may learn about the client's decision-making styles as well as his/her experiences and feelings about intimacy, belonging, and mattering.

To help clients assess their coping strategies, counselors may wish to give them "Your Coping Keys Worksheet" (Figure 5.1). This worksheet enables clients to identify strategies they currently use, as well as others they might include in their repertoire. They can ask themselves: Are there new strategies I can use to change or modify the situation, change the meaning of it for me, or change the way I manage my reactions to it?

In working with Marty, for example, we could learn how she handled her divorce, how she related to her former husband, her children, her friends and family, and also how she reached out to co-workers as a source of friendship. In looking at the meaning of her present

Here is the list of coping strategies. In the first column, check off the ones you are now using for your transition. In the second column, check off the ones you'd like to try out.

Possible Coping Strategies	*Now Using*	*Will Try*
Change/Modify Situation through Problem-Solving		
Negotiating	❐	❐
Taking optimistic action	❐	❐
Seeking advice	❐	❐
Asserting yourself	❐	❐
Brainstorming new plan	❐	❐
Taking legal action (if needed)	❐	❐
Change Meaning of Situation through Reappraisal		
Applying knowledge of transition process	❐	❐
Rehearsing	❐	❐
Developing rituals	❐	❐
Making positive comparisons	❐	❐
Rearranging priorities	❐	❐
Relabeling or reframing	❐	❐
Selectively ignoring	❐	❐
Using denial	❐	❐
Using humor	❐	❐
Having faith	❐	❐
Managing Reactions to Stress		
Playing	❐	❐
Using relaxation skills	❐	❐
Expressing emotions	❐	❐
Doing physical activity	❐	❐
Participating in counseling/therapy/support groups	❐	❐
Reading	❐	❐
Other Strategies		
_____	❐	❐
_____	❐	❐
_____	❐	❐
_____	❐	❐
_____	❐	❐

FIGURE 5.1 The "Coping Keys Worksheet." (*Source:* From L.I. Pearlin and C. Schooler, "Your Coping Keys Worksheet," from the *Journal of Health and Social Behavior, Vol. 19,* © 1978 The American Sociological Association. Reprinted with permission.)

situation, we might ask her how she would rearrange her priorities if she were promoted. She might need to practice ways to ask for help with some of her family responsibilities. Given the tremendous pressures she is under, we might inquire about the stress management strategies she uses, and suggest additional ones.

People, such as Marty, who are contemplating role changes may find it useful to consider how they handled previous changes. For example, if they moved in the past, what did they do to integrate themselves into the social fabric of the new community? When they first became engaged, how did they relate to their partner's family? Counselors can ask questions such as these in order to learn more about the relationships and coping skills of their clients.

SUMMARY

In this chapter we have identified a number of relationship transitions involving role gains and role losses, discussed three major themes of adult development—intimacy, belonging, and mattering—and looked at ways to use the 4 S's of the transition model to listen more effectively to what clients tell us about how they handle relationship changes.

Some people may have chosen to ignore or gloss over feelings generated by family transitions in the past; others may have always confronted them head on. People who cope effectively use a variety of strategies, and counselors need to listen carefully to their stories so as to help them identify and expand their repertoire of coping skills.

6

Work Transitions

Joe Jones, a 40-year-old machinist, tells a career counselor the following:

> I've been a machinist since I was 18. I learned the trade in the Army and stayed with it when I got out. I never really chose it; the Army assigned me to the training and I did well at it, so I kept at it. I'm good with my hands. I can still make a good living as a machinist, but the new technologies are changing the work. If I do have to get more training or go back to school, I don't know if I want to do it as a machinist. My boss says he'll help me pay for night school training, and my wife says I should do it. They both nag me to sign up for classes at the local community college, but I don't ever seem to make the call. I don't know what I want to do.
>
> When I was in high school, I was more interested in hanging out with my buddies than I was in studying. I graduated and went straight into the service. I was never much of a student. I don't think I could hack it today. I got married right out of the Army, and my kids are getting ready to go to college. My oldest starts this fall. I don't want them to see me struggle with what they find easy. Also, school takes a lot of time. When I was younger I worked long hours, hardly ever saw my kids, and had little time for fun. Now I have enough seniority to work the day shift. I hate to give up the time with my family and the time for myself. I have my softball team, and I like to work in the garden. My kids are almost grown and this may be my last chance to spend a lot of time with them. I hate to give that up.
>
> What I'd really like is to start my own business. I've always dreamed of being my own boss! My brother owns a neighborhood bar, and he'd like me to come in with him. He isn't making much yet, but with both of us working at it, I think we could do well. I've always gotten along well with people; that's one reason I'm tired of being a machinist. It's kind of lonely. I guess I don't really know what I'm good at. I just kind of fell

into being a machinist. I took some kind of test in the Army, and they assigned me to machinist training.

My wife stayed home when the kids were young and went back to school a few years ago to become a nurse, her lifelong dream. She has just started working full-time and is still low seniority, working the worst shifts, and not getting paid very well. She wants me to stay in my job so we can afford the kids' college expenses. She says I make good money, and that's true, but I'm just not happy. I'm 40. Soon it's going to be too late for me to change. Maybe it's too late already. I've done the same thing my whole life; maybe I'm too old to change. I've never made this kind of major change in my life. My sister-in-law changes jobs all the time, and it seems to work out for her, but I don't know if I can do that. What if it doesn't work out? Can I handle that? I just don't know. I just don't seem to be able to make a decision. I want to be sure that I'm doing the right thing. What do you think I should do?

Joe Jones's issues are typical of those of many adults in a career transition. He is questioning not only what work he does, but the place of work in his life. He is saying that work is no longer as central, or salient, as it was when he was younger. He has a sense of mastery, or self-efficacy, around being a machinist, but is unsure what will happen if he changes jobs. He wonders if he has the resilience to risk change and is unsure about how to do so—and he questions the balance between work and family life. He has changed over the years to become more family oriented, and he seems not to want to disturb this balance.

To understand Joe's *Situation* during his transition, it is important to look at the trigger, timing, source of control, concurrent stress, and his previous experience with a similar transition. As we use our transition model to analyze Joe's major issues relating to *Self*, we see that it is important to consider salience, balance, resilience, self-efficacy, and meaning-making. Joe's *Support* system includes his wife and children, his brother, and his boss. There is no mention of colleagues or subordinates, often a part of a work support system. Apparently Joe views his work as something he does alone. The *Strategies* Joe is using include exploring alternatives and seeking help from a counselor. Having used Joe's story to elucidate the above issues, we now turn to an examination of some of the other types of work transitions experienced by adults and to the strategies they may use to manage these transitions.

ISSUES RELATED TO SITUATION

Joe is not experiencing his transition in a vacuum. The world in which he lives has an impact on what is happening to him, and on the possible outcomes of his transition. His personal history makes his situation unique, as each individual's does. The following discussion covers some of the situation factors identified in Chapter 3 that are likely to play out in the life of an individual involved in a work transition.

Triggers

There is a plethora of evidence that the world has changed—that "future shock," the subject of Toffler's 1970 book, has become a present reality. Super stated that, "The rate of technological change and the shift in industrialized countries from production to service industries will mean that an increasingly high percentage of careers will not be linear . . . but will be free form or mixed form" (1992, p. 423). The introduction to a workbook designed to assist employed persons with their career development gives the following examples of the impact of these changes:

1. Specialists who have spent years perfecting a skill are told they are too narrow and limited; they must be able to perform a variety of tasks.
2. Individuals accustomed to working with facts in a structured environment find themselves in groups brainstorming activities where they are expected to be creative and use their intuition.
3. Workers who thought they had completed their education and could now concentrate on making a living are faced with the necessity of lifelong learning. (Drier, Kiss, Knowdell, Kobylarz, & Goodman, 1992, p. A-3)

The changing workplace and his boss's "suggestion" that he upgrade his skills triggered Joe's transition. He is an example of point number three. He received his training as a machinist approximately 20 years ago. Technology has changed drastically in those years, and he has not kept up with the changes. We heard him describe how he needs to retrain or get out. His boss has offered to help him with tuition, but the message is clear. He must update his skills to keep his job. And he is listening to the message.

Not all workers are so foresightful, or so lucky. Many workers do not heed the message and are forced into an unwanted transition when their place of business shuts down or downsizes and they are laid off. Other people in work transition may have very different triggers. Some individuals may be changing their area of work to avoid boredom; others may be changing due to the relocation of a spouse. Still others may be seeking increased responsibilities or better pay. There are many triggers—what they have in common is that they create change in the life of the individual.

Timing and Concurrent Stress

Two aspects of timing have an impact on Joe's transition—the state of the economy and the time in his own life. Joe is thinking about upgrading his skills or changing jobs at a time when other things are going smoothly, but one in which he needs a consistent income—remember the college tuition! He is also responding to a future need, to have more high-tech skills or a more meaningful job, rather than a present emergency such as being laid off. One individual may have a good support system and few responsibilities; another may be a single parent living far from family and also battling a serious illness. Each of these timing and stress issues is mediated by the individual's perception of them.

We not only need to consider when a transition takes place in the life of an individual, but we also must look at the state of the economy. It is far easier to cope with a work transition during economic "ups" than it is during down times. When there is full employment, new jobs are easy to find—it is a "seller's market." During recessions, even highly skilled people may struggle to find new employment. We must also keep in mind that employment conditions vary greatly by locality. In the 1980s, Michigan experienced massive automobile industry layoffs. A popular bumper sticker of the time said, "Will the last one out please turn off the lights." This gallows humor indicated a strong belief that other parts of the country had better opportunities.

It is easier to contemplate "re-skilling" when a joint union–management program prepays your tuition, your employer gives you released time, or your local adult education program is free, than it is when the costs and time are all your own. These benefits, too, often reflect the state of the economy. Joe apparently has some time to make his decision. He must upgrade to stay in his field, but the local economy seems to allow for the possibility of a successful small business. During a recession, neither of these options might be available.

Counselors may want clients to consider their values, interests, temperaments, and the like, as they make new career decisions, but clients in bad times may be too frightened to consider anything but their immediate needs for security. A public opinion survey found in 1993 that only 51% of people surveyed said that a feeling of accomplishment was what they wanted most in a job (Elmer, 1994).

The year 1993 was one of high unemployment. Career counselors often hear about a sense of urgency bordering on panic. One way to diminish that panic is to look simultaneously at immediate solutions, that is, a job right now, and long-term goals, that is work that is satisfying.

Control/Source

Dr. Mary McNeil decided to leave her lucrative surgical practice to teach surgery in a medical school. Dr. Paul Aslanian had a heart attack and could not continue the high stress and long hours of his pediatric oncology practice. For whom was the transition more difficult? We cannot answer that question without knowing a great deal more about both doctors, but we can speculate that it was easier for Dr. McNeil who was the source of the decision. In the same way people who *seek* transfers, promotions, or new career areas are likely to adjust more easily than those who have change thrust upon them—depending on their other resources.

Control can be achieved in other ways than being the source of the transition. People who can do two things will find it easier to find a new job than those who can only do one; those who can do three, easier than those who can do two, and so forth. Individuals who must change jobs have more control over the situation if they are adaptable. Similarly, they have more control over the transition if they have more education, have a good network, are healthy, and are not members of a group often discriminated against in the workplace.

Several large corporations have negotiated wage and salary contracts with their unions that include higher pay for knowing more work tasks, rather than basing raises solely on seniority. This recognition of the value of flexibility reflects a dramatic change in the needs of the workplace as well as in the goals of labor negotiations.

Many career counselors recommend that all of their clients have a "Plan B," because in today's world, it is wise to be prepared for change. Clients who take that advice when faced with a career transition have more control than those who are unprepared. Joe's foresight places him in the lucky position of managing his own career transition.

Previous Experience With a Similar Transition

Ben Franklin is credited with saying, "Experience is a dear school." The lessons from experience may be hard, but they are valuable. Consider a 60-year-old man who worked for the same company for his entire working life, who lost his job due to a merger. Consider another 60-year-old man in this same situation who has held six different positions in his working life—losing the last three to similar corporate decision-making. We might say he was unlucky to have had to handle this sort of transition three times, but we could certainly credit him with expertise in making work transitions! Furthermore, he probably has more confidence in his ability to change than man number one. After all, he's done it before.

Transferable skills are usually described as being those skills that one can carry from one job to another, such as organizational or communication abilities, or the ability to read a technical manual. Perhaps a critical transferable skill in today's global economy is that of knowing how to make changes. Just as with other transferable skills, the new task need not be identical to the old. A person can learn the skill of making changes by moving, or by working in a variety of volunteer capacities, or by being involved in a workplace that is undergoing transformation. The trick is to recognize the learning and be able to apply it in the new situation. Joe has not told us about any previous experience with a similar transition except that of mustering out of the armed services and moving into private employment. With judicious questioning a counselor may find that he has had several others. If not, his change will be that much more difficult.

Summary

As you listen to your clients in transition, pay attention to what they tell you about what has triggered their transition, the timing of it in their lives and in the world situation, and the concurrent stress they are experiencing. All this will have an impact on the meaning of the transition, as well as on your clients' ability to manage it. It is also useful to keep in mind whether or not the transition was the individual's choice, how much control your clients feel that they have over the transition, and their past experience with similar transitions.

ISSUES RELATED TO SELF

The transition model encourages us to gather information about clients' internal worlds—their selves. We will now look at four *Self* issues as they relate to work transitions.

Salience and Balance

Work is a major component of the lives of most adults—but clearly not the only component. Freud is reputed to have said that life is made up of work and love. To that duo we add play. The interplay of these domains is what we mean by balance; the place of work in one's life has been called its *salience*. Super (1980) developed a widely cited life rainbow to graphically represent this idea. The rainbow includes the life roles of child, student, leisurite, citizen, spouse, homemaker, parent, and pensioner, as well as worker. He postulated that one can ascertain the relative importance—salience-of work and other major life roles "in the life scheme of the client" (Super, 1980, p. 19).

Let us consider how the rainbow might look for a young mother, age 30, with two pre-school children. The woman, an engineer, is on a fast-track with her company, with the attendant demands of long working hours. One might speculate that her rainbow will have wide bands for work and parent, medium ones for spouse and homemaker, and narrow ones for leisurite and citizen. Let us look also at how the rainbow might look for a 60-year-old single female school teacher, with three grown children and no grandchildren. Her widest bands are likely to be worker, leisurite, and citizen, with smaller bands for parent and homemaker. For both of these people, work is an important aspect of their lives. But what of a young man, father of three, doing occasional part-time work and staying home with his children while his wife works to support the family? How might his rainbow look? Clearly it would have wide bands for parent and homemaker, a very small band for worker, and perhaps medium bands for citizen and leisurite. In his case, work is not a particularly salient aspect of life.

Hughes and Graham (1990) suggested that adults go through

cycles of initiation, adaptation, reassessment, and reconciliation in each of six life roles, similar to those in Super's (1980) rainbow: relationships with self, work, friends, community, partner, and family. We can interpret Joe's current dissatisfaction with life as being primarily caused by his dissatisfaction with his work role. It is also important to look at his other life roles and help him assess both their current salience and his current comfort level in each, considering where he is in Hughes and Graham's (1990) cycles. Is he in the process of reassessing his place in the community? Is he perhaps in the stage of initiation in his relationship with himself? It is not uncommon for people to seek a change in one life role, even though the actual source of their discomfort arises out of another role.

People frequently come to career counselors looking to change jobs, because it is "safer" to talk about career concerns than to face personal problems. A sensitive counselor needs to listen for this kind of displacement, and help adults consider whether or not they really want to make a change, and if so, in what area of their lives—internal issues, relationships, work, or all three.

Counselors may also see clients who come to their offices expressing concern about their relationships, using this to mask other issues. After appropriate trust has been established, and after the counselors have had an opportunity to hear about the concern, they may find that other issues underlie the stated problem, or even replace it in importance. Some clients may be experiencing a fear of aging, and think that a new love would cure all. Some may be avoiding their spouse's confrontation of their alcohol abuse, or they may be unhappy at work and too afraid to face the implications of that unhappiness, "blaming" instead an unsatisfactory relationship.

In their study of adults with orthopaedic and soft tissue injuries, Britnell, Madill, Montgomerie & Stewin (1992), found persuasive evidence for the salience of work in the lives of many adults. These adults, whose average age was 35, typically wanted to and did return to work with significant pain, making necessary accommodations in their leisure and family time to do so. Interestingly, even though their injuries often resulted in lesser participation in their working roles, they did not result in a reduced commitment to that role. It is important to remember the distinction between participation and commitment when an injury or other external event forces reduced work time—when, for example, a client has to care for elderly parents, or returns to school. Counselors may hear such clients' frustration with their inability to act on the work salience they feel. They may hear hopes from some that they will be able to return to full work participation in the future, or expressions of grief for the permanent loss of such possibilities. It is always important to remember, however, that some, for whom work is not particularly salient, may welcome the reduced participation.

Boylan and Hawkes (1984) studied middle-managerial men in midlife and they found that work had a lower priority for these men than it had when they were younger. A racially and ethnically diverse sample of over 1000 men aged 38–49 who worked for the California state government were surveyed, representing a cross-section of levels of midmanagement. The majority of middle managers experienced some midlife transition stress, buffered when social support—partner and friends—was both available and satisfactory. They found that career salience declined during middle age and that community service decreased, but that time devoted to personal recreation increased. Is this because midlife men were doing more of what they wanted to and less of what they thought they should? Counselors may want to listen for changes in their transitioning clients' "shoulds" and "oughts."

As counselors listen to clients in career transition, it is important to remember that for some, work is a major life role, while for others, different roles are ascendant such as home and family or leisure. Super and Nevill (1984) found that work salience was perhaps *the* important determinant of career adaptability. It is important to listen for values statements as clients describe their situations or the decisions they face. A transition may be a time to take a fresh look at values, or to consider how current values may be better implemented.

In a "personal experience" article in *The New York Times*, Scofield (1993) described his own accommodation with the realization that he, in his mid-forties, probably would not get any more promotions. He says that it offered him a freedom from considering how each act would affect his job, freedom to speak his mind at work, and freedom to spend more time with his family. He says finally, "Some would say I've lowered my goals to meet reality. I say I've exchanged career goals for a vision of life. I have never felt happier or more content. There's much more to my life today than just making a living" (p. 22). In other words, his work has become less salient, his family more so.

Anecdotal evidence of changes in work salience in midlife is extensive. As one student put it, "I discovered [through transitions and with the assistance of counseling] that my value system had been challenged and that there was more to life than chasing a career at IBM.

Family and community became more important and change seemed inevitable." He returned to college and is now pursuing a career in social work. His choice of social work, a career where he may help others in transition, is an example of looking for meaning in a career.

There are indications that for people in their 20s and 30s, family and friends come before work. "Americans' interests have expanded, meaning time for family, themselves, and their personal pursuits, crowd and sometimes overcome their commitment to work . . . 'People's view of work is not all-encompassing anymore,' says Douglas Fraser, former president of the United Auto Workers . . . 'The changes in the workplace in the last ten years are greater than any in my lifetime' " (Elmer, 1994). Achieving balance between work and personal life seems to be a growing need in our culture. One of the ironies we find here is that while downsizing of companies results in many unemployed people struggling to maintain themselves and their families, those left in the workplace are working longer hours, under more pressure, and are looking for ways to reduce their work commitments.

For Joe, also, his work as a machinist has become less salient, less central in his life. But work as a whole still seems important. He needs the income and wants the satisfaction of being his own boss and being with people. Counselors often hear this sort of reappraisal from adult clients. The oft-quoted statement that no one ever said on his/her deathbed, "I wish I had spent more time at the office," is a recognition of this common adult experience.

Resilience or Adaptability

The ability to bounce back, to weather changes without major personal turmoil, has been termed resilience. Super and Knasel (1981) proposed a new term, "career adaptability." The term was designed to focus on the balance each individual seeks between the world of work and his or her personal environment and ability to react to changing world conditions. The term responds to a world where adults make many career decisions—voluntary and forced. "One of the major reasons for the introduction of the term "career adaptability" is that it allows greater emphasis to be given to the novel, nonmaturational problems which presently confront many people" (1981, p. 199).

Until recently, career theorists have described the development of an individual's career as unidirectional, resulting from a choice and the implementation of that choice. The phrase "career maturity" has been used to describe workers' readiness to make a "good" career decision. Today's world makes such concepts obsolete for adults, as most will return to the decision-making process many times during their work lives, making new choices each time.

In developing their instrument for assessing career adaptability among young adult blue collar workers, Super and Knasel (1979) interviewed a number of Canadian workers. They culled seven dimensions of adaptability from these interviews:

(a) work values and work salience;
(b) autonomy or sense of agency;
(c) planfulness or future perspective;
(d) exploration and establishment;
(e) information;
(f) decision-making; and
(g) reflection on experience.

The interrelatedness of the concepts, discussed here (salience, resilience, and mastery) is clearly demonstrated by their findings, and as we look at resiliency, we should keep this interrelatedness in mind.

In a volume written for the Society for Industrial and Organizational Psychology, Hall (1986) suggested that adaptability is the part of the mid-career experience that focuses on work tasks and takes a long-term perspective. The other dimensions he examined are *attitude* (focusing on self in the short-term); *identity* (focusing on self in the long-term); and *performance* (focusing on work tasks in the present). Adaptability issues were defined by asking such questions as, "How can I make the changes necessary to remain on top in my field or to move into a new field?" Hall's rather complex model describes various triggers in the organization or society such as: changes in technology, changes in the work role (such as a new job), and changes in the person (such as dissatisfaction with the status quo). He goes on to say that, in the right circumstances and with the right support, these triggers lead to an awareness of choices, renewed exploration, increased adaptability, and a heightened sense of self (p. 141). Counselors are likely to hear adults facing or coping with work transitions talk about these triggers, the amount of role change experienced or anticipated, and their own feelings about the change. Again, we see the interrelatedness of all of the dimensions we are discussing.

Perosa and Perosa, studying the career changes of adults return-

ing for advanced education, found what might be called internal spurs
to change:

> From the life histories of the participants, five patterns emerged: The
> more common pattern, 73% of the sample, was for the fit between the
> individual and the first career to be "good," "excellent," or "like a glove."
> Gradually the fit broke down as it became apparent that important as-
> pects of the self were denied expression. For another group, 27%, the
> struggle was to find some other career in which they could find mean-
> ing: for them the fit had been "poor" or "terrible" from the beginning.
> (1985, p. 63–64)

Other patterns included 29% of the women who were looking for
careers to enhance new-found independence; 17% of the men looking
for careers where they could "relate" to people; 15% of the total who
were seeking a lost dream; and a scant 4% who were pursuing an
avocational interest. The student described above who made a change
from working at IBM to a career in social work clearly fits the first pattern—a good career fit breaking down as he and his life circumstances
changed. The experience of Joe Jones, whom we met at the beginning
of this chapter, could be described by several of these patterns—a "fit"
breaking down, looking to "relate" to people, seeking a lost dream, and
perhaps also looking for "meaning." Savickas, Passen, and Jarjoura
(1988) summed up the adaptability concept by saying that it "emphasizes the interaction between the individual and his or her environment
and this shifts attention from career maturity as readiness for decision-
making to career adaptability as readiness to *cope with changing work and
working conditions*" (1988, p. 83, emphasis added).

Joe's transition is triggered by a change in both his internal and
external worlds, but he is worried about his resiliency. He has little experience in managing work change and doesn't know if he can do so.
We don't know if he has weathered other transitions. That would probably be a fruitful area for counselor investigation.

Self-Efficacy

As mentioned previously, Bandura (1982) proposed a construct to explain certain behaviors such as persistence or the lack thereof in the
face of obstacles. He called it self-efficacy, the belief that one's actions
will have an impact on one's environment. He found that expectations

of success or failure were important in determining motivation; there is much reason to try if you think you will achieve your goals, little reason if you think you will not. Lent and Hackett (1987) summed up self-efficacy research thusly: "With apologies to those with literary sensibilities, if you've got the skill, support, and desire, then 'thinking you can' could light your fire" (p. 377).

To bring this concept to life, let us imagine two 40-year-old women, both forced into early retirement by the new owners of their small plant, a pickle bottling company. Both women were first-level supervisors, both had high school educations, and both had worked for the company since their graduation from high school. One of the women had overcome many obstacles in her personal life. She was married in her teens, the mother of two by the time she was 20, divorced at 25, and had been the sole support of both children since then. She also helped raise her younger sister, who was only 12 when their parents died in an automobile accident. She always believed that she could do whatever was necessary to get along. She trusted her coping abilities. In other words, she had strong self-efficacy beliefs.

The other woman had led a life with fewer challenges and fewer successes. She felt that she held her present position by virtue of luck, and that, although she got good evaluations, she performed only minimally well. She lived at home with her parents and did not believe that she could manage on her own. She felt that nothing she did could make a difference and that she would only get new work if the job counselor found it for her. In other words, her self-efficacy beliefs were very weak. With respect to self-efficacy, the first woman thus has far better resources for coping with change than the second.

In researching burnout among professional educators, DeMoulin (1991) found that low levels of self-efficacy and personal productivity may be an appropriate way to look at the burnout phenomenon. Self-efficacy enhancement is therefore a suggested "treatment" for burnout. Counselors can add to their own efficacy by listening for, and asking questions about, clients' perceptions of their ability to make a difference in their world. Requests such as, "Tell me about past transitions and how you handled them," and questions such as, "How do you gauge your chances of being successful in finding work you enjoy?" will be helpful in assessing these perceptions.

Self-efficacy also seems to be related to salience. Layton (1984) found that for college women with high career salience, self-efficacy was an important determinant of choice, whereas that was less true for women with low-career salience. Let us look at a woman with high self-efficacy beliefs who wanted to become an architect. She faced a demanding training program but was willing to put in the work because her career was important to her. Another woman who had also expressed an interest in architecture was not at all sure she could succeed (low self-efficacy) and was not willing to put in the time and effort because work didn't matter that much anyway. She therefore chose an easier program of study.

Nevill and Schlecker (1988) found that women who had high self-efficacy expectations and who were assertive were more willing to choose nontraditional occupations. Yang (1991) stated, "Women who seek traditionally feminine roles operate from an external locus of control, but, conversely, women who consider nontraditional occupations tend to operate from an internal locus of control" (pp. 353–354). Clearly, if you feel independent of other's viewpoints, it is easier to plan involvement in a nontraditional activity.

Self-efficacy also seems to have cultural determinants. Sharify (1988) suggested that for Asian Americans to be more effective in their careers, they need to increase their self-confidence—closely related to self-efficacy—and reduce their timidity. Young (1988) suggested that Asian American librarians often hamper their career progress because they need to be more flexible (resilient in our terminology) and need to reduce their fear of failure (increase their self-efficacy in our terminology). Counselors need to be sensitive to cultural variations in the meaning of what they hear from clients whose culture is different from theirs.

Halstead suggested that we keep "one primary question in . . . mind. Would my impression and understanding of this person be different if our cultural backgrounds were similar?" (1991, p. 26). Thus we may see members of groups from the nondominant culture believing that they "can't" when in actuality they are victims of discrimination. Or we may have others who gave up striving because they are tired of "knocking their heads against the wall." Still others may sound as if they lack self-efficacy when in fact they are reflecting a cultural imperative to sound modest.

Meaning-Making

As we listened to Joe Jones's story, we heard that he was feeling pressure from inside to have work that is more meaningful to him—that meets his needs for more autonomy and more personal connections on the job. Men in midlife often become more interested in relationships with people, and women often become more interested in achievement—leading to greater balance in the lives of both. The term "affective men and effective women" is more than alliterative. It aptly describes this phenomenon.

Meaning in life usually comes from multiple sources. In studying early retirees, Hatcher found:

> Many . . . did not feel that they were pushed into premature disengagement from the work force . . . Perhaps the downsizing of the company served as a "career trigger," and caused these individuals to break out of a safe routine, to fall back on untapped personal resources, and to discover new ways to earn a living and make meaningful use of their time. (1988, p. 189)

As one woman said, "I was on an assembly line. I wouldn't have had the nerve to jump off, but since I was pushed off, I am excited about the opportunities for achievement ahead of me."

Summary

The dimensions of salience, balance, resilience, self-efficacy, and meaning-making are all critical aspects of a client's work transitions. Listening for and asking about these dimensions will help counselors gain a more complete picture of a particular client's experience. One might think of them as the background of a picture, for which the client's own situation forms the foreground.

ISSUES RELATED TO SUPPORT

Counselors working with adults in transition often hear about a variety of available supports *and* the stressors that often go along with them. The following story illustrates that situation.

> Susan Rodriguez is a 55-year-old woman who is trying to balance her work as a teacher with the demands of her husband, parents, children, and church. She went back to college and completed her degree when the youngest of her five children started school. She has been teaching elementary school for 20 years, and still loves it. She managed her work and family responsibilities capably until recently, when the failing health of her mother and father led her to bring them into her home to assist

them with daily living tasks. At the same time, her oldest daughter got divorced and came back home with her two children, ages three and five. Susan is eligible for retirement, an option that her husband, soon to retire himself, wants her to exercise. She loves her job, however, and has just been asked to be a master teacher, leading a team of three in implementing a new third grade program in her school. She is excited about the changes in educational philosophy and is looking forward to the learning, growth, and recognition that will be a part of this change.

Susan's support system includes her husband, who meets her needs for intimacy and love, but who does not give her much instrumental support, and previously included her parents, although at this time they are demanding more support than they are giving. Her daughter also is in a needy time of her life, asking for a lot of emotional as well as financial support. Susan has several good friends but believes that they have problems of their own and don't need to be bothered with hers. She feels that she can occasionally talk to her teaching teammates, but there is nothing they can do to help. Susan has strong religious beliefs and is an active member of her church. She has talked to her priest, who encouraged her to join a support group for adult children of aging parents, but she doesn't think she can spare the time.

Susan has a potentially very effective support system, but she may not be using her access skills as well as she could. She also does not seem to be taking advantage of institutional support, such as agencies that might help her care for her parents. Counselors often hear adults speak as Susan does, about needing to do everything themselves—or not wanting to lean on others, appear needy, or "air their dirty laundry in public." Many ethnic groups have their own version of this mindset. Keeping a stiff upper lip is not confined to those of Anglo-Saxon origin.

Goodman and Hoppin (1990) identified some support needs particularly relevant for work transitions. They included:

(a) feeling positive about yourself (provided by people who like you and know what you can do);
(b) encouragement (provided by people who expect you to succeed, can give you positive direction, and have an optimistic outlook);
(c) information (provided by people, books, and resource materials that teach job hunting techniques and provide information on jobs and employers);

    (d) referrals (provided by people and agencies who know of help like health care or financial support available to laid off or unemployed people);

    (e) door-openers (provided by people who are willing to make contacts for you); and

    (f) practical help (provided by people who will babysit, loan money, provide transportation, or type a letter or resume.)

The support systems of people from other cultures may be quite different. Martin listed the following traditional supports for American Indians, " . . . the family, the tribe, religious beliefs, and the land itself" (1991, p. 277).

Counselors often hear people describe very limited support—like Joe's. Those who lose their jobs frequently feel that they have lost much of their support system at the same time. Statements such as, "Most of my friends were from work. They can't help me, they've lost their jobs, too" are common. Clients often see support only in terms of individuals who can meet all of their needs—a rare breed indeed. Counselors should encourage clients to think about individuals who meet some of their needs, as well as about non-people supports, such as job training centers, the public library, their faith, or their pets. Support tends to be an area in which counselors hear little and can do much.

ISSUES RELATED TO STRATEGIES

What coping strategies are Joe and Susan using? Joe is tentatively beginning the process of exploring alternatives. Susan is using the coping strategy that has worked for her in the past—doing everything herself. Clearly we have identified an area for further exploration and assistance. Counselors will want to make sure they hear about a person's past record of coping skills as well as about current strategies. Both Joe and Susan have wisely chosen the strategy of seeking help from a counselor, but their counselors are not hearing much about the strategies already under way.

Some of the strategies that counselors will hear from other clients were listed in Figure 5.1—Your Coping Keys Worksheet (See p. 136). Counselors also may hear strategies designed to change or modify the situation through problem-solving, such as negotiating. They may hear strategies designed to change the meaning of the situation through reappraisal, such as developing rituals. And counselors may hear strategies designed for managing reactions to stress, such as doing physical activity.

MOVING IN, THROUGH, OUT, AND BACK (AGAIN) INTO WORK

Counselors listening to clients engaged in managing work transitions will benefit from having a framework they can use to listen to and understand what their clients are experiencing. The following model takes an individual through a worklife cycle (see Table 6.1). A newly employed person is said to be *moving in*; a person who is fast tracked or plateaued is said to be *moving through*; a person who has been laid off, retired, or is making a voluntary career change is said to be *moving out*; and an unemployed person is said to be *trying to move in again*. As counselors listen to clients' career concerns, they need to listen to:

1. The focus of the career concern. Is the client trying to figure out how to *move into* a job or school? Is the client trying to hang in there and balance competing demands? Or is the client *moving out* of the job, school, or work force? In other words, where the client is—moving in, through, or out—influences underlying concerns.
2. The way the client handles moving in, through, or out depends on his/her resources. What comprises the client's Situation? Supports? Self? Strategies?

What then, do counselors hear from their clients during these times? In the following discussion, we will examine these issues for individuals as they cycle, or recycle, through the various stages.

Moving In

When clients secure a new job, another transition must take place. Many employers fail to provide a true orientation to new jobs. Partly as a result of this failure, as many as 50%–60% of all new hires leave their jobs within the first seven months (Leibowitz, Schlossberg, & Shore, 1991). The transition to a new job requires the worker to understand the expectations of peers, subordinates, and supervisors, and also to learn the

Table 6.1   A Model of Worklife Transitions

Work Transitions	Issues for Individual

Moving In:
 • New employees
	"Learn the Ropes"
	 • Expectations regarding
	   —job
	   —culture
	   • Explicit and implicit norms
	   • Marginality, at the edge

Moving Through: • Fast track • Plateaued • Caught in between	*"Hang in There, Baby"* • Loneliness and competence • Bored, stuck • Competing demands
Moving Out: • RIF • Retirement • Career change	*"Leaving, Grieving, Striving"* • Loss and reformation of goals • Articulation of ambivalence
Trying to Move In Again: • Unemployed	*"Falling Through the Cracks"* • Frustration • Despair

company's formal and informal norms. It often requires learning new skills and almost always requires learning new ways of using old skills. It can result in clients' feeling marginal—the feeling that they are at the edge, on the fringe. For many bicultural individuals, of course, marginality is a way of life. All of us, whether rich or poor, "minority" or "majority," feel marginal when we move into new roles. We aren't what we were, nor are we clear about who we should be and what's expected of us.

All of this comes at a time when both the individuals themselves and their families expect them to experience unadulterated joy at having a new position. One woman we know had finally moved to a long sought-after position. She loved the new work and her new colleagues, but was puzzled by her resistance to a new computer system. All of her feelings about the change had become displaced onto the unfamiliar machine on her desk. When she was finally able to recognize the magnitude of the change she had made, she was easily able to learn, and even embrace, the new system.

Moving Through

Moving through work has changed drastically in the past few decades. What was formerly a predictable series of stages, (see Super's, 1980, stages of establishment, maintenance, and decline), has become an unpredictable course—described by Gelatt (1993) as similar to the turbulent white water one encounters while river rafting.

Counselors may well hear clients' confusion and distress over navigation in the new white water and may also hear concerns about plateauing. Moving unpredictably is frightening for many, but many others are afraid of staying stuck in a dead end job—plateauing. Bridges suggests two major strategies for helping employees through that confusing, conflicting middle period. "The challenge is how to provide an interim system of temporary policies, procedures, responsibilities, and authority structures to get people through . . . creating temporary policies . . . encouraging cohesion . . . expecting old issues to surface." (1980, pp. 62–63).

The issue of plateauing was also addressed by Land and Jarman (1992) in their book, *Breakpoint and Beyond,* which looks at the process of renewal for both individuals and organizations. The researchers described a cycle of change that begins with *forming,* a period of exploration, innovation, and invention. Using examples from the physical world such as the transition of water to ice when the separate molecules forming the liquid "suddenly" line up and form a solid crystal, they postulate that after this phase a massive shift occurs, which they call "breakpoint." A person or organization then moves into a second phase, *norming.* This phase encompasses extending and improving what has gone before; the crystal grows, but does not change its nature. It is in this phase that many get stuck—plateaued one might say. If the individual or organization does not actively move into the next phase, *fulfilling,* the third phase will be a diminishment or a disintegration.

To move into a successful third stage, one must integrate the new and different. This results in a transformation that is necessary for successful fulfillment, and leads to reinventing the future. If reinventing does not happen, and they argue that it usually does not, gradual decline is the norm. As an example, they remind the reader that the development of the airline industry was not done by the railroads, which were then at the height of their success and logically placed to be leaders in the new transportation industry. The railroad industry ignored the possibilities in the infant science of flight and were left in the dust as far as passenger travel was concerned.

The parallels for individuals at midlife are obvious. Counselors often encounter adults at the breakpoint between norming and fulfilling. What they hear is discomfort, distress, and a desire to cling to the comfortable norm even while recognizing that it no longer serves its purpose. They hear confusion about what to do next and how to deal with changing demands. An understanding of the process of change itself may be useful to such clients for managing their transition, after which they will be in a better position to move back into work, at the same or a new job, with renewed commitment.

Moving Out

Bridges, conducting a workshop for people in transition, found that although the nature of their transitions varied widely, all the seminar members shared the basic experiences of: (1) an ending, followed by (2) a period of confusion and distress; leading to (3) a new beginning, in the cases that had come that far (1980). For work transitions, that ending—whether voluntary or involuntary—usually involved leaving the job.

Counselors frequently first hear about the grief that accompanies the moving-out phase. Even when a job change is voluntary, there is a process of mourning for the old ways. There may be ambivalent feelings that make it hard to acknowledge the sense of loss. When the change is involuntary, when the worker is laid off, fired, or forced into retirement, the pain is often intense. A grief period can ensue, much like that identified by Kübler-Ross (1969) relating to the death of a loved one.

A study of men whose jobs were eliminated (Schlossberg & Leibowitz, 1980) confirmed the notion that a transition can be an opportunity for either growth or deterioration. Reactions changed over time. They identified five phases—disbelief, sense of betrayal, confusion, anger, and resolution—as marking the movement in a transition process from disequilibrium following the transition to a new state of equilibrium. When the reduction in force (RIF) was first announced, many of the affected men reported feeling a sense of numbness and disbelief: "Why me?" One man said that when he was called into his supervisor's office, he thought he was going to be commended for his work or else receive a challenging new assignment; the news of the RIF stunned him. Several of the men refused to accept and incorporate the loss. Instead, they felt an unrealistic hope: "Maybe it's not true."

A sense of betrayal often accompanied the initial disbelief. Most of the employees said they felt they had entered into a psychological contract with the organization, the terms of which were, "If I am loyal and competent, the organization will take care of me." The RIF represented a breach of that contract, a "slap in the face," a "kick in the pants." One man who was within three months of being a career veteran was especially bitter about the betrayal: "If an RIF must be done, it should be based on a man's production."

Once they had recovered from the initial shock and their immediate sense of having been dealt with unjustly, the men began to accept the reality of the situation. At this point, many began to panic: "What do I do now?" They tended to be immobilized, waiting for some "magical" solution to occur. Around this time, a special program of career assistance was started, giving rise to some ambivalence. On the one hand, the men were dismayed at being fired; on the other hand, they were grateful to the organization for the help and support it offered. They wanted to be able to put the blame somewhere but could not find a suitable object. Their emotions fluctuated from anxiety and anger to excitement and anticipation. Some men contradicted themselves in a single statement. For instance, one man began by talking about the problems created by the reduction in his income—but then immediately after spoke with great excitement about his plans to move to Florida.

Among those employees who could not resolve their confusion, the natural progression was to *anger*, usually directed at themselves or at the organization. Often, the anger was expressed in inappropriate ways by "bad-mouthing" or "dumping on" the organization. In other cases, anger was directed elsewhere, for instance, at the veterans-preference provision in the Civil Service regulations or at the computer which had actually selected the men to be fired. Sometimes the anger took a very concrete form: 14 of the 53 employees affected by the RIF filed formal grievance complaints against the employer. One man articulated his anger by saying, "I'm going to appeal this case and become a thorn in somebody's side."

By the time of the three-month follow-up interviews of the 53 men, 19 had been reassigned to other jobs in the organization, 9 had decided to retire, and the remaining 25 had found new jobs. In virtually all cases, they seemed to have resolved their reactions to the transition.

It is important to note that these positive reactions resulted from the fact that the men were all helped to obtain new jobs. This positive resolution was not as easily achieved during the late 1980s and early 1990s, when the increasing number of job losses was coupled with the decreasing number of jobs. Job loss during that period often resulted in continued anger and increased depression.

Another schema that provides a useful description of the grief process was proposed by Spencer and Adams (1990). They identified a series of stages that included losing focus, sinking into "the pit," and a search for meaning. Of particular interest to counselors working with the newly unemployed is "the pit"—a time when adults experience paralysis, even hopelessness, of ever emerging from this despair. Counselors often hear tales of depression or inaction from adults in the midst of the job search that counter the logical expectations of maximum effort. Clients themselves may be as puzzled as their family members as to why they are not "looking harder." Some people may spend months in the pit! Counselors often find that all they can do for these clients is listen, be supportive, and help them begin to visualize an end to their pain. Developing job search strategies is probably premature in this situation.

The Schlossberg and Leibowitz study (1980) does not address the issue of making meaning of the pain caused by the RIF. Scofield, who wrote the personal article in the *New York Times*, and the student who left IBM for a career in social work, are good examples of that search for meaning. Scofield found it in spending more time with his family; the student found it in doing work that he felt mattered. Adults who tell counselors that they have used their involuntary leisure to develop closer relations with their families or who now volunteer their time to help other newly unemployed people, are additional illustrations of this principle. In recognition of this phenomenon, as well as in response to his own spiritual beliefs, Bolles (1993) added an extensive section on finding your mission to his classic, *What Color is Your Parachute?*

Stephan (1989) wrote a self-help book entitled, *Finding Your Life Mission* to help individuals with this phase of the transition process. She presented ten "creative paths" that can help in this process. The paths include:

(a) clearing your mind: allowing yourself a period of time each day to eliminate distractions and enjoy silence and serenity;

(b) eliminating negative thinking: substituting positive thinking or affirmations;

(c) anticipating the unusual: letting go of some control to allow surprises into your life, tapping your creativity, seeing old things or ideas in new ways;

(d) visualizing solutions: practicing visualizing places and circumstances; imagining how your life will be when you find your mission;

(e) inquiring within: asking yourself questions and listening to the answers; being in tune with your body and paying attention to the signals it sends;

(f) risking daily: risks can be intellectual and emotional as well as physical.

In helping people learn how to take risks, for example, she provided practice steps such as, "Know what you want from your risk, take a private risk, rehearse your risk, share your fears, accept failure as part of the risk, and recognize the risks you have already taken" (pp. 101–102).

Families of the unemployed may also develop useful strategies for coping with job loss. In one family where the husband had been unemployed for 18 months, the wife reported three major coping mechanisms. First, the family kept trying to modify the situation by continuous, systematic job hunting. In fact, their phone bills averaged $400 a month, indicating that the husband was working on networking and contacts. Second, they tried to control the meaning of the problem. They joined a support group, made up of others with the same problem, that focused on the economic aspects of structural unemployment as well as job search strategies. They also identified the positive aspects of the situation; for example, the father was now able to be involved with the children on a more regular basis. In this way, they took the blame away from themselves personally. Third, they utilized responses that helped to manage stress by keeping busy with a rental property, running, and gardening. Obviously, moving out raises many issues for counselors to attend to. What about moving in?

Moving In Again

When we examine moving in again, we can benefit from research done by Peterson, Sampson and Reardon (1991) on the needs of career decision-makers. In developing a system for helping students at their career center, they discovered that they could divide clients into three groups of people, each of which presented themselves with differing "stories" which led to different helping strategies.

They found that some clients who came to their center were decided—that is they knew what they wanted to do and only needed help in knowing how to get there. Those people would tell counselors that they needed academic advising, job search assistance, resume writing, etc. For those students who needed instrumental assistance and information, workshops could be offered to address specific needs. A series of workshops on job search, for example, might include networking, writing a cover letter, writing a resume, identifying job openings, learning how to "ace" an interview, and learning follow-up techniques.

Another group of students were undecided. They talked about the pros and cons of various possibilities and wanted assistance in sorting out their priorities, interests, and values. These students could also be served in a group format through a structured career development program. The group discussion could focus on identifying values, interests, and temperaments; learning about the world of work, labor market information; looking at life style choices; learning decision-making strategies; and developing an action plan.

A third group, most challenging for counselors, were the indecisive. These students presented more complex issues and often had some personal issues that blocked their ability to make decisions. Like Susan Rodriguez, they may have been in too great turmoil to focus appropriately on career decision making. For these students, individual counseling was usually the "treatment of choice." Each student had to be helped to work through individual issues before they could move to making career decisions. A successful outcome of counseling for those students might be to move into group one or two.

GENDER DIFFERENCES

Many researchers have looked at gender differences and work, considering differences on such variables as attitudes toward job and career, drive to achieve, and work-related behavior. Often such approaches involve analyzing these differences on the basis of early socialization patterns.

Notwithstanding changes in recent years, many girls in our society are still often brought up to be passive, dependent, and nurturing, whereas boys typically are brought up to be active, independent, and aggressive. Thus, many women come to be inculcated by the "vicarious achievement ethic" first identified by Lipman-Blumen and Leavitt in 1976. Such women define their identities not through their own activities and accomplishments but through those of the dominant people (usually men) in their lives: at first their fathers, later their husbands, still later their children. As a corollary of this tendency, many women perceive themselves primarily in such roles as wife, mother, and homemaker; even those with jobs outside the home may devalue or deemphasize their role as worker. Men, on the other hand, are governed by the direct achievement ethic and tend to base their identities on their career achievements. They are "success objects," whose value as human beings is measured by their ability to provide for their families.

There has been increasing attention in recent years to women's career development (e.g., Astin, 1984; Betz, 1989; Farmer, 1985; Fitzgerald & Weitzman, 1992). Gutek and Larwood (1989) summarized the research and stated the reasons why they believe women's careers are now, and will remain for the near future, different from men's:

1. There are differential expectations for men and women regarding the appropriateness of jobs for each sex . . .
2. Husbands and wives are differentially willing to accommodate themselves to each other's careers, with wives more willing to move or otherwise adapt to a husband's career needs than vice versa . . .
3. The parent role is differentially defined for men and women; the mother role requires substantially more time and effort than the father role . . .
4. Compared to men, women face more constraints in the workplace, including discrimination and various stereotypes detrimental to career advancement. (p. 10)

Women face two kinds of barriers to success in work—external and internal. Although the situation is improving, women do not yet receive equal pay with men for comparable jobs. Neither is there yet full access to certain occupations or certain levels of responsibility—the so-called glass ceiling effect.

Some of these patterns were reflected in a classic study of women in middle-management and top executive positions (Hennig & Jardim, 1977). Most of the women in the sample had made their career decision (defined as "a conscious commitment to advancement over the long-term") ten years later than is generally true for men. For some of these women that decision was in a certain sense a passive one, something that "just happened" when the woman suddenly realized that she was probably going to be working the rest of her life. These managerial women were inclined to attribute their success to luck or to the kindly intervention and encouragement of a superior. Nonetheless, most of them believed that further advancement would come about through their own efforts at self-improvement and their development of competence on the job. What these women lacked, according to Hennig and Jardim, is "a sense of the organizational environment—the informal system of relationships and information sharing, ties of loyalty and of dependence, of favors granted and owed, of mutual benefit, of protection—which men unfailingly and invariably take into account" (p. 12).

This difference is attributed in part to men having learned early in their lives to play games such as football, which involve teamwork, the long-range goal of winning, and the use of short-term strategies with a view to reaching that goal. Women have little exposure to such team sports, concentrating instead on such activities as swimming, tennis, and gymnastics, that focus more on the display of individual competence and do not involve working with team members. Women's failure to recognize the team-sport aspects of the managerial career may lead them to behave in certain ways that decrease their chances of success in the organization.

Hennig and Jardim specified the following behavioral differences between men and women in management. First, the sexes interpret "risk" differently: women see only the immediate negative aspects (the danger of failure) and men see not only negative but also long-range positive aspects (the opportunity for success and advancement). Second, in deciding on what style to use in playing the role of subordinate—helper, follower, junior colleague, equal, friend—men are more aware of the expectations of others, especially the boss, and choose a style that will satisfy those expectations, whereas women are inclined to adopt a take-me-as-I-am attitude. They are less skilled at dissembling than men are, again because they lose sight of the long-range goal of winning the (career) game. Finally, men take a more instrumental view of human relationships in the corporation and are thus more willing to work with people whom they may not like personally. On the other hand, women often view human relationships as an end in themselves; they cannot accommodate themselves so easily to the demands of working with people they don't like and thus lay themselves open to the charge of "overemotionalism" on the job.

While this study is almost 20 years old, we suspect that many of the gender differences discussed hold true even today. Indeed, more recent research indicates that similar variables are still influential in women's lives. Roberts and Newton (1987) described what they called women's "split dream," where the focus shifted between careers and family—for some women career first then family, for others family first then career. Many researchers have described this difference in career sequencing between women and men. Goodman and Waters (1985) described it as the out-of-sync career commitment curve.

As we have already noted, Gilligan made the point that though sex differences are identified and discussed, they are not incorporated in most models of human development. We must recognize that gender differences are critical in understanding the transition process.

SUMMARY

We have presented a multiplicity of issues related to the kinds of experiences, thoughts, and feelings that have an impact on adults engaged in work transitions. We have discussed what counselors might hear from the perspective of the 4 S transition model, and have added to that the proposition that all transitions involve moving in, through, out and back in again. We hope you keep these examples in mind as you read Part III, What Counselors Do.

Part III
WHAT CAN WE DO WITH WHAT WE KNOW AND HEAR?

INTRODUCTION

In the last section we looked at transitions from the perspective of clients, as they tell us about their individual, relationship, and work transitions. We intended that those chapters would prompt you to ask questions about what you can do to help clients cope more effectively. This section is designed to respond to some of those questions. Written from the counselor's point of view, it is intended to give you ideas and suggestions for helping clients expand their coping resources.

As you read this section, remember that counselors have differing theories and approaches to individual and group counseling. A discussion of those theories is beyond the scope of this book, but interested readers may consult books such as Corey (1991) or Corsini and Wedding (1989), that compare major counseling theories. Remember also, that in order to be effective, you will have to adapt the ideas we present to fit your own style and approach. You will also need to consider issues of cultural diversity as you work with clients whose cultural background is different from your own.

We will discuss techniques for using the transition model to facilitate change in clients individually, in groups, and through other means. We revisit some of the clients whose transitions were described in Part II, and consider what we can do to help them, and other adults, improve the balance of their resources to deficits.

Chapter 7, which focuses on individual counseling, blends the transition model with the process guide to helping, developed by Cormier and Hackney (1993). Chapter 8 begins with a discussion of the value of group counseling in providing both information and support for adults in transition. It draws on the classic work of Irvin Yalom (1985) in identifying curative factors in group therapy, and the research of Robert Weiss (1976) who developed a model of groups for people in transition. In addition to seeing adults in transition individually or in groups, counselors may also be involved in noncounseling arenas. Chapter 9 invites readers to look beyond their office doors at activities that include working with self-help groups, consulting, and developing programs and workshops to assist adults in transition. The final section considers the role of counselors as advocates, helping to affect changes in organizations and society, which may make the environment more supportive for adults in transition.

7

Individual Counseling

The transition model provides a framework—a mental structure if you will—for counselors to use as they help their adult clients look within themselves, their relationships, and their work. Our approach is simple: help clients assess and enhance their resources for coping—their Situation, Self, Support, and Strategies.

Levinson described a successful outcome of a midlife transition in his case study of John Barnes, biologist:

> He had given up the image of himself as a youthful hero going out to save the world, but had not yielded to the threatening specter of the dried-up, dying old man. He accepted himself as a middle-aged man of considerable achievement, experience and integrity—and of serious shortcomings. He felt privileged to be able to do work he enjoys, and he was content to make a modest social contribution as parent, concerned citizen, scientist, teacher and mentor to the younger generation. He had a sense of well-being. (1978, p. 277)

How did John Barnes reach this state of resolution? How can we help other adults in transition achieve the same peace? Cormier and Hackney (1993) presented a particularly useful road map for counselors to follow when helping clients work through problematic transitions. We clearly cannot in one chapter present all that you need to know to become a counselor, but the following overview should provide a way to tie your counseling knowledge to the framework of the transition model.

CORMIER AND HACKNEY'S COUNSELING MODEL

The Cormier/Hackney model is based on the premise that the counseling relationship is developmental in nature. Although each of their five stages is not truly discrete from the others, and clients and counselors may move back and forth among the stages, the process can be described in a linear fashion. The stages are: (a) relationship building, (b) assessment, (c) goal-setting, (d) interventions, and (e) termination and follow-up. We will discuss each of these stages briefly and then concentrate our attention on what we call the action stages—assessment, goal-setting, and interventions.

Relationship-Building

The first stage, relationship-building, is often called developing rapport. It requires the counselor to demonstrate what have been called the "core conditions" of empathy, genuineness, and positive regard or respect (c.f., Rogers, 1957). Most theorists, even when they are not proponents of Rogerian person-centered therapy, agree that these conditions are useful in developing a positive relationship with the client. In order to demonstrate these conditions, and in general to help clients see that you are interested in them and able to help them, you need to use certain skills.

As Cormier and Hackney present these skills, they remind us of the issue of cross-cultural differences in how clients and counselors communicate. For example, eye contact, considered a necessity of communication in Western middle-class society, is considered intrusive by some groups. The authors summarized their discussion of culture, "With so many variables to consider, . . . it becomes apparent that being aware of the potential impact of cultural characteristics is the real objective for the beginning counselor" (1993, p. 50). We would add that even seasoned counselors must stay alert for multicultural issues, especially when their clients are from a group with whom they have had little experience. All counseling relationships depend on:

1. Demonstrating empathy. Counselors can use nonverbal attentiveness, verbal attentiveness, paraphrasing and reflecting client messages, and reflecting client feeling.

2. Conveying genuineness. Counselors can use supporting non-verbal behaviors such as direct eye contact, smiling, interested facial expression, and leaning toward client while seated. Counselors can also use congruence, openness, and self-disclosure. (One way to manage potential cross-cultural differences in expression of genuineness as well as the other core conditions is to use "nonverbal behaviors that parallel or are in synchrony with the client, particularly in the initial stage of helping" [p. 57]).

3. Conveying positive regard: Counselors can use nonverbal behaviors similar to those used in conveying genuineness and enhancing responses—"those that comment on some positive aspect or attitude about the client and provide encouragement to the client in some fashion." (p. 63)

Assessment

The second stage, assessment, makes use of the techniques of clarifying questions—open-ended and closed. Some of the information that one might want to acquire in an intake interview includes: identifying data; range of problems; current life setting; family history; personal history—medical, educational, military, vocational, sexual, and marital. Be careful not to act as an FBI agent with one closed question followed by another. These should provide information necessary to lead into a problem–definition analysis that includes (a) components of the problem—cognitions, behaviors, and interpersonal relationships; (b) patterns of contributing events; (c) intensity of the problem; and (d) client coping skills, strengths, resources (pp. 96–98).

Because assessment can have positive and negative effects on clients, it is important to use care and sensitivity during the assessment portion of the counseling interview. If well done, clients feel understood, relieved, hopeful, and motivated. If not well done, clients feel anxious, interrogated, vulnerable, and evaluated (pp. 92–93). Counselors can avoid some of these negative reactions by taking care to intersperse relationship-building techniques such as reflecting thoughts and feelings, and by being sensitive to the client's reactions during the assessment phase.

Goal Setting

The third stage, goal setting, responds to counselors' and clients' need to know where they are heading. Goals have motivational, educational, and evaluative functions. Agreeing on the desired outcomes of counseling can keep the sessions on track; agreeing on how the counseling will proceed is an appropriate aspect of entering into any counseling relationship.

Of course, both outcome and process goals may change during counseling. As counselors help clients deepen their understanding of themselves and their situations, they may abandon earlier goals and set new ones. The important point is to make these changes as explicit as possible. When setting goals, counselors may also use the techniques of confrontation, imagery and visualization, and role enactment. Language work such as completing sentences like, "I want . . . ", "I do not want . . . " may also be useful at this stage.

Interventions

Cormier and Hackney's fourth stage—interventions—is clearly the meat and potatoes of the counseling meal. Selecting appropriate interventions reflects the counselor's theoretical orientation. Let us express a hope here that you will be flexible in choosing interventions, basing your choice on your client's needs as well as your own predilections; that you will consider your client's learning style and the characteristics of the problem as well as your own experience and comfort level. Most counselors adhere to one of the following four major theoretical orientations: (1) *Affective interventions* are designed to help clients focus on feelings. Some strategies used by affectively oriented counselors include listening for and reflecting feelings, focusing, (c.f., Gendlin, 1981), and helping clients integrate or change feeling states. Some other techniques that may be used come from the gestalt literature, for example, the empty-chair technique, or dream work. (2) *Cognitive interventions* are designed to help clients change their belief system—their thinking. Strategies include: (a) Ellis's (e.g., 1984) A B C process for challenging irrational beliefs; (b) transactional analysis (c.f., Berne, 1964); (c) postponement strategies; and (d) cognitive restructuring—shifting from self-defeating to coping thoughts. (3) *Behavioral interven-*

tions are designed to help individuals replace a maladaptive behavior with a more desirable one. Some strategies include: social modeling; role play and rehearsal, systematic desensitization; and self-management techniques, for example, self-monitoring, self-rewards, or self-contracting. (4) *System interventions* are designed to change the system in which individuals find themselves. They are based on the beliefs that: (a) all elements in a system, for example a family, are interrelated; (b) change in any part of a system, for example in an individual, will lead to alteration of the entire system; and (c) systems have inertia and therefore resist change. This leads to the conclusion that it is difficult for individuals to change without a concomitant change in the system in which they are involved, usually their family. Systems interventions, or family therapy, are beyond the scope of this book, but they are often appropriate for people in transition, especially if the transition is one that involves the family, like a job loss or the birth of a child. Some of the systems interventions mentioned by Cormier and Hackney (1993) include altering communication patterns, altering family structure, and using the family genogram. (For more information on systems interventions, see Minuchin & Fishman, 1981, or Haley, 1976.)

Termination and Follow-Up

Stage five, termination and follow-up, is a process that begins when either the counselor or the counselee decide that the counseling relationship will end soon. Reasons for termination vary widely, ranging from a projected move, to lack of funds, to dissatisfaction with progress, or to such satisfaction with progress that there is a lessening need to continue. Regardless of the etiology of the decision, progress should be assessed by client and counselor, and generalized when possible into other areas of life. Follow-up should be planned and should include referral if necessary. Finally, the relationship should end.

An alternative termination strategy uses the metaphor of the periodic check-up. Goodman (1992) suggested that the "dental model," with its expectations of regular check-ups and routine maintenance, is an analogy that can be applied to helping in the 90s and beyond. In the more traditional format, we, as counselors, often distinguish ourselves from many of our mental health colleagues by saying that we use an educational rather than a medical model. Instead of diagnosis, treatment, and cure, counseling emphasizes teaching students and clients the necessary skills for developing satisfying and productive lives.

The premise behind the dental model of counseling is regular check-ups, closer together at first, but lengthening eventually, to see how things progress. In those meetings, counselors and their clients will check out the effectiveness of the maintenance activities they had agreed upon, for example, mood-altering exercises or support utilization. They would make a determination about the effectiveness of current levels of functioning, and work together to plan the future. In this model, final termination would be a rare event; rather, each check-up would include decisions about future sessions.

THE TRANSITION MODEL AND THE CORMIER/ HACKNEY MODEL: AN INTEGRATIVE APPROACH

The following figure illustrates the integration of Cormier and Hackney's stages with the transition model, showing how it can be used by a counselor working with an individual in transition. Figure 7.1 correlates illustrative counselor behaviors for each stage of the Cormier and Hackney model with each area of the transition model.

Counselors' behaviors during the relationship-building and termination stages of the Cormier and Hackney model are not likely to vary, regardless of the area of the transition model being addressed. In relationship building, counselors strive to build rapport—to get to know their clients better. During termination, counselors strive to help their clients evaluate their progress and make plans for their futures. However, counselors can enhance their work in the assessment, goal setting, and intervention stages by using their understanding of the 4 S's of the transition model. The figure can be used as follows: (Italicized words here identify terms used in Figure 7.1.) Suppose a counselor is at the *intervention* stage of counseling with an adult who, during the *assessment* stage, identified the *self* as an area of need, and during the *goal-setting* stage, expressed a desire to return to a *sense of equilibrium.* You might use the intervention of a *positive asset search* to help that adult rediscover strengths and identify internal resources to use in coping. The rest of the figure can be used in a similar manner. The balance of this chapter provides more detail about using the assessment, goal setting, and intervention stages of the Cormier Hackney model with each of the com-

Stages in the Cormier Hackney Model:	The 4 S Transition Model:			
	Situation	Self	Supports	Strategies
Relationship Building	Counselor Uses Basic Listening Skills			
Areas to Assess	Client's Environment	Internal Resources	External Resources	Current Repertoire of Coping
Sample Client Goals	Modifying the Environment	Return to Equilibrium	Increasing Support	Developing an Action Plan
Possible Counselor Interventions	Reframing, Assertion Training	Positive Asset Search	Referral to Support Group	Problem Solving Strategies
Termination Follow Up	Counselor Helps Clients Review What Has Happened and Plan Next Steps			

FIGURE 7.1 Counseling adults in transition: Combining the Cormier/ Hackney and the 4 S transition models.

ponents of the transition model—the Situation, the Self, Supports, and Strategies.

Assessment

The goal of the assessment phase is to help both counselors and clients gain a better understanding of the issues that brought the client to counseling in the first place. During this phase, they jointly assessed the clients' balance of resources and liabilities. For example, Jack Williams, discussed in Chapter 4, questioned his identity and lifestyle, the lack of opportunities he saw in his small town *environment* (his Situation), his *internal resources* (his Self), his perception that his wife did not understand his current concerns and his lack of perceived *external resources* (his Supports). Although the *current repertoire* of coping strategies he had considered were not likely to be effective, his willingness to confront his life and seek help represent a good beginning.

The other cases presented in Part II also illustrate the importance of assessment. Examples include Marty Smith, who "mattered too much," Joe Jones, the frustrated and perhaps technologically obsolete machinist, and Susan Rodriguez, the master teacher in a career stage different from her retired husband's. With each of these clients we would depend primarily on listening skills for our assessment.

Assessing situations. To understand a client's Situation during a transition, a counselor must explore the transition's triggers, timing, source, control, role change, duration, previous experience of the client with a similar transition, and concurrent stress. These describe aspects of the transition that are particular to the individual. As mentioned, a dozen adults experiencing the same transition, such as getting divorced, all operate in a context that makes each of their situations unique. These areas should be discussed with clients as you work jointly in the assessment phase of counseling because talking about them will help clients gain greater understanding of the nature of their transition. Let us look at two divorced women to examine how clients facing similar transitions can differ.

> Shu Fen Lee, a 40-year-old homemaker, recently divorced her husband of 20 years. She worked as a receptionist in a law firm for 3 years after graduation from high school, then married and spent full time at home raising her 5 children, who now range in age from 7–18. Although she is receiving child support, she must return to work to support herself and help support her children.

In working with her to assess her Situation, her counselor helps her to look at the context in which the transition is happening. On the positive side, she is staying in the family home, which she now owns without a mortgage. Her ex-husband is reliable about paying his child support. Her health is good. Her elderly parents live with her, and her mother can help with child care for brief times, if necessary. On the negative side, her ex-husband hardly sees his children, her father's health is rapidly failing and her mother will probably soon need help in caring for him, and her secretarial skills are out of date—she has never touched a computer.

> Ivana Wilson, also newly divorced, came to this country two years ago to marry her husband, whom she met when he was working in Hungary. She speaks very little English, has never worked in the United States, and

is still waiting for her citizenship papers. Her parents are dead, and the rest of her family is scattered, none near her. Ivana's situation is clearly very different from Shu Fen's.

Counselors can use an environmental scan as a strategy for helping clients assess their Situations. This scan is often referred to as "developing contextual awareness," that is, being aware of the context in which one lives (Watts, personal communication).

Locke and Parker identified five areas of cultural assumptions and values for counselors to think about as they work with clients. They are:

1) Activity. How do people approach activity? How important are goals in life? Who makes decisions? What is the nature of problem solving?
2) Definitions of social relations. How are roles defined? How do people relate to those whose social status is different? How are sex roles defined? What is the meaning of friendship?
3) Motivation. What is the achievement orientation of the culture? Is cooperation or competition emphasized?
4) Perception of the world. What is the predominant world view? What is the predominant view on human nature? What is the predominant view on the nature of truth? How is time defined? What is the nature of property?
5) Perception of self and the individual. How is self defined? Where is a person's identity determined? What is the nature of the individual? What kinds of persons are valued and respected? (1994, pp. 42–43)

We suggest that you keep these questions in mind as you read the rest of this section. Be aware that you don't need to know all the answers; often the best way to find out your clients' values is to ask them. Given the variety of values within even the dominant culture, it may be important to ask such questions of all clients, as the answers may affect the meaning of their transitions.

Some clients may need to be taught how to look at the environment in which they find themselves. They may need to be encouraged to watch the news on television, listen to it on the radio, or read the newspaper, with an eye on issues related to the one they are facing. Often "news magazines" on air or in print, provide the in-depth coverage that provides this kind of awareness. Others may gain an awareness of the world around them by listening to friends, acquaintances, and work colleagues discuss their lives—again listening for information that will help them understand the context of their personal transition.

It is important to remember that clients' cultural environments are also a part of the context. People have differing ways of looking at goals and decision making, defining roles, viewing the world, or valuing competition or cooperation. Both counselors and clients need to understand the implications of these cultural mediators as they strive to assess their transition situations.

For transitions related to the individual, the environment may include others engaged in similar searches for meaning. The women's and men's movements are good examples of this. Knowing that others are experiencing transitions like one's own provides a kind of emotional support. As we look at relationship issues, the relevant context may be a family situation, including the changing customs of society. Consider, for example, the difference between 1950 and 1990 in how someone might react to the transition of becoming a grandparent via an unwed daughter. In 1950, many people lied to the neighbors, refused to acknowledge the child, and a few even severed relations with the daughter. In 1990, many more would come to terms with the situation and maintain close ties with both daughter and grandchild.

Ivana and Shu Fen share the overall environment of the United States, but they may well be in different minienvironments created by where they live or the belief system of their cultural group. Contextual awareness may help laid-off workers avoid shame at their plight and increase understanding of the societal forces that caused the company to reduce its size. In all of these examples, contextual awareness may also lead to political action—empowering clients to change the context.

As counselors help clients assess their environments, it is important to help them develop a reality base—seeing their situations as they really are, not as they perhaps wish or fear. We are reminded of a client who had lost her ability to drive because of failing eyesight. She determined that asking friends for rides was her only option, a position she found extremely demoralizing. Her counselor was able to help her discover both public and private transportation designed for physically challenged people. As she was able to accept herself as being "one of them," she was able to expand her view of the environment in which she was now operating.

Traditional assessment techniques may also be used in examining clients' situations. In assessing Joe Jones's situation, for example, the counselor could have Joe describe his family and community obligations, and have him begin to learn about the world of work and opportunities for education and training. The technique of information interviewing (see Azrin & Besalel, 1980) is an effective way for many adults to conduct this exploration. Others may find it helpful to read about occupations in such publications as the *Occupational Outlook Handbook* (1994).

Assessing the self. We believe that the most effective way to assess clients' internal resources is by listening as clients tell their "stories." By using the basic counseling skills of attending, reflecting thoughts and feelings, and asking open and closed questions, we get to hear these stories from the client's perspective. In the discussion that follows, we will first examine some methods of assessment, then we will focus on two particular areas of the self—"hardiness" and "self-efficacy." For any one individual, we will want to target certain areas of the self. In Joe's case, for example, one might give him an interest inventory or an ability test. These would help Joe expand his knowledge about what he likes and what he can do. Further, these kinds of instruments often tie interests and abilities to job titles, so Joe might be able to consider a wider range of opportunities. Or one might help him use a card sort technique to identify occupations of interest while recognizing the necessity to set priorities and make choices.

A career counselor could have Joe compose a work autobiography to observe his transferable skills and his past decision-making/problem-solving approaches. Systematic assessment instruments are also helpful. For example, counselors may use *The Salience Inventory* (Super & Nevill, 1985) to help understand the importance of work in an individual's life. They might use Krumboltz's *Career Beliefs Inventory* (1991) to help individuals become aware of and confront beliefs that may be blocking their progress.

Computer-aided career development programs such as Discover for Adults (American College Testing Program, 1989), Discover for Retirement Planning (American College Testing Program, 1990), or SIGI (Katz, 1975), are particularly geared to the needs of adults. They provide a way for clients to integrate their interests, values, and preferred work environment with job titles and descriptions and to gain information on required training or education for each. (It is beyond the scope of this book to describe these instruments and programs in depth; for more detailed information, see books like Kapes, Mastie, and Whitfield, 1994, or Zunker, 1994.)

Hardiness. As we begin assessing an individual's ability to manage the transition at hand, we might consider looking at hardiness, a concept that provides a way of looking at an individual's stress resistance—the way people view themselves and their situations (Kobasa, Maddi, & Kahn, 1982). Dailey (undated), expanding on this work, described several dimensions of a hardy person:

1. Openness to change. Looking to the future rather than to the past, seeing opportunity rather than barriers, accepting, and perhaps even enjoying, challenge. The simplest way to assess openness is to ask individuals questions such as: "What do you fear and what do you look forward to as you think about the future?" and "What positive consequences can you see coming from this transition?" It is important not to devalue clients' suffering if the transition is painful. Rather the goal is to help them see that there is a future for them, albeit a different one from what they had anticipated. A new widow usually does not see her transition as positive, but she can be helped to see that her future may still contain happiness.

2. Commitment. Sense of purpose, seeing "life events as part of a self-chosen life course . . . [feeling] responsible to a larger social context or community" (Kobasa, 1980, p. 6). Clients who feel that they matter, to individuals and to society, usually have a stronger sense of purpose than those who don't; clients with clear goals are often better able to focus on the future than those who wait for events to happen to them. In a slightly different way, Egan (1994) discussed commitment to the counseling process as a predictor of success. Perhaps the clearest way to define commitment is to say it is related to the amount of energy the client is willing to invest in achieving goals. Counselors can assess commitment by considering such factors as whether clients keep appointments, do assigned "homework," or whether they seem willing to experience some pain in exploring and gaining understanding of their internal world. Counselors can help clients achieve commitment by identifying incentives—rewards—to achieving counseling goals. Rewards can come from adding something positive to life, for

example, developing talents, or minimizing something unpleasant, like reducing pain.

3. Control. Believing that one has control over how one will respond to life events is the opposite of a sense of powerlessness. One may still express deep feelings; we do not believe that keeping "a stiff upper lip" is always, or even often, the best course to follow. One may control one's response by choosing to grieve deeply and publicly over a loved one, crying (or raging) frequently, and allowing oneself to feel and express all of one's pain. Another person may, however, choose to express his or her grief by maintaining a dignified quietness, using the energy of grief to work for cancer research, or by becoming involved in action-oriented groups such as Mothers Against Drunk Driving, or by supporting gun control legislation.

4. Confidence. Feeling personally valuable and believing that rejection does not mean worthlessness. Although we should never underestimate people's insecurities, confident people approach transitions with a distinct advantage. We can assess global confidence in a variety of ways: with formal self-esteem measures; by asking our clients how confident they feel; by looking at their nonverbal behavior and making our own estimation of confidence. We can also ask them questions that reveal how accepting they are of others, knowing that confident people accept their own imperfections and therefore tend to be more accepting of the imperfections of others.

When judging confidence, we must be aware of cultural differences in how confidence may be expressed or hidden. Many cultural groups have taboos against speaking positively about oneself; others have taboos against eye contact or assertive speech patterns. It would be a mistake to assume that people who have these taboos lack confidence because they differ from white Western male patterns. In addition, people often hide lack of confidence under an attitude of bravura; counselors need to be able to see beneath such surface presentations.

Not all lack of confidence is internally based and therefore "curable" through attitudinal change. A person may be reacting realistically to a situation that is indeed discouraging and perhaps beyond his or her ability to fix. Watts (personal communication) stated that counselors have an obligation to help clients learn about the relevant sociopolitical-economic causes of their transition so that they can separate their own responsibilities from those things over which they have little or no control. An example of this is provided by You (undated), discussing the problem of finding work experienced by new Korean immigrants to the United States. You stated, "A significant number of immigrants lower their self-esteem in response to the dissonant situation of no jobs and even no vocational qualification, despite their previous work experience and former job status. In order to adapt themselves to the reality of the lower immigrant status, immigrants generally have low expectations regarding their future vocational situation" (unpaginated).

In a related vein, we are encouraged to think about Seligman's (1990) definition of optimistic and pessimistic persons. In the assessment phase, we need to listen for "half full/half empty" viewpoints. Seligman provides a "test" of optimism that clients can take if additional evidence is needed to determine where they fit on this dimension.

Self-efficacy. Bandura (1982) found that expectations of success or failure were important in determining motivation. This construct is useful in assessing an individual's internal resources. The phrase "self-fulfilling prophecy" reflects a commonsense understanding of the relationship of self-efficacy to helping adults in transition set goals and plan their futures. Clients who believe that their own actions can influence their environment will be more motivated to set goals and work toward them than those who doubt their effectiveness.

To assess self-efficacy, we may ask clients if they believe that they can influence their world, their situation, or their fate. Do they feel that most of the control for what happens to them comes from themselves? Do they feel capable of meeting the challenges that they face? Krumboltz's *Career Beliefs Inventory* (1991) provided this information concerning career efficacy.

Assessing supports. How do we help clients assess this area of their life? We need first to ask them to describe, or list, the external resources they have available to them. Who is "in their corner?" Who, in Kahn and Antonucci's (1980) terms is part of their convoy?

The people in our clients' support systems may also be the same ones that create stress for our clients. We are reminded of the dualistic concept of nourishers versus drainers. This concept is perhaps best described by using an analogy that compares our emotional sense of satisfaction to the water level in a bathtub. If we imagine life's nourishers as filling our "tubs" with water, and life's drainers as allowing the water to flow out, we can see that for our clients to be "full," they need to have or create enhanced flow in—nourishers—and diminished flow out—drainers. This may mean avoiding situations that are confidence draining, avoiding people who are negative or pessimistic, and spending more time in positive situations and with positive, encouraging people. In the assessment phase of counseling, we can determine how full our client's tub is—and who and what are the nourishers and the drainers.

We may also want to assess clients' abilities to add to their support system, to make connections. This skill has been identified with hardiness, as people who know how to access support are more able to do so in times of stress. Getting a "reading" on clients' abilities to make connections will help counselors decide what strategies they may need to teach.

Assessing strategies.

Assessing strategies. Many adults have experienced prior transitions that they navigated successfully. The strategies they used then may be expanded. This is what might be called a base for growth. Helping clients remember past useful strategies can be accomplished in a variety of ways, some of which depend on whether you, as counselor, are primarily affectively, cognitively, or behaviorally focused. An affectively oriented counselor, for example, might ask Marty, the overcommitted client, to describe when she felt more in control of her life. A cognitively oriented counselor might encourage her to think about the irrational beliefs that led her to think she must take care of everybody and make them all happy. A behaviorally oriented counselor might encourage her to keep track of how many times each day she says "yes" to her family members and to try saying "no" to each of them twice a day.

Pearlin and Schooler (1978) delineated three coping responses that represent a systematic way to examine Strategies for managing transitions. Their list, which is reflected in Figure 5.1 (p. 136), includes:

1. Changing the situation through negotiation, optimistic action, advice-seeking, and exercise of potency—used synonymously with self-efficacy.
2. Controlling the subjective meaning of the situation by positive comparisons, selective ignoring, and substitution of rewards.
3. Managing the stress of the situation by emotional discharge, self-assertion, and passive forbearance.

We must always consider, however, those strategies that were successful in the past but which no longer are in the client's best interest. A classic example comes from the adult children of alcoholics literature (e.g., Black, 1987; or Wegscheider, 1981). A child may have become the "good kid" to help survive in a chaotic alcoholic family. That good kid may have hidden all feelings, especially negative ones, eventually not being even aware of them. Virginia Satir (1972) used the dramatic phrase, "brave response for survival," for strategies that helped one cope in childhood with difficult situations. For example, one might have learned to repress feelings in order to cope with the pain of being abused by an alcoholic mother. The response may no longer be useful, and the conditions that spawned it no longer in existence. Similarly, a person raised in a tough neighborhood may have had to be ready to fight at all times; that pugnacious attitude is probably not helpful as he/she faces adult transitions. Sorting out useful strategies already in our clients' repertoires from those that may be counterproductive is therefore another useful assessment arena.

Goal Setting

If we agree that a primary goal of assessment is to help the client have a basis for goal setting, then we can see clearly that the self-appraisal fostered by the above strategies is an essential starting place. Let us look then at goal setting in light of the transition model.

In Egan's (1994) terms, goal setting helps discover a scenario for a better future. There are three parts to goal setting: conceptualizing possibilities; using questions like, "What do you want?"; choosing realistic possibilities and turning them into viable goals (1994, p. 31).

Each aspect of the 4 S model can be considered in assisting clients in setting goals.

Goals related to the situation. Clients working with internal transitions may set a variety of goals—goals that help them to have a different cognitive understanding of the situation, goals that relate to a deeper understanding of their own psychological dynamics, or goals that relate to changing their behavior. Clients may set goals that change the way they perceive a particular situation, or they may want to change the situation. We call this *modifying the environment.* Clients struggling with transitions involving relationships may set goals that help them redefine the relationship, change the ways they relate to significant others in their lives, or grieve for lost relationships. Clients involved in work transitions may want to enter a particular work situation or may be forced to leave it; they may want to plan changes within a work situation or they may have goals related to formal or informal education or training. Or they may want or have to choose an entirely new occupation.

Goals related to the self. Even when a transition is desired or well accepted, we often still want our feelings to "return to normal." Sometimes we just want to come to peace with the transition. "Talking it out" is the commonsense phrase for what helpers know is an important process of expressing rather than suppressing feelings. Frequently clients will use a transition experience as a spur to pursue other therapeutic goals. Unresolved conflicts from earlier times in life may be addressed; long-standing problems such as depression may be brought to the counselor's office. Behavioral issues such as phobias may be confronted.

Transitions, be they events or non-events, or of short, long, temporary, or permanent duration, create a disequilibrium. In more idiomatic terms, they "upset the applecart." Psychologically as well as physiologically, human beings share with the rest of the physical world the tendency to return to homeostasis, to return to equilibrium. Clients express this tendency when they say things like, "I wish things could just stay the same," or "I wish things could go back to the way they were." Often dynamic self-understanding is the first step to a return to equilibrium.

An impetus for personal growth, what has been called the "teachable moment," sometimes occurs during times of disequilibrium. It may be expressed by questions like, "What did I do to get myself in this mess?" "How come I always get involved with alcoholics?" or "I seem to be overqualified for every job I get. Am I doing something wrong?" These questions help clients set goals for change. Goals related to the self then usually involve a search for emotional relief or personal growth, in counseling terms, dynamic self-understanding.

Goals related to support. Generally people in transition find that their support systems either have diminished or have been overwhelmed by the new demands placed on the members of their system. These people need then to *enhance or increase support*—as shown in Figure 7.1 earlier in this chapter. Marty Smith exemplified an important exception.

Marty, you will remember, mattered too much, to too many people.

What might be viewed as her support system was actually functioning more as a stress system. Marty needed to get support by adding other sources. She needed to add "nourishers" and to find ways to protect herself from "drainers."

Former supports often fail to meet an individual's current needs. For example, many newly divorced or widowed people find that the couples who were an important part of their support system while *they* were a part of a couple are no longer interested in being a part of their new lifestyle. And even when they are willing, the support they used to provide may no longer be what the newly single person needs. Similarly, new parents may find that old friends, if childless, do not understand the complexity of their lives. These friends may have trouble understanding the need to plan all social events well in advance and to never be sure they won't have to change plans at the last minute.

Goals related to strategies. Clients often come to counseling because the strategies they have been using in the past are now not successful. Furthermore, they are often at a loss about what else to do. Helping them develop more, or better, strategies is often an important immediate goal of counseling. In reality, clients often wish to move directly to strategizing, and counselors have to "slow them down" to look at other issues before they move to action. *Developing an action plan* is an appropriate goal, after enough self-understanding has been created to make the plan likely to be a success.

A Case Study

Let us use an example to make some of the preceding discussions come to life.

> Chuck Danto, a 33-year-old, single, recovering alcoholic, finds himself flooded with feelings he doesn't know how to handle. He stopped drinking two years ago with the help of Alcoholics Anonymous's 12-step program, and thought that after two years of non-drinking he was "home free."
>
> Suddenly he finds that he is reacting to everything—his family, friends, and colleagues say overreacting. He feels sometimes out of control emotionally. He will react with rage to a minor irritation, and he finds himself crying at little things. The irony in all of this for Chuck is that, as far as he remembers, he never "fell apart" like this while he was drinking.

Chuck's goal is to *return to the equilibrium* he has recently been feeling, without returning to drinking. His counselor helps him articulate another goal—to develop a *dynamic self-understanding,* in other words to get a better handle on what's happening to him. The counselor tells Chuck that it is common for drinking to be used unconsciously or consciously to stifle feelings, and assures him that the flooding emotions he feels now are also common. As Chuck develops an understanding of the family patterns and personal predilections that led to his drinking, he will be able to better manage these unaccustomed emotions.

Chuck also decides to set a goal of changing some of the places and people with whom he spends time—*modifying the environment.* He is finding that his increased sensitivity makes his job as an assistant principal in a junior high school more difficult. Specifically, he finds himself empathizing too much with the students and finds he is less comfortable imposing discipline on them. He decides to add career decision-making to his list of counseling goals. He also realizes that although he stopped seeing his drinking buddies when he joined AA, and although he still attends weekly AA meetings, he has not developed new friends. This has meant relying on his family for most of his social life, a situation that is not satisfying for him. *Increasing support,* then, has become another of Chuck's goals, meaning, in his case, looking for new relationships.

As all of these goals are developed and agreed upon, Chuck and his counselor recognize that the final step will be to *develop an action plan* that will enable him to master strategies such as reframing, selective denial, and developing hope and optimism. Employing these strategies will help him complete his transitional journey.

At this point, you have worked with your clients to assess their current status, and have set mutually acceptable goals for counseling. What do you do next? Your interventions will vary, reflecting both your own preferred counseling approach and the needs of your particular client.

Interventions

Individuals often need help in identifying options. The story of a 36-year-old man who became a paraplegic as the result of an automobile accident illustrates this point. After the initial physical battle to survive, he became preoccupied with how to live. Not surprisingly, at first he saw no options. Before the accident he had been a construction worker.

Clearly he would be unable to continue that activity. His first attempt to build a new life was aborted when his application to law school was rejected. After exploration it became clear that this application had been a response to the influence of his mother, who was a lawyer. A year after the accident, and before he clarified his vocational goals, he wrote his mother, "I want to share with you the perspective I now have on my future. Because of your love and support I am facing the future with courage, hope, and curiosity." The word *curiosity* showed that on a deep level he was going to make it, that he was going to create options, that he was going to be in control. And, in fact, soon afterwards he applied and was accepted in a school of architecture, which continued his interest in building and took account of his disability. He created an option.

Fifty clerical workers at the University of Maryland (Charner & Schlossberg, 1986), were asked to identify a significant transition. The transitions fell mostly in the family category, followed by geographical moving and work. When asked, "Generally, in change situations, how do you perceive options?" Ninety-four percent saw more than one. However, when asked, "For this transition, how many options did you perceive?" Thirty-four percent saw only one. This indicates that individuals in transition usually see options, but under stress or when in the midst of a transition which has significantly altered their lives, they often "freeze" and can see only one option.

The concept of options also explains the difference between those who have a midlife crisis and those who experience a midlife transition. Everyone has a midlife transition, that is, a time when he or she begins to see time until death instead of time from birth. But only a few run off, as did Gaugin. Those having a "crisis" probably see limited options.

It is in the interventions stage that we see the greatest differences among counselors who take different theoretical stances. Following is a discussion—organized around types of interventions—affective, cognitive, and behavioral that will illustrate how those approaches can be used in helping clients work with Situation, Self, Support, and Strategy issues.

Affective interventions. Affective interventions are often the most appropriate for those issues relating to identity, autonomy, and meaning-making. The *active listening* techniques used in establishing a relationship are useful in beginning the process of helping clients identify and clarify their feelings. Strictly client-centered therapists may use these techniques almost exclusively throughout their counseling sessions. Often the discomfort that arises from transitions involving the self stems from the fact that one is not aware of why one is feeling ill at ease. Labeling the feelings and discovering their normality may provide relief. Some clients, however, will find it difficult to identify any feelings; some will be blocked only on some categories of feelings. Although it is an overgeneralization, we have found it useful to be alert for women who have trouble identifying angry feelings and men who find it difficult to recognize their frightened or sad feelings. Early socialization messages like, "Nice girls don't get mad," and "Big boys don't cry" do carry forward into adult life. These prohibitions are often so strongly internalized that the adult is not even aware of having them, let alone willing to express them.

Many other techniques have been developed to help people recognize and express feelings. These include bibliotherapy, focusing, and gestalt techniques. Some affectively oriented helpers believe in delving into childhood experiences to explore sources of current feelings. These explorations may lead clients to change the way they feel about current events or situations.

One man experienced acute anxiety as he faced his 50th birthday. His wife encouraged him to begin financial planning for retirement, which he resisted mightily, calling it the "R" word, and refusing even to discuss it. As he explored the meaning of this birthday, he found that he felt well physically, was at a comfortable place in his career, and was looking forward to the easing of the family's financial burdens when his youngest child completed college in two years. His anxiety was a puzzle to him.

His counselor encouraged him to think back to his childhood and how he viewed 50-year-old men at that time in his life. He then "remembered" that his father, in his early 40s when our client, an only child, was born, had a major stroke a few weeks after his 50th birthday. His father lived as an invalid for many years after this time, and the family never expressed its grief for its loss of a healthy father and husband. The young boy came to be referred to as the "man of the family," and indeed took on many responsibilities much earlier than he otherwise would have.

This awareness enabled the client to do several things. He began to grieve for his father and for his own "lost" childhood. In the process of doing that, he was able to learn to feel and express other emotions, a development that greatly enhanced his sense of well-being and improved his relationships with his wife and children.

In addition, he now could separate his own life from that of his father, understand the care he took of his health, exercising and eating sensibly, and give credence to his doctors when they said he was at a low risk for a stroke. He could plan for the future with some confidence that he would live to have one. His anxiety was diminished, and he faced the future with optimism.

Ivey described one affective intervention—a positive asset search. The function of this intervention is, "to identify and emphasize client strengths" (1994, p. 141). It is a "useful method to ensure a more optimistic and directed interview . . . to find good things about the client and things he or she does right. Emphasizing positive assets also gives the client a sense of personal power" (p. 144).

Using active listening skills as a base, the counselor conducts a positive asset search by asking such questions as: "What went on this week that you feel good about?" Some clients respond well to checklists of strengths (c.f., Goodman & Hoppin, 1990) or to looking at transferable skills. Reframing, discussed below, can also be a useful tool in identifying positive assets, particularly when your clients see themselves primarily in negative ways.

An important function of affective interventions for people in transition is that of validating and clarifying their feelings. Adults often feel alone with their feelings, especially their fears. Adults in transition often think that the people around them "have it all together," and that others know what they want and how to get there. Tentative efforts to express their concerns to friends or family members may be met with sympathy, or they may be brushed off. Many of these others may be uncomfortable with feelings in general; and, if they are family members, may in addition be afraid to see weakness in someone they depend on. They may feel anxiety about a transition that could or already is affecting them.

For instance, Jack Williams's wife (from Chapter 4) may not be sympathetic to Jack just because of what his potential change may mean to *her.* Jack, however, may well find relief by having a counselor truly listen and help him understand what he is feeling. Marty Smith, likewise, may find it helpful to list the positive aspects of her situation and look at her own strengths in that context. She may then be able to articulate her feelings to her husband in a way he can hear, but first she must be clear herself about their origin. She might find, for example, that she felt angry about always deferring to her first husband and that she is afraid that she is repeating a pattern.

Joe Jones, whom we met in Chapter 6 as he faced retraining or unemployment, will probably find it useful to express his fears of failing in school. He will also benefit from conducting a positive asset search before he decides which path to follow. Exploring his feelings may also lead him to better understand his wife's and brother's feelings, and to understand why they have differing ambitions for him. He may begin to see that he is procrastinating and that in doing so he is allowing circumstances to make his decision for him. If he loses his job because he does not get the retraining he needs, or if his brother gets another partner for the bar, his choice will be taken away. A counselor might help him to see that in a way he wants that to happen—to avoid responsibility. But he may also see that giving up control of his future is perhaps not getting him what it is he really wants.

Cognitive interventions. Many counselors find that cognitive interventions are a useful way of helping adults navigate transitional experiences. We do not mean to imply that the distinctions are always clear. Often cognitive work is combined with affective, and/or behavioral work.

Reframing can be described as the process of looking at a situation from a different point of view. The oft-used example of seeing a glass as half empty is an example of a situation ripe for reframing. The goal in this case would be to help the client see it as half full.

Consider the following example. A 40-year-old woman has recently been left by her husband of 20 years. After she took some time to ventilate some of her fear, anger, and grief, and after the counselor had gained some information about the marriage, she was asked, "Could you imagine yourself thinking that he did you a favor?" As her life progressed and she began dating, she was finally able to reframe what she had seen as desertion and relabel it as a chance for her to create a new and happier life. Her counselor had helped her to reframe the events and therefore change their meaning.

Hof (1993) described a process of instilling hope and optimism. He suggested that counselors use their full range of skills in doing this, but added suggestions for some specific hope-fostering techniques. Although geared to couples, they offer useful suggestions for counselors working with anyone in transition. Five of his suggestions are presented:

1. Counselors can provide support, nurturing, and empathy. They can also help clients see that "It is okay and normal to learn/ change in steps or stages" (p. 225). Helping clients understand what they can and cannot control can be a very powerful intervention indeed. Consider an unemployed aerospace worker who was laid off because of a reduction in the defense budget. Before this person can complete the grieving process and move on in life, the frustration around being fired must be "let go" and focus placed on what is controllable—personal decisions and planning.

2. Hof's second technique, relabeling and reframing, turns negative views around and corrects clients' cognitive distortions. This may include helping clients see positive aspects of their situations, silver linings if you will. Not all events, however, have positive interpretations. For example, a man adjusting to the deaths of his wife and son in an automobile accident would be hard pressed to see anything good in this tragic event. Helping him gain hope that he can still have a positive future is appropriate; telling him that there is a silver lining would be cruel.

3. Ivey's positive asset search is designed for the purpose of implementing Hof's third technique, "identifying . . . strengths and the expression of them, or of positive potentials" (1994, p. 226). People undergoing work transitions may also find it helpful to look at their technical and transferable skills. (See Bolles, 1993; or Goodman & Hoppin, 1990.)

4. Helping clients identify and use their spiritual or transcendent beliefs, values, and resources is Hof's fourth technique. Because many religions, life philosophies, or ethical creeds offer encouragement and hope in times of trouble, the use of those beliefs, values, and resources can infuse some hope in a time of difficulty, pain, or even despair. Shame and guilt cause many individuals and couples to turn away from their religious and spiritual supports, just when they need them the most (Hof, 1993, p. 226). Spirituality is often enhanced, or embraced for the first time, in midlife. This phenomenon makes Hof's suggestion even more appropriate for counseling adults in transition.

5. Hof's fifth technique involves using absurdity, humor, and laughter. Hope can be increased when clients recapture, or learn for the first time, childlike playfulness and creativity. The

physiological effects of laughter can be healing in themselves; psychologically, humor can help clients keep their problems in perspective.

Seligman suggested that optimism, too, is learnable. He suggested that blind optimism might be a mistake, but that choice is the goal. "[We] will give you a choice about how to look at your misfortunes— and an alternative that doesn't require you to become a slave to blind optimism" (1990, p. 208). He suggested that a risk analysis helps one determine if optimism is the right course. If the risks are too great, one should perhaps be careful. (We do want our pilot to be pessimistic and de-ice the plane one more time!) But in navigating a transition, counselors can help their clients learn to choose when to take an optimistic stance—when to have hope.

Ellis (1984) proposed a step-by-step process for challenging a client's view of a situation. The process, often known by its acroynym A-B-C-D-E, includes (a) discovering the Activating event, b) identifying the client's Belief system, c) identifying the emotional Consequences of the event, d) Disputing the client's existing beliefs, and e) arriving at new Effects. This A-B-C-D-E process is geared toward changing clients' thinking about events, beliefs, and consequences. A key element in this approach is the disputation or confrontation of irrational beliefs.

Using the analysis developed by Ellis (1984), Seligman suggested that people use one of the following techniques to change irrational beliefs:

1. *Distracting oneself.* Some ways to do this are:
   a) Think of something else. Counselors can help clients plan ready substitutes for disturbing thoughts, and clients can learn to use them. For example one might ask newly laid-off workers to practice thinking, "I am worthwhile" whenever they start to think, "I am useless." Thought-stopping, closely akin to thought substitution, focuses on *not* thinking about a particular person or event. (See *How to Survive the Loss of a Love*—Colgrove, Bloomfield, & McWilliams, 1991).
   b) The imaginary umbrella stand. This technique involves leaving one's worries in an imaginary umbrella stand at the door of one's home or workplace. The premise is that it is easier

to let go of troublesome ideas if they can be reclaimed when convenient. A related technique is to list disturbing thoughts to think about later.

c) Physical reminders. Many people find it helpful to have a concrete reminder, for example, a rubber band around the wrist that can be snapped as a reminder when one starts to think troublesome thoughts.

2. *Disputation.* This technique teaches clients to argue with their own beliefs and, we hope, win the argument. A recently divorced woman who wanted to date again but believed she was too unattractive to interest any man kept a log of any compliments she received or heard about herself. She enlisted a few trusted friends to help her and soon had a satisfyingly long list. These "facts" effectively disputed her beliefs, and she soon was able to change, or at least modify, her beliefs.

3. *Looking for alternative explanations.* It was said that the great actress Helen Hayes always felt sick to her stomach before a performance. Clients who experience nausea when anxious about an upcoming event, a job interview for example, can tell themselves that they are preparing for a performance in the same way a great actress did.

4. *Decatastrophizing.* Going off a diet one evening doesn't mean being out of control forever. Nor does one bad grade mean flunking out of school. Many people need help in becoming aware that their catastrophic expectations are unlikely to materialize.

Suppose, for example, you are trying to help a woman who moved across the country with her newly transferred husband. She is having trouble settling in and making friends. She says, "The neighbors are all snobs. I called on the woman across the street and she never even called me back. I know I'll never make any friends here." Assisting her to identify her irrational beliefs can help her to reopen her efforts at making friends.

Or take the adult who begins a session with her career counselor with, "This time I want to make the right decision. I want to get training in a field that I am sure will have opportunities for me and that I will enjoy and be able to stay with for the rest of my working life." Waiting for that kind of certainty—a near impossibility—could paralyze the client. Challenging the irrational belief may help the individual engage in effective career planning.

Transactional analysis (c.f., Berne, 1964) is another cognitive process useful in working with adults in transition. The strategy involves helping clients identify the aspects of themselves that derive from *parental* messages (often negative ones), remnants of *childish* thinking, and their rational *adult* parts. They can then make new decisions about what to think based on an understanding of what is real and true today. The recently transferred spouse described above may have been told as a child not to go where you are not wanted. This belief makes her even more prone to give up her attempts at making friends.

Cognitive restructuring, another thought-based approach, uses an analysis of self-defeating thoughts and behavior as the precursor to changing how one deals with the world. Cudney (1980) proposed a system in which he invited clients to examine their self-defeating behaviors and to choose between what he called the life road and the death road—metaphors for ego-affirming and ego-destroying feelings, thoughts, and actions. Times of transition seem to call forth a particular need to rethink one's thought patterns, as previous ones may no longer fit new circumstances.

Teaching networking, another way to help clients manage their need for support during work transitions, is based on the fact that approximately 80% of jobs are found through some personal contact. Networking, often touted but rarely taught, teaches clients how to identify potential contacts, write a script, rehearse telephone calls, develop a recordkeeping system, and follow up on commitments. Learning how to network results from a cognitive intervention; actually networking is a behavioral change.

Meichenbaum (1977) used a cognitive analysis to develop behavioral interventions. His stress inoculation training is based on the belief that people will cope more effectively if they understand the situation they are in and if they know and use techniques to reduce their anxiety. Ritter (1985) used Meichenbaum's concepts to help clients develop and rehearse a repertoire of self-statements designed to help them prepare for, confront, and cope with stressors. Counselors can help clients formulate statements such as:

- You can develop a plan to deal with it, don't worry.
- Don't try to eliminate the fear entirely; just keep it manageable.
- One step at a time.

- Relax, you are in control; take a slow deep breath.
- Keep the focus on the present; what is it you have to do?
- It worked; you did it; it wasn't as bad as you expected. (p. 43)

Behavioral interventions. Behaviors can be defined to include thoughts, but here we will focus on overt actions. We believe behavior change is important, and also that there are occasions when affective and cognitive change occur as a *result* of behavioral change.

Modeling, role play, and rehearsal. These closely related techniques provide ways for clients to see others or see themselves performing desired behaviors. Imagine that you are working with a forty-year-old man who is having difficulty adapting to a new marriage. After his parents were divorced, he had little contact with his father. Twenty years of living on his own makes him unsure how to be part of a couple. He tends to make unilateral decisions about activities and is then puzzled at his wife's resentment. His counselor suggests the following strategies:

1. Watch other couples and observe what the husband does, particularly in regard to decision making about how they will spend their time (*social modeling*);
2. Act out with the counselor a situation in which he is not sure how to behave. He will play his wife and the counselor will play him (*live modeling and role play*);
3. Act out the above scenario playing himself (*role play*);
4. Act out a real situation that he expects to face in the near future (*rehearsal*).

When using each of these interventions, the counselor needs to provide feedback about the specifics of what is being done. It is also helpful to begin with easier behaviors and move up to more difficult ones. In the case described above, we might want first to have our client practice asking his wife's advice before he makes dinner reservations, eventually discussing with her his career plans and long-term goals.

Imagery training. A special case of rehearsal, imagery, allows people mentally to practice handling situations. Commonly used by athletes and performers, imagining oneself successfully behaving in the desired manner can be helpful in actually attaining the desired behavior. It has several advantages over rehearsal: it can be done alone, at any time; it applies in situations for which rehearsal is impractical; and it encourages clients to become self-directed, not depending on the counselor to play other roles or provide feedback.

Many people need practice in imagining a specific situation, but keep in mind that even though for the majority of people imagery is visual, for many it is auditory or kinesthetic. Ideally, it combines all three elements. Thus, a person preparing for the first day on a new job may want to "walk through" the day beforehand, imagining preparing for work, arriving there, seeing the worksite, hearing its sounds, feeling its atmosphere, performing the job duties, managing breaks and lunch, and ending the work day. Additional elements may be added as necessary and appropriate. When helping people with poor work records, for example, you may want to encourage them to imagine all the barriers that might prevent them from getting to work or completing the assigned tasks. Strategies for overcoming these barriers can then be identified and rehearsed.

Assertion training. One way of helping clients change their situations is by teaching them some assertive skills—communications techniques that provide for the rights and dignity of others while maintaining one's own rights and dignity. Being assertive is an alternative to being passive or being aggressive. Counselors can help their clients integrate assertive approaches by examining the socialization messages they received as children. Many people heard things from their parents that they interpreted, rightly or wrongly, as, "You don't count," or "What you want doesn't matter." Or they may have heard "rules" like: "Don't make waves!" "Don't make trouble!" "Don't draw attention to us!" People in vulnerable positions, for example women and members of some ethnic minorities, may have had such "rules" foisted on them even more firmly. People who received these kinds of messages tend to be passive more often than is useful to them. On the other hand, some people heard messages such as, "The squeaky wheel gets the grease," or "Might makes right." These people may tend to use an aggressive communication style.

Adult children of alcoholics often hear strong messages concerning keeping family secrets. Being truly assertive may require telling the truth about another's drinking or other "skeletons in the closet." It may be difficult for such clients to recognize that they have as much right to help as their family member has to the secret. In this case, assertiveness training may be a necessary prelude to any other helping interventions.

For assertion training to be useful, it must be translated into behavior. Clients are typically given an opportunity to practice difficult behaviors during the counseling sessions—role play and rehearsal—and then given "homework" that requests them to practice the behaviors in real situations. They then return and discuss what went right and what didn't, and perhaps practice again and try again in "real life." Most people who need assertion training are too passive, but there are some who can benefit from it who are too aggressive. These people, too, need new interaction skills and behaviors. Because of the increased potential for feedback, assertion training is often particularly effective in a group format.

Anxiety reduction techniques. Affectively oriented counselors may ask nervous clients about their feelings during anxiety-producing experiences. Cognitively oriented counselors may ask nervous clients about their thoughts. Behavioral counselors generally identify symptoms and focus on reducing the physical manifestations of anxiety or fear, often relying on progressive relaxation and systematic desensitization to help clients experience less anxiety. Although it is beyond the scope of this book to give instruction in implementing these behavioral strategies, they are often a useful beginning to any intervention where anxiety is debilitating or blocking other change. We have found progressive relaxation often to be a useful beginning to a counseling session, allowing the client to be more fully present.

Combination interventions. Few counselors adhere strictly to one type of intervention. Client needs differ and counselors must be able to vary their approach accordingly. Some interventions we find particularly helpful with adults in transition do not fit neatly into any of the above categories.

Problem-solving interventions. Force field analysis, originally developed by Kurt Lewin in 1943, provides a method for analyzing the steps needed to reach a goal. The steps include: (a) stating a goal or desired outcome, (b) identifying all of the pathways or methods you now know to reach the goal, (c) identifying all the actual or potential barriers that may prevent you from reaching your goal, (d) picturing the pathways and barriers as forces or vectors operating in opposite directions, and (e) discussing ways to increase the pathways or reduce or overcome the barriers. Many clients find this to be a helpful way to approach an action plan or solve a problem. And, as mentioned earlier, identifying barriers makes it more likely that a person will have the resources to manage them if and when they arise.

This approach was very successful with a rural displaced home-maker, Marie. She wanted to be a nurse's aide, but the community college was 60 miles away. Although she had a grant to attend school, was sure of her career goal, and very much wanted to be self-sufficient, all she could see were problems in attaining the goal. She listed innumerable barriers, including external barriers such as no child care if her children were home sick from school, potential bad weather in the winter that might make driving difficult, and no private place to study at home. She also identified several internal barriers such as fear of failure, occasional bouts of depression, and a history of not following through on commitments.

Force field analysis allowed Marie to visualize this on paper. She then added, with the help of her counselor and a positive asset search, her ability to learn new things, her genuine delight in helping others, a new maturity, and a determination to make this change a successful one. She identified a few new barriers also, including lack of funds for books and materials and a sister who thought she was nuts to work so hard and told her so frequently. She was then able to do the following: (a) make contingency plans for the external barriers, for example, find a neighbor who could handle child care in a pinch, (b) learn some assertion techniques to get her sister "off her back," (c) identify a person in her displaced homemaker support group to call when she got depressed or anxious, (d) investigate further grant funds from the college to help pay for books and materials, and (e) set aside a small corner of her bedroom for a private study place. Although new problems may well arise for her, she has learned a way of analyzing them.

Many people find other problem-solving strategies useful. For some, concrete, sequential, decision-making activities fit their personal style. DECIDES, the easily remembered acronym for the step-by-step approach developed by Krumboltz and Hamel in 1977, has become a classic. They suggest that clients:

1. **D**efine the problem: What is the decision to be made?

2. **E**stablish an action plan: How will I make this decision?
3. **C**larify values: What is most important to me?
4. **I**dentify alternatives: What are my choices?
5. **D**iscover probable outcomes: What is likely to be the result of following each alternative?
6. **E**liminate alternatives systematically: Which alternatives won't fit my values and situation? Which have the least probability of success?
7. **S**tart action: What do I need to do to make my plans a reality?

Other people suggest more intuitive decision-making approaches. H.B. Gelatt's (1991) positive uncertainty theory suggested that if you wait to be sure, you will never decide; if you decide too firmly, you won't be flexible enough to change as needed. His plan was based on two attitudes: (1) accepting the uncertainty of the past, present, and future, and (2) feeling positive about that uncertainty. It includes four paradoxical principles: (1) "Be focused and flexible about what you want, ... (2) Be aware and wary about what you know, ... (3) Be objective and optimistic about what you believe, ... [and] (4) Be practical and magical about what you do" (p. 12). For readers who want more examples of decision-making strategies, Richard Sharf (1992) outlines a number of them.

Solution-focused brief counseling. Another problem-solving strategy (Walter & Peller, 1992), it is based on the premise that maintaining a solution focus helps clients avoid playing "ain't it awful?" (Berne, 1964), and move to looking for new thoughts, feelings, and behaviors. Clients: (a) identify what they want—stating their goals in positive terms, (b) discuss what's working—exceptions to the current unproductive behavior, and (c) identify what could be hypothetically happening—if a miracle occurred.

Play therapy. Typically considered an intervention for children. Frey (1993), however, made a case for using play therapy with adults. It is especially effective for adults who did not play much as children, or for those who have reached some sort of therapeutic impasse. Because play is naturally illogical, it frees people to break away from the way things have been and see what could be. Perhaps it taps into different parts of the brain than other approaches. Regardless of the mechanism, it seems to work with many clients. Much has been written about using humor in helping, a closely related technique to play therapy, (e.g., Moody, 1978; Mosak, 1987). This, too, used with delicacy, can help adults in transition see their problems in a new light.

Developing rituals. Certain transitions, for example weddings, births, or retirement come with attached rituals that ease the passage. Others, such as divorce, job loss, chronic health problems, or failing to get a promotion are ignored. Furthermore, the rituals that often were a part of life before the transition may be accessible no longer. For example, three couples who were all married on the same date, in different years, developed a tradition of celebrating their anniversaries jointly, making it a special event. When one of the couples got divorced, the tradition continued with the other two. Not only did the former husband and wife lose a cherished celebration, but they also felt left out of an important ritual.

A ritual can help with the "betwixt and between period" to connect you to your former roles, assumptions, relationships, and routines, and to move you to your new ones. Myerhoff (1984) discussed the importance of rituals in helping people deal with marginal periods when they are shifting from one phase of life to another, that is, when they are in transition. Housewarming parties are a commonplace example of this. Originally these events provided a way for people to acquire the goods necessary to set up housekeeping; for most people today, they are a ritual to connect old friends with one's new locale.

Non-events, in particular, are rarely ritualized. Counselors can use Myerhoff's suggestions to help clients develop new rituals. For example, a couple who have decided not to have children may celebrate the decision with the purchase of fragile glassware, and invite their friends for an "exhibition." A man who has realized that he will never be promoted to upper management may take his family on a vacation to "celebrate" the lessened work commitment that results from this awareness.

CONCLUSION

The foregoing has been an attempt to summarize some of the techniques you might use in helping an adult client cope with transitions, using the Cormier/Hackney and Transition models in combination with other techniques. We have discussed counselor techniques to be used in the assessment, goal-setting, and intervention stages of the model, as appropriate in helping individuals increase the balance of deficits to resources in the areas of Situation, Self, Supports, and Strategy. We have also indicated how counselors from different theoretical orientations might use this schema to help their clients.

8

Group Counseling

Eleven years ago I totally lost my zest for life when my wife of a lifetime was killed . . . Soon, with the help of some young people I discovered group psychotherapy. . . The most helpful idea I found to combat acute depression came from a young woman I met through the group. She said that my pain of depression came because the "arrow" of my thrust in life, my attention, my energy was turned inward. Unless I turned the arrow around, outward, and forward in time, the pain would remain . . . To turn the arrow around, I found, was not easy. At age 63 there is, looking back, a trodden path easy to discern, easy to reminisce about. But looking forward there is untrodden ground, new trails must be broken constantly—that takes effort. (Bergman, undated)

In the statement above, taken from an article entitled, "Fresh Currents in the Stream of Life," the author wrote poignantly of the effects of group counseling on his search for identity and meaning in his life. He also talked of the role of the group in helping him develop appropriate strategies for coping with a major loss.

This chapter focuses on techniques counselors can use to work in groups. Groups are complex, requiring counselors to combine individual counseling and group management skills. We begin this chapter with some general information about the value of groups for adults in transition and a typology of groups. Then we describe a variety of groups and specific techniques designed for adults who are experiencing different kinds of transitions—some individual, others involving relationships or work and career. In that way, the three major parts of this chapter correspond to the three chapters in Part II. The final section examines the value of groups in helping people assess their assets and liabilities in each of the 4 S arenas.

GROUP COUNSELING AS A MODALITY

It is tempting to start this section by saying that the keys to success in working with adults in transition are support, support, and support. Whether the transition is a temporary one or a permanent one, whether it represents a role gain or a role loss, whether it comes "on time" or "off time," people experiencing major changes in their life often benefit from a better understanding of what they are going through, and from realizing that "I'm not the only one that's got it," and "I don't have to handle it alone." Stated differently, adults in transition need information and support, both of which can often be provided most effectively through group counseling.

Curative Factors in Group Counseling

Let us consider how Yalom's (1985) discussion of the therapeutic factors in group therapy applies to adults in transition. He identified 11 curative factors: imparting information, instillation of hope, universality, altruism, the corrective recapitulation of the primary family group, development of socializing techniques, imitative behavior, interpersonal learning, group cohesiveness, catharsis, and existential factors.

Imparting information. We can hardly overestimate the value to clients of gaining information about the transition they are experiencing or anticipating. Regardless of whether that transition involves confronting a change in family status or a career change, or whether it is an event or a non-event, obtaining information about the change helps individuals gain some sense of control. Yalom noted that information often "functions as the initial binding force in the group until other curative factors become operative" (1985, p. 11).

Instillation of hope. People in a group who have "been there," that is, people who have experienced a similar transition and are further along in the process of moving through it, can instill hope in people who are moving into the transition. The same curative factor can operate whether the group is designed for returning learners, dislocated workers, or people who have just learned they are HIV positive. People who are reeling from the impact of the transition can benefit from seeing people who have begun to cope with it, or who have integrated the transition as part of their lives. For example, people who fear losing their sight, or have been told that they will, can receive tremendous inspiration from watching people who are blind function. A major strength of many of the 12-step programs, such as Alcoholics Anonymous, is that at each session people who have experienced the particular problem and are in the process of "recovering" tell their stories to inspire others.

Universality. As they move into or out of any particular situation, adults can benefit from discovering their commonalities, from realizing they are not alone. Such a realization, referred to by Yalom as a sense of universality, typically comes when people in a group learn that many others have shared similar experiences and feelings.

A group of older adults, meeting at a senior center, arrived at such an awareness in an unusual way. One member of the group reported on his discomfort as he reflected on the large holiday dinner at his daughter's house the previous week. "I don't understand," he said, "why I always feel so much more comfortable when our daughter comes to our house than when we go to hers." As other members of the group reported a similar preference for being hosts rather than guests, they realized that they were seeing relocation of the holiday dinner as a signal of decreasing abilities. It became a metaphor for their fears about becoming dependent on their children. As they discussed this with their counselor, several members of the group realized that while fear of becoming a burden was an understandable and shared concern, it was counterproductive to let those fears—that anticipation of a possible future transition—interfere with current pleasures.

Capuzzi and Gross (1992) asserted that seeing one's problem as an example of a more general pattern may serve to demystify and deintensify the problem. Such a realization can also lay the groundwork for action steps to deal with the problem. It can help people mobilize their energies to help themselves and each other, and perhaps seek social redress, attempting to change the situation.

Altruism. Helping each other relates to Yalom's fourth curative factor, altruism. He observed that clients benefit "from the intrinsic act of giving . . . they offer support, suggestions, reassurance, insights, and share similar problems with one another" (1985, p. 14). When people experience major transitions, their self-esteem often plummets. The opportunity to be helpful to others by providing support and/or information may help to reverse the downward slide in self-esteem. Consider the case of a recently divorced woman who is seeing herself as an unlovable failure. If she is able to provide some support to another group member, and gets a smile in return, it may help her see herself as "worth being with."

Corrective recapitulation of the primary family group.

In Yalom's view, a major value of therapy groups is that they help patients relive and correct problems stemming from their original family groups. Early issues, such as sibling rivalry, can surface and become topics of discussion. Although such a "correction" can be very valuable for certain clients, most groups for adults in transition do not spend time reviewing early experiences in their family group. When such assistance seems necessary, a referral for individual or specialized group therapy is appropriate.

Development of socializing techniques.

Groups can serve as a meaningful laboratory for learning social skills. Consider, for example, the widower who relied on his wife to make social engagements with friends and nurture family relationships. His actual or feared ineptness in such situations may keep him from reaching out for the sociability and intimacy he now needs. In getting feedback from other group members about how they perceive him, he can develop "outsight" as well as the insight that can come from individual counseling. The group can help him identify and acknowledge the social skills he does have, as well as help him develop additional strategies.

Imitative behavior.

In groups, members have an opportunity to model themselves after the group leader and/or other members. They also can learn vicariously as they observe interactions between the counselor and other group members as well as among members themselves. Pearson (1992) noted that in groups "members can 'catch' functional attitudes such as hope, perseverance, concern for others," and can also learn "specific coping strategies such as asking for help, publicly admitting failures, and substituting constructive for destructive behaviors" (p. 98). Groups for people diagnosed with a particular disease, or for their family members, are clear examples of adults in transition who can benefit from modeling or vicarious learning.

Interpersonal learning.

Yalom contended that group experiences can enrich the insight provided by individual counseling. He talked of the group as a social microcosm in which clients can display their maladaptive behavior, learn how others perceive that behavior, and come to take responsibility for the impact they have on other people. In groups, leaders and members can identify ways in which individuals are employing self-defeating or life-giving approaches (Cudney, 1980). Such feedback can facilitate learning for people who are trying to adapt to life changes. For example, a woman whose child was killed in an accident while she was out of town may continue to berate herself for leaving. The group can help her identify the many things she had done for her child, and try to stop her from dwelling on the "if onlys."

Cohesiveness. According to Yalom, "cohesiveness in group therapy is the analogue of relationship in individual therapy" (1985, p. 48). Members of cohesive groups are more accepting of each other, more supportive, and more likely to self-disclose. Such cohesiveness can be encouraged by skilled leaders who help people talk about their transitions and give each other appropriate feedback. Capuzzi and Gross (1992) suggest, "The actual benefit of self-disclosure and feedback relates to how these processes generate empathy among members. Empathy, or the actual experience of being understood by other members, is what catalyzes personal growth and understanding in the context of a group" (p. 19). Being part of a cohesive group can also supply the support and motivation that people in transition need in order to take constructive action on their own behalf.

Appropriate humor can add to group cohesiveness. Sometimes humor involves using a paradoxical approach. For example, a counselor can ask group members to brainstorm strategies that will guarantee that the transitions they are contemplating will lead to disaster. A paradoxical instruction might be: "Think of as many ways as possible to 'not listen' to friends, family, and co-workers!" or "What could you do to turn off people in your support system?" People who have recently assumed a management position can be asked what they could do to make staff meetings as dull as possible. Once the laughter subsides, the group can often help members develop appropriate strategies.

In the article quoted at the beginning of this chapter, Bergman described some of the efforts he made, including returning to school, becoming a writer, taking up dancing, and traveling to Europe by himself. Paradoxically, one of the major actions that helped Bergman cope with the transition of being widowed was embarking on several other transitions. The support and encouragement he received from the group seemed to inspire these new directions.

Catharsis. Many people experiencing transitions have a lot to be angry, sad, or frightened about. Yet they may be reluctant to express their feelings to their family or friends for fear of further burdening them. Similarly, people experiencing some transitions may be reluctant to let work associates know of the situation, or their feelings about it, for fear they may be considered less valuable as an employee.

The movie *Philadelphia* captured the agony of an attorney with AIDS who feared telling his law firm of his disease. One woman, recently recovered from cancer surgery, had difficulty deciding what to tell potential employers about her health. She saw her recovery and desire to get on with her life as a reason she would be a conscientious and loyal employee, but feared employers might view her as emotionally unstable or an insurance risk. Groups provide a safe and supportive environment in which people can share such concerns, and achieve catharsis.

Group counselors must constantly make decisions about how to handle such sharing of concerns. Expressing concerns is cathartic up to a point. If the goal of the group, however, is to help people develop strategies for dealing with their transition, then counselors must be aware of when and how to redirect clients in the direction of action steps, to help them move from "Ain't it awful" to "What can I do?" How that is done may depend in part on the theoretical orientation of the counselor and on the type of group.

Existential factors. Acknowledging that the term is hard to define, Yalom related it to "the central features that make us human—that is purpose, responsibility, sentience, will, values, courage, spirit" (1985, p. 94). Such concepts may be helpful to adults in transition even when they are not discussed directly. For some people contemplating or experiencing difficult transitions, the realization of their own ultimate responsibility for their lives may be both reassuring and challenging.

Cautions About Group Counseling

Although group work can be extremely valuable, it is clearly not appropriate for everybody. Gazda (1985) noted that the same factors that make group counseling potent may also add risk. When several clients are present, the counselor has less control, and some clients may be ostracized or pressured by other members. Clients may also experience "sibling rivalry" and worry about breaches of confidentiality. Such concerns underline the importance of group counselors being well trained in group management as well as in counseling skills. These cautions also argue for a carefully thought-out selection and orientation process for group members.

As part of that process, Corey (1995) suggested that group leaders warn prospective members about particular risks. For example, "members should be made aware of the possibility that participating in a group (or any other therapeutic endeavor) may disrupt their lives" (p. 34). Corey noted that even changes that are constructive in the long run may create crisis and turmoil along the way.

Another major risk of group counseling is that confrontation may be misused. "Intrusive interventions, overly confrontive leader tactics, and pushing of members beyond their limits often produce negative outcomes" (Corey, 1995, p. 36). To reduce this risk, Corey recommended that leaders model effective and nonjudgmental behavioral feedback.

Gladding (1991) observed that research on the impact of group counseling is less sophisticated than evaluations of individual counseling. He summarized some of the methods that can be used to assess group members' progress on a variety of dimensions (1991, p. 336). Since groups are not the treatment of choice for all clients, we strongly urge practitioners to build evaluation procedures into their programs whenever possible.

Several authors have identified categories of people who may be inappropriate for groups. Brown (1988) suggested that people who are paranoid, obsessively self-centered, out of touch, suicidal, highly hostile, aggressive, or in crisis may not be good candidates for a group experience. When considering older adults, Burnside (1984) recommended excluding people who are disturbed and prone to wandering, incontinent, manic-depressive, psychotic, deaf, or hypochondriacal.

On a more practical level, we believe that groups are not the best method for people who are preoccupied with their own problems to the extent that they find it difficult to listen to others or to "take turns." An orientation session may provide an opportunity for the group counselor and each potential member to make an informed decision about the appropriateness of the group.

Types of Groups

Gazda (1989) identified three major types of group work— group guidance, group counseling, and group psychotherapy. In his schema, guidance groups are designed to be preventive and growth engendering, psychotherapy groups are seen as remedial; while counseling groups are both preventive and remedial. All three types can be helpful to people anticipating or experiencing transitions—if there is a good match between their needs and the content and process of the group. In addition, self-help groups, which are not part of Gazda's typology, can be extremely valuable.

Group guidance programs are generally offered in an educational format, where a major task of the leader is to disseminate information. In some guidance groups, members have an opportunity to personalize the information, so the experience moves toward group counseling. Group counseling is designed for individuals experiencing problems that information alone cannot solve. Usually, the topics covered in group counseling are developmental or situational in nature. Gazda includes T-groups, sensitivity groups, organizational development groups, encounter groups, and some structured groups in this category.

Group psychotherapy, on the other hand, is targeted toward people who have serious problems, often of long duration. As a major goal of such groups is remediation or personality change, they are generally not needed for adults in transition unless the transition brings to the surface much deeper issues.

A major need of adults in transition is often for training in social skills. Such training can be provided by all three types of groups, depending on the orientation of the group. For example, a stress-management program that focuses on explaining the sources of stress and giving information on stress-management techniques would be considered group guidance. A group that combines provision of information about stress with opportunities for group members to practice stress-management techniques with each other, and to give and get feedback, would be group counseling. If the goal of the group is to "uncover" reasons members experience various events as stressful and to attempt psychodynamic interventions, the group would be more therapeutic in nature.

Pearson (1992) also discussed the contribution of group counseling programs to increasing member coping resources, or what he calls effective self-enhancement. In his view, this comes from a combination of (a) consciousness-raising or awareness of a need for change, (b) strengthened commitment to take action, and (c) empowerment or development of knowledge or skills required for self-enhancement.

Remembering Cultural Diversity

Although Pearson's three objectives can be a guide for group counselors in many situations, it is important to realize they may not be effective for all counselees. Many potential clients come from less individualistically oriented cultures than the dominant one in this country. As indicated by Locke and Parker (1994), clients from different cultural backgrounds may also have different perceptions of themselves and different motivations.

In a provocative article on cross-cultural considerations in group counseling, Newlon and Arciniega (1992) challenged counselors to consider the cultural implications of traditional counselor approaches in working with members of minority groups. They noted, for example, that "Afro-American [sic] group members may come from situations in which they feel powerless, hostile, and lacking specific direction . . . Therefore, Afro-American members may want concrete responses from the group leaders much like they would receive from respected family members or friends" (p. 290).

Similarly, they stated that even though acculturated Hispanics may respond to traditional group counseling, "traditional immigrants, or first generation, are going to be more hesitant to accept participation in group approaches that rely on individual responsibility and abstract thinking. They will more likely respond to the group leader as an authority figure who will help interpret the system" (p. 291). They also asserted that Southeast Asians are more likely to want a leader who will "take an active, directive role and give them explicit directions on how to solve problems and bring immediate relief from disabling distress" (1992, p. 293).

A Taiwanese student expressed frustration, explaining that his advisor thought him unqualified to be a counselor because he always held back his personal feelings in group discussions. "He did not understand that we seldom 'confess' our 'personal stuff' to someone else" (Chin, 1993, p. 2). People with this kind of a background may have difficulty with many personal growth group experiences, and may benefit more from a highly structured group or from individual counseling.

Characteristics of Effective Groups

Robert Weiss did some of the earliest work conceptualizing the needs of people in transition and setting up groups to test his model. In a seminal article, Weiss (1976) suggested a useful system for classifying three different types of situational distress: crises, transition states, and deficit situations. He defined a crisis as a sudden, severely upsetting situation of short duration that requires individuals to mobilize their energies and resources. Examples might be a serious accident or the sudden onset of a major illness in the family. The crisis may end with a return to normal or with a changed situation. In the case of a serious illness, the individual may recover, become permanently disabled, or die. In either of the latter cases, surviving family members enter a transition state involving relational and personal changes.

The end of a transition state is usually marked by a new life organization and personal identity. If the new life situation is not satisfactory, then the individuals are in a deficit situation. For example, widowed persons with dependent children may find continuous difficulty in raising children as single parents.

In Weiss's view, people in each of the three states benefit from different forms of assistance. Individuals in crisis need both support and services to help them through the crisis; those in deficit situations need continuing, problem-focused support. Those in transition experience a void because their habitual patterns have been disrupted and they have not yet developed alternative ways of handling their lives. To help fill this void, people in transition need a cognitive framework that orders and explains their experiences and a temporary community of others in the same situation. Individuals in transition states are particularly likely to benefit from counseling as the decisions they make at this time may affect the rest of their lives.

Effective transition programs include three kinds of helpers:

(a) the expert who has studied the underlying issues connected with a particular transition;
(b) the veteran who has successfully negotiated a similar transition; and
(c) other group members who offer the immediate understanding that comes from being in the same boat.

In Weiss's view, each kind of helper can assist individuals in transition as they struggle to establish a new emotional equilibrium.

Weiss's research also speaks to the importance of designing groups to meet the needs of people experiencing different transitions. For example, he found significant differences in what worked for groups of separated and widowed people. Separated people found discussions of the nature of separation helpful while bereaved people found that discussions of the nature of grief evoked a great deal of pain. He also found that mixed-sex groups were valuable for separated people but not for widowed people. The separated people came to understand their former spouses better as a result of hearing from other men or women. Widowed persons had no need to understand things from their spouse's viewpoint.

Weiss's findings on the importance of tailoring subject matter to meet the needs of different groups have wide applicability. Let us look at two groups in transition: first semester graduate students and newly promoted supervisors. Both groups can benefit from "cognitive information" about their transition, as well as from the support of veterans and peers. Information about the transition *process* would help both groups, but members of each group would need information specific to their particular transition. A major job of the expert here is to identify underlying issues that are relevant for each group.

Weiss' model can apply to intrapersonal, interpersonal, and work-related groups. The following discussion begins with an examination of transitions that may bring clients to group counseling and then moves to a description of representative groups and sample activities.

GROUPS FOR PEOPLE FACING INTRAPERSONAL TRANSITIONS

Intrapersonal transitions are often triggered by existential questions such as "Who am I?" or "Where am I going?" Often these questions stem from non-events, realizations such as "I am not the person I expected to be," or "I took a long look at my life, and saw all the things that did not happen."

Intrapersonal Transitions that May Bring Clients to Groups

Decade birthdays or other marker moments may precipitate intrapersonal transitions as reflected in the following newspaper column headed, "At 40, at midday, a time for change":

> Coasting toward my 40th birthday . . . I was half-listening to National Public Radio when a man mentioned the birth of a baby—"a baby," he said,

"at the dawn of its day" . . . the voice inside my head said, "If a baby is at the dawn of its day, where at 40—am I?" The light is changing in my life. Although several hours of sunlight remain, and the evening holds it own allure, my morning is gone. High noon passed and I didn't even notice. (Ager, 1994)

Sometimes intrapersonal transitions are triggered by external events that leave individuals feeling very much alone. Such was the case of Gregory Bergman, whom we met at the beginning of this chapter, whose internal transition was triggered by his wife's sudden death.

For many adults, a major internal transition may be suddenly defining themselves as old or older. This redefinition may be triggered by seeing an "old" face in the mirror, by thinking that "I sound just like my mother when she was old!"; by receiving a letter stating that at 35 one is no longer part of the "junior congregation" at church, or by being offered a senior discount. Groups may provide a good opportunity for adults to discuss their feelings about their aging, to identify ways to seek support, and to consider strategies for garnering more control.

Illustrative Groups and Techniques for Intrapersonal Transitions

In the 1960s, prompted by the resurgence of the feminist movement, counseling centers around the country developed a variety of group counseling programs to help women—and sometimes men—explore, understand, and cope with issues of identity, autonomy, and life meaning. Under different rubrics, and with different approaches, many of these programs have continued. A sampling of personal-growth workshops, some carried over from earlier years, reflects the variety of groups.

Investigation into identity. The Continuum Center of Oakland University in Rochester, Michigan, originally designed a program to help women think about who they were, apart from their roles as wives and mothers, and how they could most effectively broaden their roles and their views of themselves. To encourage such exploration, the program provided opportunities for women to identify personal goals, analyze conflicting responsibilities, and develop strategies for improving communication skills with family, friends, and co-workers (Continuum Center, 1978). Similar programs, under different names, have continued into the 1990s, and now attract men as well as women.

This program, and others like it, combine provision of information by a professional counselor with opportunities for participants to personalize the information in small groups facilitated by a peer counselor. Given its combination of information, group support, and role modeling of peer counselors, the program taps into many of the curative factors identified by Yalom and Weiss.

At many sessions in this program, group leaders use structured exercises to stimulate discussion. For example, the counselor may explain Virginia Satir's (1972) models of poor communication giving examples of placating, blaming, overly logical, and irrelevant behaviors. Then participants consider which of the behaviors they are most likely to use when transitions have created stress in their lives. Group members also talk about and practice becoming more honest or, in Satir's terms, more "real."

The four S's in the transition model also provide a focus for counselors. Group members can define their particular transition, identify the resources and deficits they bring to it, and consider alternative ways to access support and develop new strategies. For example, Jack Williams, the man from Chapter 4 who is considering going into business for himself, might learn that his awareness of "time left" is understandable in terms of what we know about adult development. He would likely gain support from realizing that other group members are struggling with similar concerns, and he might become familiar with other ways to "be a man." Group leaders could help him identify the many areas in his life in which he had experienced success, urge him to consider how he had managed that, and encourage him to think of ways to utilize his skills in new arenas. He could also use the group to "rehearse" strategies he might employ when talking to his family about his concerns.

Hitting your stride, good news about women in midlife.

This group, based on the book of the same name (Cohen, Coburn, & Pearlman, 1980), is designed to help women reframe their views of middle age. Ager, whose article about her 40th birthday was cited earlier, might be a good candidate for this workshop. The following anecdote illustrates the potential of the group.

At one session, group members were asked to complete a series of questions including: (a) As a child I knew people were middle aged when _____; (b) I first started to think of myself as middle aged when _____; (c) I use my age as an excuse for _____; and (d) Middle age has expanded my opportunities to _____. Processing these questions helped group members identify concerns about aging and the extent to which some members had internalized age bias.

One 50-year-old strongly objected to the presence of a 35-year-old. After considerable exploration, the counselor and the group helped her realize that her objection seemed to be, "If someone 35 is middle aged, then I, at 50, must be approaching old age." And she was not ready to give herself such an identity. The discussion not only highlighted the extent of age bias present, but also provided an opportunity for counselors to use some reframing techniques.

Life mission: The essence of you. Cecilia Peters (personal communication, 1993) developed a workshop, based on the book by Stephan (1989), discussed in Chapter 6, that leads participants through an internal intuitive process to help them identify what they really want in life. The program examines ways to respond to a personal "calling" through a career, a pastime, a cause, or anything in between.

To help group members with self-exploration, counselors ask them to list, and discuss, 25 words or more that describe themselves, preferably not in relation to other people. They are also asked to list their fears, then to recast their statements in terms of how their life would be without those fears. In terms of the Transition Model, these are techniques counselors can use to help people learn more about their views of themselves and their situations and to begin to identify what is supportive to them. Throughout the workshop, a variety of visualizations and meditations are used, some of which can then be recast in terms of alternative strategies. In this group, spirituality is included as an important element as members explore the meaning—and mission—of their lives.

In the Life Mission workshop, the leader uses the group to encourage self-acceptance and acceptance of others, and sees group support as an essential ingredient of the program. In Yalom's terms, the workshop serves to instill hope and involves many of the other curative factors. Such a group may appeal to people who are "right-brained" in their approach to life, and may be helpful to people who need to deal with unresolved developmental task issues, such as achieving autonomy. The workshop is, therefore, an example of a psychotherapeutic group appropriate for people in transition.

Groups for persons with particular illnesses. Coping with a major illness is obviously a significant transition. Livneh and Sherwood-

Hawes (1993) discussed the value of group counseling for persons who have sustained heart attacks, and suggested cognitive, affective, and behavioral goals for participants. Cognitive goals include using information about cardiac impairment to realistically assess their strengths and limitations; affective goals focus on provision of support, relief of tension, and reduction of depression; and behavioral goals include development of skills to promote independent functioning, utilize appropriate exercise and relaxation techniques, and access interpersonal and community resources. They suggested that groups be conducted in an inpatient setting so that members can "practice strategies for coping with problems, and achieve a less complicated transition from the hospital or rehabilitation center into the external community" (1993, p. 57). The authors recommended groups that are educationally based and focus on coping skills rather than on development of insight alone.

A special challenge with this population is that persons who have sustained a heart attack may deny that they have heart disease or acknowledge the presence of the disease but deny its seriousness. "Three strategies that may be used to undermine the impact of denial are the raising of awareness, mild confrontation, and the inclusion of successfully coping veteran participants in group meetings" (p. 60). This recommendation fits well with those of Weiss.

Life review groups. Since Robert Butler first articulated the concept, life review groups have become increasingly popular as a counseling intervention with older adults (Capuzzi,Gross, & Friel, 1990; Moody, 1988; Waters, 1990). Although people of all ages periodically take stock of their lives, often at times of transition, this activity has special meaning in old age. At that time, the existential questions people ask themselves may also involve a look backwards, and become not just "Who am I?" but "Who have I been?" and "How did I do?" The answers to these questions may affect how people feel about themselves in terms of integrity vs. despair, the developmental task of old age identified by Erikson (1950). Having such discussions in a group underlines the value of the 11th curative factor identified by Yalom, existential factors.

Doing a life review can help older adults decide what to do with material and emotional legacies. Singer, Tracz, and Dworkin (1991) concluded that life review groups can encourage socialization, lead to a sense of self-worth and life satisfaction, and help alleviate loneliness, hopelessness, and depression. Sherman (1987) compared topic-focused reminiscence groups with those that added a focus on feelings and found that the latter had a more positive impact on the emotional quality of participants' lives. "Not only did they report that the present was enlivened by their memories, but for most there appeared to be a newer, more open, and accepting or integrative attitude toward the past" (1987 p. 572).

Counselors can trigger life reviews in many different ways, depending on the needs of particular clients and groups. For example, if group members need to activate supports in their lives, group counselors can ask them to think about various periods of their lives and to identify the people and activities that were most important to them at each stage. Counselors can then encourage participants to think about how their support system has changed over time and what they did to access support in the past. Several techniques for helping older adults learn from their past are described in Waters and Goodman (1990).

In guiding a life review, counselors can help group members gain a sense of pride from looking at the people they have influenced and the crises they have weathered. Such recollections may also serve as an excellent vehicle for encouraging people to identify past coping strategies and to consider how they can be adapted to fit new transitions. Many different groups have developed programs for stimulating life reviews. For example, AARP has a program entitled "Reminiscence: Finding Meaning in Memories" and offers a *Reminiscence Training Kit* (1989) for potential group leaders. Bi-Folkal Productions has developed a series of reminiscence packages to stimulate memory sharing. Packages, which include photographs, music, stories, and old household items to use as triggers, are available in many public libraries.

Although most life reviews involve talking, a variety of props—such as old magazines and newspapers, political buttons, greeting cards, or photographs—can be used to stimulate memories and discussions. People whose transitions involve a reduction in cognitive functioning may find such stimulation valuable. Music works particularly well in such cases. In many long-term care settings, older adults who have difficulty with conversations may be seen singing and dancing to songs from their past. This kind of success experience may help to strengthen the coping resources of people whose balance of assets to deficits is declining.

In discussing techniques for counseling people over 60, Stachow (1993) urged counselors to consider the extent to which clients are experiencing fears of, or actual, loss of control over mind, body, spirit, finances, environment, or relationships. In her view, a goal of counseling is to help people realize that change is possible and worth pursuing at any stage of life. To help older adults regain a sense of mastery, she recommended asking such questions as:

(a) How has your life changed recently?
(b) What do you think is happening to you?
(c) Have you ever felt this way before?
(d) How did you cope with it (or other difficulties) before?
(e) Why can't you do that now?
(f) What would you like to do about this situation?

Questions like these can be used in individual or group counseling. In a group situation, they might provide an excellent opportunity for group members to provide feedback to each other, to share resources, and to take advantage of many of the curative factors identified above. Such factors also operate in groups for people facing transitions in their family or with other close relationships.

GROUPS FOR PEOPLE FACING FAMILY/ RELATIONSHIP TRANSITIONS

When we think of groups for people in transition, those involving interpersonal relationships are often the first that come to mind. A glance at the community services section of many newspapers reveals a variety of groups for people moving into or out of relationships.

Common Transitions Bringing Clients to Groups

Relationship transitions may be triggered by one's own decisions or actions or by those of somebody else. Reflecting this difference, those in groups for divorced persons often somewhat ruefully identify themselves as a "dumper" or a "dumpee"; just as in couples groups, some may consider themselves to be the "dragger," others the "draggee." Whether a person is the instigator of a change or the reactor to it, drastic changes in the pattern of relationships are often the impetus for people to seek counseling.

A variety of transitions can bring to the surface recurring themes having to do with intimacy, belonging, and mattering. Adults worry about intimacy as they consider what kind of love relationships they want to establish, and wonder if they will ever meet an appropriate life partner or develop friends as close as the ones they left behind. If they are ending a relationship, a major fear may be of being alone the rest of their lives. Additionally, many people experience a lack of intimacy within an established relationship. Different groups are needed for each of these considerations. Thus we have groups for engaged couples; for widowed, separated or divorced persons; and for marriage enrichment. People who have moved and miss close friends may also want to find supportive groups in their new locale.

Questions of where we "belong" often surface after a transition. This can be particularly true of widowed or divorced people whose social life revolved around couple activities, but it is also true of parents who spent many hours in parent–teacher organizations and in volunteer work for their children's school. Do they still belong there after their children graduate?

Similarly, we know of one woman who developed a close relationship but was reluctant to marry because she didn't want to give up her leadership role in Parents Without Partners. That was the place she felt she most belonged. People whose identity, or sense of belonging, is tied to being, say, an officer in a union or a member of a city commission, may feel abandoned if their term ends, or worse yet, if they are not re-elected. Adults who have to leave a softball league or other team because of an injury may feel similarly bereft.

Immigrants from one country to another may experience serious emotional as well as geographic dislocation, clearly related to issues of belonging. Moving often takes people away from close friends and extended families. Hoffman's (1990) book, *Lost in Translation,* an account of trying to "belong" in a different language attests to this. Although not as dramatic a change, people who move from one part of the country to another, or from one neighborhood to another, may also experience feelings of marginality. Many people find it helpful to discuss issues such as these in personal growth groups like those described above, while others will profit more from specialized groups, some of which are described below.

The need for support is life-long, but an individual's existing support system can often be one of the "casualties" of a major life transition. Ironically, we may have most need of a support system as we are moving into or through a transition that may disrupt that very system. Frequently this is true in cases of a geographic move. The same problem may arise when a job change, retirement, or illness takes us away from co-workers who were close friends.

Illustrative Programs and Techniques

Because there are so many different types of group counseling programs for people dealing with changing relationships, the following descriptions provide only a limited sample.

Groups for couples and families. Couples groups may be targeted to engaged couples, married couples, or gay and lesbian partners. Some religious groups require that couples receive counseling, often from a member of the clergy, before they can be married in the church.

Books often can provide a focus for group discussion. For example, in her book, *You Just Don't Understand: Women and Men in Conversation,* Tannen (1990) described typical gender differences in communications patterns and approaches to problem solving. Couples reading this book can often laugh at the illustrations she gives, and in the process gain a better understanding of their own differences. Corey and Corey described a number of exercises they use in couples groups. For example, group members may be asked to complete sentences such as "The thing I'd most like to change in myself [or my spouse] is . . . " or "My greatest fear concerning our relationship is . . . " (1982, p. 266). The stimulus for couples to enroll in such groups may be events, such as one partner's thinking about or having an affair, or non-events, including a general feeling that the relationship could be better.

Similar concerns may bring gay and lesbian couples to counseling. According to House and Tyler (1992), gay and lesbian couples typically bring up issues such as differences in background, communication problems, jealousy, and concerns about health and finances, just as do people in heterosexual relationships. They add, "lesbian and gay couples, however, face other relationship problems related to their sexual orientation" (1992, p. 196). For example, they may differ as to whether or when to "come out" to family, friends, and work associates. Gay and lesbian couples have fewer role models than do heterosexual couples and may benefit greatly from knowing how other couples deal with their daily lives.

The authors suggested that "Because many of the issues facing gay and lesbian couples are related to being male or female in our society, same gender leaders are apt to be most appropriate for these groups . . . Gay couples tend to experience competition as a difficulty in relationships, whereas lesbian couples frequently have difficulty with fusion and separation" (1992, p. 196).

Sometimes family counseling is indicated because of concerns about an older member of the family. Gwyther (1986) noted that families who are dealing with a transition such as the illness of an older member may resist "therapy," but may be willing to come for a meeting or for interpretive information. She also observed that the focus in working with older families "is generally on coping, not on correcting long-standing maladaptive personality styles or relationships" (p. 42).

Lustbader and Hooyman (1994) suggested an interesting technique for delegating tasks at family meetings. Counselors ask each family member to make a "wish list" as to how they would like to see a particular situation handled. Counselors then instruct members to trade lists so they can identify areas of conflict and agreement and attempt to arrive at a distribution of tasks that seems fair to all.

Rituals and metaphors can be used in family counseling to help some families face transitions. Sand-Pringle, West, and Bubenzer (1991) described an innovative intervention using gardening activities to help a family allow a son to leave for a halfway house. He planted some seeds in the family planter to symbolize his continuing place there and took a separate planter with him to his temporary home. The mother, who needed to be empowered in the family, was cast as the master gardener.

In this case, the family was the group with many of Yalom's curative factors operating. The plants symbolized hope, the joint efforts led to some cohesiveness, and family members were able to express some of their pent-up feelings. In the typology of groups, this is an example of a psychotherapeutically oriented group.

Groups for separated and divorced people. Even though approximately 50% of marriages in this country now end in divorce (U.S. Department of Commerce, 1993), divorce continues to be among the most stressful of life's transitions. Whether a marriage is cut short by divorce or death, survivors must relearn skills of singlehood after they work through coping with grief and trauma. Groups can be particularly helpful to people in the process of working through that pain.

Many groups for divorced persons, such as the well-known Parents Without Partners, are self-help groups (to be discussed in Chapter 9). Others are led by professional counselors. In a review of the literature on groups for separated and divorced persons, Zimpfer (1990) talked of the importance of understanding stages in the divorce process in order to determine which kind of group work is most appropriate for particular individuals. Recently divorced and panicky people may benefit from short-term and crisis-based counseling, while people who have made some adjustment and are concerned with what to do with the rest of their lives may do better with long-term group work.

Most divorce groups described in the literature were structured, combining education and counseling. Halpern (1994, personal communication) used a structured activity, called an "obstacle checklist," which enumerates common problems. The list, which includes such issues as letting go of the former spouse, making new friends, forgiving the former spouse, sleeplessness, mood swings, and concerns over sexual involvement, helps the group focus on specific discussion topics and serves as a progress report for each person. Members use the list to record insights or ideas on how to handle each problem. Some of the checklist items apply to widowed persons, as well as divorced persons but the groups are seldom mixed. Widowed persons, who are working on not deifying their late spouses, may find it much too difficult to listen to people who are vilifying their "exes."

Groups for widowed persons. In a chapter on groups for people experiencing major losses, Vernon stated, "Although the bereavement process involves common feelings and stages, group members get the most benefit from a group that addresses their specific kind of loss" (1992, p. 269.) Being widowed, for instance, arouses innumerable feelings, some of which are difficult to discuss with family and friends. For example, a widow who is left with limited resources and seemingly unlimited responsibilities may be angry with her spouse for dying and guilty or depressed about her anger. It may be easier for her to discuss these feelings with other people in the same situation rather than with her children who are grieving themselves.

The opportunity to express such feelings, and hopefully gain some catharsis, is an important aspect of groups for the bereaved. On a more tangible level, members can also exchange ideas on ways to handle various aspects of their lives, from finances to sexuality.

Vernon described the flow and sequence of one structured group. During the first three sessions, members focus on the past. They tell their stories of losing their partners, discuss loneliness and aloneness, and consider the areas in their lives in which they feel most deprived. The counselor can stimulate such discussions by asking members to bring in photographs or by asking questions about what people miss most and least about their mates. By the fourth session, counselors can encourage members to discuss the new things they are learning to do and areas in which they may now be experiencing growth.

About halfway through the workshop, group members begin to address pragmatic changes. "By this stage, group cohesiveness will probably allow participants to share information and advice on new roles and responsibilities such as finances, child care, household responsibilities, settling an estate, or disposing of personal effects" (1992, p. 272). As the group moves to a discussion of the future, the counselor can encourage members to talk about how their lives might be in six months or a year. Counselors can ask members about where they might be living, how and with whom they might be spending their time, and what kind of feelings they might be experiencing. As the group terminates, members need an opportunity to express appreciations and regrets and to say their good byes. They also need a chance to discuss strategies they can use to continue to get the support provided by the group.

Counselors can use reframing techniques to help clients move from despair to hope. A widowed teacher who talked about missing her husband and the activities they enjoyed together was encouraged to begin appreciating the freedom she now has to write books, travel with friends, and adhere to her own schedule. Another widow was feeling resentful and overwhelmed at having to take over her husband's business until a group helped her redefine this as a challenge and an opportunity to apply some of her communication and administrative skills in a different arena.

As mentioned, AARP is a major resource for those interested in establishing groups for widowed persons. Based on the work of Silverman (1980, 1986) and her associates at Harvard University, AARP established the Widowed Persons Service (WPS). In 1989 WPS sponsored over 200 programs in the United States. A trained group leader, herself a widow, reaches out on a one-to-one basis to new widows before they attend their first group session.

AARP launched a special program for widowed Chinese in Phoenix, Arizona, staffed by bilingual volunteers. As reported in the Newsletter for AARP Volunteers, "Normally, the grieving process is very private to the Chinese . . . But Maggie Eng, director of the Chinese Senior Center, saw needs in the members who had left their native country and no longer could rely on large extended families for support at the time of their loss" ("Widowers overcome," 1991, p. 1). Volunteers, who translated into four dialects, provided instrumental help with social security and housing arrangements, and also encouraged widowed persons to begin socializing again.

Groups for caregivers. As people live longer, more older adults need caregiving from spouses, adult children, friends, and/or paid caregivers. The mix of love and frustration that often accompanies having major responsibility for a parent or other older adult is well documented. Fortunately, the need for help is becoming more widely recognized, and groups for caregivers are springing up at hospitals, nursing homes, senior centers, family service agencies, religious organizations, libraries, and community centers.

Counselors who work with caregivers need to be familiar with a variety of community resources, which can serve as formal supports. Counselors also need to understand the feelings of caregivers, who may be emotionally drained and physically exhausted—sometimes by family conflicts as well as by their caregiving responsibilities—and yet are often reluctant to use available external resources. In dealing with people suffering from severely disabling illnesses, particularly dementia, caregivers may find that "the mourning process may be even more debilitating when the lost loved one is still alive" (Dobson & Dobson, 1991, p. 188).

Family members of persons with Alzheimer's disease may need to be separated into groups based on the stage of the individual's disease. In the early stages, family members may be into denial and reluctant to associate with other group members because such an association may lead them to lose hope.

In the early stages of the disease, the patients themselves may benefit from groups if they are able to understand what is happening to them and can express themselves. Typical topics might include: feelings of being abandoned by friends, concern that family members don't really understand that their impairments are due to illness, and an awareness of the stigma of their illness. Co-therapists are recommended for patient groups, both for therapeutic purposes and to deal with such situations as a wandering member.

Johnson (1990) developed a useful concept that helps caregivers understand the difference between giving up and letting go. It is a graphic presentation of the Serenity Prayer used in many 12-step programs:

> God grant me the serenity to accept
> the things I cannot change, the
> courage to change the things I can,
> and the wisdom to know the difference.

	(1) Can Be Controlled	(2) Cannot be Controlled
A) TAKE ACTION	MASTERY	CEASELESS STRIVING
B) DO NOT TAKE ACTION	GIVING-UP	LETTING-GO

FIGURE 8.1 Achieving mastery: the action/decision model. (*Source:* Richard P. Johnson, PhD, "Back to the Basics." *Co-op Networker: Caregivers of Older Persons, 6* (1), © 1990, Mercy Family Practice Center, St. John's Mercy Medical Center, St. Louis, Mo. Used with permission.)

Using the graphic form (Figure 8.1), group members are asked to distinguish between situations that can be controlled and those that cannot be. In all situations, they have to decide whether or not to take action. If the decision is one that can be controlled and they take action, they are achieving mastery; if they do not they are giving up. For example, if an older person wishes to stay in his or her home, and assessment indicates that this is possible with appropriate support, then the caregiver is achieving mastery if she or he arranges for adult day care and appropriate home care.

On the other hand, there are decisions that cannot be controlled. For example, if a parent, whom the adult child thinks is depressed, absolutely refuses to consider counseling, then the daughter who continues to bring up the issue is engaged in ceaseless striving, or "banging her head against a wall." With assistance from the counselor, group members can often help each other make appropriate decisions and "let go" without guilt.

GROUPS FOR PEOPLE FACING CAREER-RELATED TRANSITIONS

Counselors hear about many different work-related transitions—looking for jobs, changing jobs, being promoted or laid off, not securing a desired job, or retiring. In most such situations, clients may have to "let go" of dreams or expectations or establish new goals. As they do this, the line between career transitions and other parts of an individual's life often blurs.

Transitions that May Bring Clients to a Career-Related Group

As we have seen, transitions are sometimes internally triggered, stemming from a person's desire to initiate a change. At other times, a transition may be thrust upon the individual. The context in which transitions arise affects the type of group experience which is most helpful. For example, counselors working with people who are angry about being laid off or forced to take an early retirement must attend to the anger before they can expect group members to begin career planning or a job search in earnest.

Several studies (e.g., Amundson & Borgen, 1988; Kivlighan, Johnsen, & Fretz, 1987; Mawson & Kahn, 1993) attest to the value of group procedures in career counseling. In evaluating various kinds of group interventions, Spokane (1991) gave a more cautious assessment. He reported that re-analysis of several studies suggests that group interventions of six to seven sessions are about as effective as individual interventions of one or two sessions. Therefore, program planners may need to carefully consider whether groups are truly cost-effective.

Counselors must also consider the match between individuals and the type of group. According to Spokane:

> It now seems that nonsocial, shy, or withdrawn individuals will not fare well in group interventions. In those cases, care must be taken to supplement group with individual counseling or to screen members for appropriateness before the group begins . . . pre-counseling expectations may affect the client's preference for and progress in group versus individual treatment. (1991, p. 153)

Spokane expressed concern over the high incidence of dropouts from career programs and suggested that counselors address issues of low self-esteem, which seem to contribute to the drop-out phenomenon.

Client reactions to a career program may change over time. At the conclusion of a two-day workshop, adult women clients reported that the affective aspects of the group experience, particularly measures of Yalom's therapeutic factors of universality, catharsis, and cohesiveness, were most important. In a follow-up study two months later, participants still valued the affective aspects of the workshop, but reported that cognitive factors, such as information on resources and occupations, and on self-understanding, were the most tangible benefits of the group (Mawson & Kahn, 1993).

Career counselors can enhance the impact of group processes "by sequencing activities, choosing exercises, and structuring client participation to ensure the appropriate balance of attention to task (cognitive factors) and members' feelings (affective factors)" (p. 245). Readers are encouraged to keep that balance in mind as they consider situations that might bring their adult clients to career groups.

Career-related changes, whether made by choice or necessity, are apt to raise concerns about mastery, competency, balance, and identity. These recurring themes can be addressed through groups that combine providing career-related information with opportunities for group support. Peer counselors can also serve as supportive "veterans," an important element recommended by Weiss (1976). Several union/management-sponsored groups use this approach. Former union workers, who have already made a transition to retirement or other employment, facilitate small groups.

At times of career transition, the need for support can become enormous. Adults making career transitions frequently need an opportunity to talk to others who are "in the same boat" or further along in the process. They need friends who know what they can do, who can provide appreciation and encouragement. They also need information, door openers (people willing to make contacts for them), people with whom to have fun, shoulders to cry on, and practical help that might include lending money, providing transportation, or babysitting.

As many people struggling with career decisions or trying to find a new job are reluctant to ask friends and co-workers for assistance, their usual sources of support may be cut off. Therefore, the support of members of a career counseling group may be particularly important and may serve as a model encouraging people to seek support from others.

Many of the coping strategies necessary for success in career deci-sion-making, job search, job retention, and retirement planning can be taught and practiced in groups. For example, members can learn to set goals and develop action plans for achieving them. Groups can be par-ticularly valuable in encouraging compliance with the action plan. Mem-bers who might procrastinate on commitments made to themselves will be less likely to do so when they have made a promise to other group members.

Being able to identify and talk about one's values, skills, interests, and accomplishments constitutes important strategies in planning a ca-reer and searching for a job. The modeling and role playing opportu-nities in a group make group counseling a valuable modality for honing these strategies. Similarly, networking is a key strategy needed by job seekers. The process can begin in a group, where members frequently suggest contacts to each other.

Shared experiences make it easier to laugh at otherwise difficult situations, and humor can be a valuable strategy to make looking for, retaining, or leaving a job easier. For example, in both job search and post-retirement planning workshops, people who need time to pursue their paid or unpaid job search can laugh together over the "honey, do" lists developed by partners who think the unemployed individual now has limitless time to perform chores. Many of these strategies are taught in the sample programs described below.

Illustrative Career-Related Programs and Techniques

Career counseling groups for adults in transition are offered through schools and universities, at the workplace, and in community settings. Examples of programs in various settings are discussed below.

Career planning programs. Zunker suggested a model for de-veloping career-counseling programs for adults in transition that includes such strategies as identification of experience, interests, and skills; clari-fication of values and needs; planning for education, training, or occu-pations; and movement toward a plan for life learning (1994, pp. 326–328). He then suggested techniques and specific tasks for each strategy.

For example, he recommended using interviews and autobiogra-phies to help adults identify their experiences. Specific tasks include such items as: "identify and evaluate previous work experience . . . assess familial relationships . . . identify reasons for job change . . . identify ca-reer satisfaction variables" (1994, p. 326). According to Zunker, such specific tasks are important because adults in transition often overlook skills they have developed in other contexts. His model included techniques for teaching decision-making skills, a central part of many career counseling programs.

Another group approach uses quilts as a metaphor "to more effectively see and portray events and meanings in women's lives and work . . . quilts and quilting offer a new way of thinking about careers that overcomes the weaknesses of devaluing women's experiences and splintering their lives" (Sagaria, 1989, p. 13). Counselors ask group members to describe their quilts and give each other feedback based on such questions as "How is this quilt like Susan?" or "How does what Susan told us about her quilt fit with what she has told us about her career goals?" The quilts reflect the importance of relationships and serve as a vehicle for helping group members recognize their commonalities.

Another useful technique, storytelling, "serves a powerful function in career counseling, because storytelling enlightens the narrator and the audience" (Jepsen, 1992, p. 3). The stories, complete with what Jepsen called the "trouble" or the drama that keeps our attention on a story, provides an interesting way to discuss career decisions and career problems. "The audience (counselors, peers, group members) helps shape several aspects of the story . . . the special skills of a counselor are critical to a full telling of a career story" (1992, p. 7).

Some career planning groups are targeted at people facing particular transitions. One program designed for displaced homemakers, offered by the Jewish Vocational Service (JVS) of Detroit, is publicized with an attractive brochure entitled "When It's Time to Start Over." Inside the brochure, the description explains the value of the group in a simple manner. "First there's support . . . then there's hope . . . then there's work." This program adds job club services and monthly women's network meetings to the usual career-planning topics.

A more specialized JVS service, designed to assist Russian refugees, includes assessment of work-related English and explanations of the American work culture, along with sessions on job search techniques. Many of the immigrants have difficulty understanding that in this country people compete for jobs and need to sell themselves. In the former Soviet Union, they were assigned to jobs. According to the director of the program, "The concepts of productivity and efficiency are totally foreign" (Moxley, Personal communication, 1994). At the same time, women immigrants may find it hard to understand that in this country there is no subsidized day care or standard paid maternity leave.

The information, support, and modeling aspects of a group can be helpful in both pre-retirement and post-retirement planning. Some of the issues brought up by pre-retirees and post-retirees are the same, others are different. Our experience has been that in working with people before retirement, it is essential to start with the financial aspects of the transition. Until people know how much money they will have and what their benefits will be, they are not ready to discuss changes in their relationships or how they will spend their time. Such concerns are absolutely crucial to the successful navigation of this major transition, and comprehensive group programs are available. AARP offers a variety of publications and workshops—some for people in general, others especially designed for women or single persons (AARP 1991, 1993b, 1990). A computer-based program, Discover for Retirement Planning (American College Testing Program, 1990), is based on the transition model. Each section of the program offers users an opportunity to take stock of their resources and to develop plans based on their assessment.

People who come to post-retirement groups may already have a good handle on the financial aspects of their situation, and be more concerned about what they are going to do with the rest of their lives. The "honeymoon phase of retirement" identified by Atchley (1983) may be over. Post-retirees may have completed the necessary household repairs, put the family pictures in albums, and begun getting under a spouse's skin. The "need for space," which some 30-year-olds with commitment phobia talk about, may resurface in retirement. Partners may need help in negotiating the amount of time they spend together and apart. A panel of retirees who are living very different lifestyles may add some inspiration and information to both pre- and post-retirement groups.

Counselors face special challenges when leading groups of people with physical disabilities who want to return to work or cope more successfully with their work situation. A combination of information about the disability and support designed to restore damaged feelings of competence and self-esteem seems to be essential. In addition, special skills may be needed for particular disabilities. For example, silence in a group is likely to be very upsetting to blind participants, so the counselor may need to explain what is going on when one member is thinking. Clients with a hearing impairment are likely to become passive, so assertive skills may be an important component of their career planning groups (Livneh & Pullo (1992). When working with people with physical disablities or from different cultures, it is important for counselors to listen carefully for the values and assumptions of the individuals.

Job search groups. Many adults in transition already know what they want to do or "be," but need help in putting their plans into action. Typically groups for job seekers teach participants how to identify their strengths and abilities, analyze an employer's needs, and attempt to identify a fit. Goodman and Hoppin (1990) developed one widely used, competency-based program that included useful strategies for self-assessment, decision-making, planning a job-search campaign, communicating with employers, interviewing, retaining the job, and preparing for the next one.

Losing a job and having to look for another one can be particularly traumatic for older workers. Barclay and McDougall (1990) put it this way: "If who we are is what we do, what happens to our identity when we don't do that anymore? Such is the dilemma of the growing number of participants in older worker programs: dislocated workers, displaced homemakers, terminated employees, or even recipients of 'voluntary' early retirement" (p. 53). The authors described the services of Operation Able, a national network of organizations that promote the interests of older workers. One of their workshops, the ABLE Institute, is a seminar on job-search techniques. In it "participants learn about the hidden job market and how to gain access to it, develop 'age-proof' resumes, practice positive approaches to interviewing, and discuss the transition back into the work force" (p. 54). The support that older job seekers give each other is of particular importance to the success of this workshop, as it is for all the groups we have described.

USING THE 4 S MODEL WITH GROUPS

When working with groups, as well as with individuals, counselors can integrate the Cormier-Hackney counseling model with the transition model. This integrated model, shown in Figure 7.1 (p. 175), fits well with the four stages of group development—exploratory, transition, action, and termination—identified by Gazda (1989).

During the exploratory stage, counselors help members get acquainted and begin to assess their problems and needs in view of their life changes. In the transition stage, they set goals and begin to move to action. In the action stage of groups, counselors intervene to help members develop new coping strategies. Whether working with individuals or groups, counselors should view the termination stage as the appropriate time to assist clients in evaluating their progress and making a commitment to follow-up.

In almost any groups designed for people considering, anticipating, or experiencing a transition, the first step is to encourage them to describe their transitions. What happened or may happen? The major job of counselors after that is to encourage group members to assess and improve their resources for coping in each of the four areas of the Transition Model.

Although we talk about the 4 S's separately in the following discussion, it is important to remember that the lines among them blur. In some ways, the situation of any individual includes aspects of the other three S's. Each individual's personal environment is unique. Thus, four women in the same returning learners' group may have very different resources in terms of socioeconomic situation, support systems—friends, extended family, work colleagues, spiritual resources—and coping strategies. An effective group can help each member identify and enhance his/her unique available resources.

For example, a woman who has lost her job and is feeling helpless in terms of finding another may get useful feedback from other group members who help her realize how successfully she has weathered other transitions. The group may also help her see her network of supportive friends and her ability to take care of herself as assets in her present situation. A group can help one woman who is financially able to be unemployed for a short time see this as an asset in that it enables her to be more selective about other jobs. At the same time, the group may be able to persuade another woman, whose financial situation is tenuous, that it is appropriate to accept government assistance to tide her over.

The Situation

In groups, members can explain how, from their point of view, the context in which they operate affects the impact of the transition. They can also discuss the extent to which the transition alters their life style, what we have earlier called their roles, relationships, routines, and assumptions. As the other group members offer feedback, each of the group members can realize that although they may all be experiencing a similar transition, their individual situations differ.

The Self

Under a skilled leader, a group may be particularly valuable in helping members assess Self factors. For example, individuals concerned that they do not have the psychological resources to cope with major losses may be reassured to learn from other members that their degree of turmoil is normal. They may also profit from hearing ideas as to how people experiencing similar transitions gained some measure of control over their lives.

Many transitions, particularly those involving role losses, lead to a drop in self-esteem. People who feel they are no longer needed can benefit just by having group members glad to see them each week. When members share resources, their ability to contribute to someone else may positively affect their view of themselves.

One activity, which is part of a job-seeking workshop developed by Goodman and Hoppin (1990), illustrates the value of group feedback. To demonstrate the concept of transferable skills, the leader asks one member to come to the front of the room and write the title of a recent job on a simulated theater marquee. The marquee has the words "Star of the Roxy" at the top. The "Star" explains the job and, with the help of other group members, lists as many skills as possible involved in that job. Then the group discusses ways in which the skills and personal characteristics of the group member can be transferred to other jobs and settings. Frequently "stars" leave with a more positive view of their skills and abilities, and a more optimistic outlook about finding another position. This activity also helps members prepare for their job search, with positively identified skills they may have taken for granted.

Group counselors can maximize the effectiveness of feedback by encouraging interaction and humor. For example, to enliven the discussion of transferable skills, the counselor can tell the story of a man who, with no background in the field, got a job in labor relations. He convinced his employer that as a former basketball referee he knew how to make quick decisions and take the heat!

Support

By their very nature, well-functioning groups provide support. In addition, they can encourage members to explore and enhance their individual support systems. Regardless of the type of transition, clients need to consider who or what has been supportive for them in the past, and how they have accessed that support.

Pearson (1990) developed a model for using social support-oriented concepts and procedures in counseling practice. The first step is to identify the strengths and deficiencies in an individual's support system. If this assessment indicates that client-based barriers, such as withdrawal, ineptness, or alienation, are the major causes of the problem, then the task of the counselor is to help the client make some changes. Depending on the theoretical orientation of the counselor, client-based interventions might focus on restructuring attitudes or changing behaviors through modeling and communications skill training. Opportunities to practice new skills in a group can be particularly valuable.

If initial assessment suggests that the barriers lie more with other individuals or the larger social context in which the person operates, then interventions must focus outside the individual. These can range from counselor contacts with the client's network to political advocacy.

Using Pearson's model, a useful group activity for the assessment stage is to have people evaluate their own support systems. The idea of a support system can be explained to most clients in words like, "people who are there for you" or "in your corner." To facilitate self-evaluation, counselors can use a worksheet listing such needs as acceptance, self-esteem, peers, guidance, and role models. Next to each need is a brief description of the type of support provided. For example, to meet our need for acceptance we need people who like us, to meet our need for peers, we need people who *are* like us. In a blank column on the worksheet, clients fill in the name of the person or group who supplies that type of support to them. (Waters & Samson, 1993; see also the surveys in the appendix of Pearson, 1990).

Another approach is to use a version of the convoy worksheet, (Figure 3.2, p. 71), based on the work of Kahn and Antonucci (1980). Group members can fill out this sheet, entering the names of their personal supports in the appropriate concentric circle. These kinds of assessments help group members to identify the strengths and "holes" in their system. Once the resources and deficits have been identified, group members can help each other develop strategies for shoring up those deficits stemming from internally created barriers. Strategies may include ideas on how to meet new people, investigate community resources, or learn to ask for help.

Asking for help is difficult for many people. "Knowing how to take care of yourself is a sign of adulthood" we say to ourselves, or "If he loved me he'd know what I need." Explaining the concept of cosmic accounting, mentioned in an earlier chapter, may help group members be a little more willing to ask for help. The term "cosmic accounting," developed by Uhle (personal communication, 1988), refers to the tendency of people to keep mental records of what they give and receive. Many of us have in our heads an accounting system that deals with simple exchanges such as who owes whom a dinner invitation or a favor. Cosmic accounting represents a more complicated exchange in that people may "pay back" somebody else, rather than the person who helped them. An example may bring the concept to life.

Three women, dressed in business suits, were on their way to a conference in a new car that blew a tire. As it was such a new car, not even the owner knew where the jack was. The three were standing forlornly by the side of the road, trying to figure out what to do, when a passing motorcyclist stopped. He not only changed the tire, but also gave the women instructions on how to change it themselves in the future. When he finished, the owner asked if she could pay. "Oh no," he said, "just promise me that the next time you see someone who needs help you'll stop." The notion of "passing a favor along" is a key element of cosmic accounting. Stories like that one often make it easier for group members to understand the concept and may trigger a realization that they already have a number of "credits" in their cosmic account on which they can draw.

To return to Pearson's (1990) model, if the problem with the support system seems to lie outside of the control of the individual, then the counselor can help group members work in a larger context. Sometimes this involves linking informal supports with formal ones. This may be particularly important with some of the caregiver groups discussed above. In other situations, working in a larger context may mean that clients and/or the counselor move to advocacy.

Strategies

Throughout this book we have mentioned three types of strategies for coping with a transition—those aimed at modifying the situation, those designed to change the meaning of the situation, and those serving to help individuals manage the stress of change. Groups can help in all three areas.

Coping effectiveness training. Folkman and her associates developed a pilot program of Coping Effectiveness Training for groups of 8 to 10 people infected with the Human Immunodeficiency Virus, commonly called HIV. The program is based on "cognitive-behavioral principles to improve people's skills in appraising, coping, and obtaining social support in stressful situations" (Folkman et al., 1991, p. 250).

The first step, appraisal training, teaches people to break down global stressors into specific problems. The global stressor of being infected with HIV is overwhelming. It may be more manageable to think about such specifics as not having enough energy to work a full day, having to tell close friends and relatives that one has HIV, or the demands of a treatment schedule. Each of these stressful contexts can be narrowed further to specific stressful situations. For example, "not having enough energy . . . to put in a full workday might be narrowed to the specific incident of requesting a transfer to a less taxing job" (p. 252). The task of the counselor is to help participants be as specific as possible about their stressors so they can establish goals for coping with them.

The next step is training people to expand their repertoire of coping skills. Based on the Lazarus Folkman typology, group leaders teach the difference between problem-focused and emotion-focused coping. The former tend to be more useful with situations that are amenable to change, the latter with situations that cannot change. In problem-focused coping, participants are taught how to apply decision-making skills to manage problem situations more effectively. Emotion-focused training is designed to reduce distress through application of cognitive and behavioral strategies. Examples of cognitive strategies would be selective attention, reframing, humor, and the use of spiritual or religious resources. Behavioral strategies include exercise, relaxation, and engaging in activities the person finds pleasurable.

Another component, social support training, helps people identify the kinds of support they need and develop strategies to obtain and maintain the support. These skills are taught in three parts, which the program developers call "Choosing it," "Obtaining it," and "Keeping it."

In designing the program, Folkman and her associates included brief didactic lectures, modeling by the group leaders, and opportunities for participants to practice skills. They also developed a workbook that summarized key points of each session and presented homework exercises. "To keep the workbook from being too serious, material . . . tends to be humorous, and cartoons are used throughout. The humor may be more effective if it is tailored to issues that are relevant to the group, as we did with the workbook we developed for use with gay men" (p. 251).

Comparisons of treatment and control groups indicated that treatment groups improved in terms of coping skills, particularly a reduction in self-blame. After six weeks, the treatment group exhibited less depression and more positive morale than the control group. While their model was piloted with persons with HIV, the authors expressed a belief that it "holds a promise as a brief intervention to help people in diverse settings manage the stressful demands of daily living" (p. 257).

Other stress management programs. Stress management programs are of particular importance to adults in transition because stress is often associated with change. In groups, clients can share both their sources of stress and their stress relievers. Such sharing can help members better understand why they may be feeling stress, as well as broaden their ideas about what might help relieve it.

Counselors can help group members realize the tremendous variability in terms of what is stress producing and what is stress reducing. This very difference often constitutes a source of stress in families and among friends. If one person's stress reducer—be it big parties, skiing, or political discussions—is a stress producer for his/her partner, negotiations are clearly needed. The group counselor can help members develop their negotiating strategies.

Group counselors can also introduce exercises, such as those suggested by Tubesing and Tubesing (undated) to help members develop more stress management techniques. Stress Bingo is one that works well in groups. Bingo-like cards are made up with a variety of possible stress relievers—such as listening to music, taking a hot bath, walking in the woods, reading a novel, or calling an old friend—printed in the boxes on the cards. Group members are instructed to talk with each other and to ask others to put their initials in the boxes that contain relievers they actually use. In addition to getting their cards filled up with signatures, group members are able to get ideas on how various people use the stress relievers. Typically, Stress Bingo leads to much laughter, which is itself a tension reliever, as well as to a productive exchange of ideas.

Assertiveness training. Like coping effectiveness training and stress management, assertiveness training focuses on skill development. Assertiveness training workshops are designed to help participants modify their behavior and develop new communication patterns or strategies. They can be useful for adults of all ages who are experiencing or anticipating changes. They can help to change the situation, change the reaction to it, or modify stress.

Many assertiveness programs are based on Lange and Jakubowski's (1976) now classic book. The authors stated:

> Assertion training incorporates four basic procedures: (1) teaching people the differences between assertion and aggression, nonassertion and politeness; (2) helping people identify and accept their own personal rights as well as the rights of others; (3) reducing existing cognitive and affective obstacles to acting assertively; and (4) developing assertive skills through active practice methods. (p. 5).

When such training is done in a group, people who tend to be passive or aggressive can see for themselves—and get feedback on—the effect their behavior has on other group members. Individuals can also practice assertive communication with a variety of people in the group. In terms of Yalom's curative factors, assertiveness training helps people develop improved socializing techniques, benefit from imitative behavior, and achieve some interpersonal learning.

Lang and Jakubowski's (1976) book includes many suggested exercises for use in women's groups, men's groups, and mixed sex groups. Women's groups may be designed to help women accept and use their personal power while men's groups may help men accept their vulnerability, listen more effectively, and express affection. Moore and Haverkamp's (1989) research suggested that structured group interventions can indeed help men become more emotionally expressive.

Assertiveness training is often helpful with older adults. One such program entitled, *Growing Older Bolder,* (Waters, McCarroll, & Penman, 1987) combines consciousness-raising activities with structured exercises. Participants are taught to make "I" statements and encouraged to practice giving and receiving compliments. To enhance the impact of group support, group leaders urge participants to take a mental picture of members exchanging compliments. They can recall this image, which is a group version of the positive asset search, when they need support as they confront present and future transitions.

SUMMARY

In this chapter, we have discussed the value and limitations of groups for adults in transition, described a number of group counseling workshops and specific techniques, and talked about how to use the Transition Model in group settings. In groups, clients have opportunities to hear about a variety of sources of support and coping strategies used by others. When we ask adults what has helped them survive, we most often hear about a sense of humor, support from special people, and faith. All our discussions underlined the importance of group support, the idea with which we began this chapter. We hope that the explanation of specific programs and techniques will give you ideas you can use in your settings, and we also hope you will consider advocacy and other ways you can help your clients. They are discussed in Chapter 9.

9

Consultation, Program Development, And Advocacy

When we hear the word *counseling,* most of us envision a professionally trained helper working face-to-face with one or more people considered clients. Indeed, individual and group counseling is what we are trained to do and what most of us like to do. But it is not the whole story. Increasingly, counselors are being called upon to act in other ways to assist adults in transition.

Some counselors now work in the corporate world, and others are community organizers; some counselors design programs in colleges and universities, while others develop workshops for senior centers; some walk the halls of legislatures as lobbyists, while still others talk about preventive mental health on talk shows. For some counselors, these broadened roles represent an exciting challenge, for others they are an intrusion or a necessary evil.

As part of their training, counselors are taught to be supportive, encouraging, and accepting. In contrast, advocacy and legislative efforts may involve controversy and adversarial relations. A random sampling of mental health counselors expressed limited interest in learning how to lobby more effectively or provide psychoeducational services to clients (Wilcoxon & Puleo, 1992), probably because such activities take counselors out of their comfort zone.

No longer can counselors be merely good listeners. As consultants, trainers, advocates, and program developers, counselors have opportunities to make organizations and systems more responsive to the needs of adults. If clients are to look for available supports in the community, those supports must be there. And counselors can play a role in putting them in place. In some cases counselors' efforts can help create structures that favorably tip the ratio of resources to deficits for adults in transition.

It is our opinion that although counselors should not impose their own values on their clients, counselors should act on their values to bring about needed societal changes. In this chapter, we talk about a variety of ways counselors can do this, including working with self-help groups, consulting, developing programs, and advocacy.

WORKING WITH SELF-HELP GROUPS

The last half of the 20th century has been described as the era of the self-help or mutual-aid group (Harvard Mental Health Letter, March, 1993). This report estimates that in the United States at least 6 million people participate each year, and that 12 to 15 million Americans participate at some time during their lifetime.

> Members of these groups are people with a symptom, disorder, situation, or experience in common who unite to fulfill a need, overcome a handicap, or cope with a crisis . . . The main purposes of self-help groups are mutual solace, education, and personal change. By talking to others with similar problems, members heighten their own understanding. They see how their actions affect others and how others cope with troubles similar to their own. (p. 1)

Some observers and researchers (e.g., Lieberman, 1990), distinguish between self-help groups, support groups, and other mutual-aid groups. However, in this chapter we are treating as self-help groups all those that generally fit the description given in the Harvard Mental Health Newsletter. Most self-help groups are designed for people experiencing or anticipating a variety of transition events or non-events. The groups can be extremely helpful to people who need support as they look at themselves in their changed roles, analyze their situations, and look for new strategies to help them navigate the transition.

There is general agreement among researchers that self-help groups are becoming ubiquitous, at least with certain segments of the population, but estimates of the number of people involved differ. Combining data from three surveys, Lieberman and Snowden (1993) estimated that 7.5 million adults participated in a self-help group during

1992. They stated, however, that the use of such groups for mental health problems is a predominantly white, middle-class phenomenon.

Using a very broad definition of support groups, Wuthnow said that "4 out of 10 Americans belong to a small group that meets regularly and provides caring and support for its members" (1994, p. 4). The title of Wuthnow's book, *Sharing the Journey: Support Groups and America's New Quest for Community*, articulates his basic belief that such groups represent a major trend in American society. He wrote: "For as long as most Americans can remember, our society has been described to us as being composed of individualists . . . But the standard wisdom now needs to be challenged. Bible studies, prayer fellowships, self-help groups, twelve-step gatherings, therapy sessions, recovery groups—all have been gaining increasing importance in recent years, as both sources of emotional support and settings in which millions of Americans are seeking spirituality" (p. ix).

Advantages and Limitations of Self-Help Groups

Among the special strengths that Wax attributed to self-help groups, he singled out their ability to "transform adversity into bonding . . . [and] stigma into honor. Members learn to stand up and say, 'I am an alcoholic' in increasingly public places. The gradual desensitization makes a badge of honor out of what had been a curse" (1985, p. 2).

In the view of some analysts, self-help groups also pose a danger as lay people may be involved in dealing with serious mental health issues. Others fault self-help groups and their members for being too tied up with their own needs, or for encouraging people to stay "stuck" in their situations rather than moving on. In her book, *I'm Dysfunctional, You're Dysfunctional*, Kaminer (1992), suggested that self-help groups encourage simplistic thinking. She criticized many of the groups for stressing somewhat rigid techniques and devaluing complex ideas or uncertainties.

Wuthnow underlined the divergent opinions about the value of support groups. He observed that while proponents see them as a way of saving American society, and redeeming individuals from destructive addictions, critics deem such groups artificial, "contributing more to a narcissistic obsession with self than to a more responsible society" (1994, p. ix).

Frank Riessman, one of the founders of the self-help movement, and his colleague (Riessman & Bay, 1992) acknowledged that in some quarters "self-help is seen as a diversion from social change, emphasizing instead individual or psychological change—substituting personal therapy for social action" (p. 28). The authors asserted, however, that some self-help groups have used their shared sense of identity to boost political activism. They cited a number of self-help groups, such as Victims for Victims, Disabled in Action, SHARE and other breast cancer groups, the Gray Panthers, and the National Black Women's Health Project, that are explicitly oriented toward social change.

In Riessman and Bay's view, "the trend of self-help groups empowering individuals and leading to political activism can be seen in the women's movement, which began in the 1960s with small consciousness-raising groups, and gradually emerged as a full-fledged social and political movement" (p. 29). They saw a similar progression in movements for disabled rights and gay rights. "The internal identity-strengthening dimension of self-help served as a critical first step that enabled the groups to move outward and engage in social and political action" (p. 34). Even AA, which has taken a position against political action, has spawned political changes. In the view of the authors, the creation of the National Institute on Alcoholism and Alcohol Abuse was a by-product of the AA movement.

In the same journal, a community organizer in the South articulated a clear need for grassroots organizations that would allow people to express their self-interests along with their political principles. After describing the key role women's support groups have played in her life, she said, "We've got to help people understand the connections between their personal needs and their political realities . . . We've got to consciously build a social-change movement that offers safe space and celebration, validation and support" (Okun, 1992, p. 48).

Some organizations sponsor both self-help and political action groups. For example, a community mental health center in an ethnically diverse community sponsors a variety of self-help groups including Alcoholics Anonymous and a Grandparents Group. In a different vein, it also sponsors T.R.A.I.N. (Taking Responsibility And Initiative Now), a group for residents who want to work together to improve the community through grass roots organizing and advocacy efforts (*Newsbrief*, 1994, pp. 4, 5).

How Counselors Relate to Self-Help Groups

Mental health professionals can play a variety of roles vis-à-vis self-help groups. Wax (1985) suggested that helping professionals are in a good position to provide logistical support, start-up assistance, help with organizational and group development issues, consultation, reciprocal referrals, and help with political action, advocacy, and public education. All such cooperative efforts, of course, require sensitive communications and patience on the part of both counselors and representatives of the group.

In some situations, counselors and other helping professionals may initiate groups as they see a need for their clients to have peer support. A well-publicized example would be the host of support groups for family members of persons with Alzheimer's disease sponsored by the Alzheimer's Association (Barnhill, 1994). In various parts of the country, professionals have helped organize groups for grandparents who are raising their crack-addicted children's children (Trupin, 1993; R. Waters, 1994).

Sometimes groups are organized by lay persons who then seek professional assistance. Such was the case of a group for families and partners of people with HIV/AIDS in a rural setting (Anderson & Shaw, 1994). In this instance, the conservative nature of the community led to a great deal of secrecy about the group. After 14 months of meeting on their own, members sought the group leadership services of a trained mental health worker—someone who had worked with stigmatized populations and with grief issues and who was not a native of the community. The latter characteristic was deemed important to preserve the privacy of the group's members.

Despite the fact that the trend toward formation of self-help groups came, in part, as a rebellion against the formal and threatening mental health system, the relationship between counselors and self-help groups has a long history (Riordan & Beggs, 1987). The authors noted, for example, that during the last century, social workers assisted immigrants in forming mutual aid societies.

Riordan and Beggs also observed that as the self-help movement grew in this country, the suspicions that lay people and leaders of self-help groups had toward professionals were by no means one-sided. "For their part, professionals initially reacted with dismay that ranged from clinical hostility to ambivalence. The recent literature now reflects not only a receding ambivalence but a strong trend toward symbiotic cohabitation . . . the group is encouraged to remain autonomous while having access to professional help as desired" (1987, pp. 427–428).

Many counselors refer their own clients to self-help groups as an adjunct to individual counseling, or as a source of support when they terminate a client. Counselors may also help with "recruiting" for self-help groups if they give public talks about transitions and mention the value of self-help groups to people approaching, moving through, or moving out of a transition.

In addition, some counselors train facilitators and/or group members who lead self-help groups. For example, one of the authors of this text (Waters) has worked with P-FLAG (Parents and Friends of Lesbians and Gays). Members of this group come together to support each other as they deal with a variety of transitions, such as realizing their child is gay or facing the non-event of missing out on becoming a grandparent. At the request of one of the members, the counselor originally offered a workshop to train group facilitators in basic communications and group management skills. She had them practice active listening, effective questioning, and caring confrontation. Since then she has consulted informally on issues such as how to handle "difficult" group members, particularly those who withdraw from or dominate group discussions.

In training facilitators, a key element is to make the training experiential. It is also important to help facilitators appreciate their skills and understand their limitations so they know when to refer group members to professionals with different training. Any of the applied counselor training models (e.g., Brammer, 1993; Cormier & Hackney, 1993; Egan, 1994; or Ivey, 1994) can be adapted for use with facilitators of self-help groups. There are also training manuals especially designed for use with paraprofessionals. In Great Britain, professionals train parents who lead telephone-contact groups for other parents of children with special needs (Hornby, 1988). Donner and Fine (1987) at Georgetown University have written a guide for developing self-help, advocacy groups for parents of children with serious emotional problems.

Peer counseling programs for older adults, a form of self-help group, have become widespread, with facilitators typically trained by professional counselors. Bratter and Freeman (1990) stated that "Careful selection of the trainer/supervisor is integral to the quality and longevity of the program . . . A trainer conducting classes in a 'participatory learning' model exemplifies a nonauthoritarian figure and thus provides an important role model for them as counselors" (1990, p. 50).

Another model for professionals and senior peer counselors working cooperatively is provided by an Oregon group, Volunteers Involved for the Emotional Well-Being of Seniors (VIEWS). In that program, professional counselors screen inquiries from older adults and refer those deemed appropriate to peer counselors (*Aging Today*, 1993). We urge readers to consider the various roles that counselors can play in interacting with self-help groups as they read the following discussion which gives additional views on the value of self-help groups as well as examples of different types of groups.

Types of Groups for People Experiencing Various Transitions

A glance at the community activities section of any metropolitan newspaper attests to the variety of self-help groups. People experiencing individual transitions will find groups where they can search for meaning in life, sometimes with an emphasis on spirituality. Here, too, are the host of groups for persons learning to cope with various disabilities from shyness to cancer, and the variety of 12-step programs, such as Alcoholics Anonymous or Gamblers Anonymous. A hallmark of the 12-step programs is that people are always defined as in transition, they are "recovering," not recovered.

Sometimes groups are gender-specific. Ever since the publication of *The Feminine Mystique* (Friedan, 1963), there have been consciousness-raising groups for women. More recently, such groups for men have sprung up. Hassan said that self-help groups offer men, who typically lack intimacy, "a sanctuary in which they can share their emotions without fear of being disdained" (1992, p. 18).

Among the most popular groups are those for people who have experienced, or are anticipating, *family or other relationship-related transitions*. Groups for singles include some individuals wishing to change that status and others wishing to find friendships and intimacy while remaining single. There are also self-help groups for divorced and bereaved people, expectant and new parents, parents of teenagers, parents without partners, and children of aging parents, as well as caregiver groups.

An unusual support group, Aftermath, helps families of criminals cope while the offenders are in prison (Dawson, 1993). Its founder "spends most of her time with women whose husbands, brothers, or fathers have committed murder, rape, or other sexual offenses. Discovering that someone they love has committed a hideous crime devastates most people" (p.12). Negative publicity, friends who desert them, and neighborhood hostility can add to the pain of an already difficult transition. An indication of the need for such a group is that five years after its founding, Aftermath had branches all over Great Britain.

Self-help groups for people experiencing work transitions may involve displaced homemakers, people searching for jobs, those considering or coping with retirement, or those being hired into positions that are nontraditional for their gender or ethnic group. Thus there are groups for male nurses, women in the construction trades, and black business owners. Counselors can be involved in helping to establish such groups or helping them increase their effectiveness once they are under way.

In our electronic age, support groups do not always involve face-to-face contact. *The New York Times* (Lewis, 1994) carried an interesting story of a murder victim who was mourned by his family and "grieving friends . . . in the electronic community called cyberspace. [These friends lamented his death] with an on-line wake that lasted weeks" (Lewis, 1994, p. A1). They communicated with each other, expressing their reactions to his death, through their computers. The article went on to discuss a wide array of computer-based relationships, formed by people seeking both information and emotional support from their networks.

Even in cyberspace, there are gender differences. In the cover story of *Newsweek* (Kantrowitz, 1994), "Men, Women and Computers," several writers discussed the different ways men and women approach their computers, and the information networks that link them. They also wrote of difficulties women may experience such as being electronically stalked or made the butt of inappropriate jokes. "What really annoys women is the flaming [flooding a mailbox with nasty messages] and the people boasting—the things that annoy women are things that men do all the time (Kantrowitz, 1994, p. 51)." One flaming victim "retreated into her own galaxy by starting the all-female Starfleet Ladies Auxiliary and Embroidery/Baking Society. The private electronic forum, based in Houston, now has more than 40 members, including psychologists, physicians, students and secretaries" (p.48). Because many networks are considered sexist, counselors referring their women clients to the support and information available on computers need to be familiar with women's networks. Gender-specific networks can be a particular source of support to women who can use electronic mail to discuss work and/or family issues without having to leave their desks.

Articles about the role of technology in support groups can be found in journals of many different professional groups. Writing in the

American Journal of Nursing, Sparks discussed the value of ESGs (Electronic Support Groups) in which "participants share problems, solutions, miracles and miseries" (1992, p. 63). While ESGs lack the immediacy of face-to-face contact, they offer more privacy and can be called on 24 hours per day. In some cases, the electronic sharing may be a stimulus for members to seek face-to-face counseling.

Rounds, Galinsky and Stevens (1991) described a group based on less sophisticated technology, a telephone conference call. The model program for people with AIDS living in rural areas was designed to provide both information and social support. The six-session program employed a semistructured psychoeducational approach. Beginning with a get-acquainted session, the agenda moved from giving information on medical and social care systems, friendships and support networks, to more personal discussions of feelings, safe sex, and concerns about dying. The authors noted that people with AIDS in rural areas face two kinds of barriers—geographic isolation and concern about being locally stigmatized. Telephones are familiar and offer privacy. The value of privacy was underlined during a discussion of masturbation when one of the men said, "I'm glad everybody don't see me now because I'm blushing" (p. 15). Telephone support groups serve only a small number of people (three or four members is considered the maximum number that can effectively engage in a telephone group), but they do represent a way of reaching those who may otherwise be left groupless.

Self-Help Groups: A Summary

Clearly, the self-help movement is a significant force in current American society, involving at least six million people per year. There are groups for people experiencing intrapersonal, interpersonal, and work-related transitions. Many of the topics self-help groups focus on are also discussed in counseling groups. The difference is that the former are led by group members who share the "problem," whatever it may be; the latter are led by professional counselors, who may or may not be in the same situation. While they do not generally lead self-help groups, professional counselors can be involved with self-help groups in many ways including recruiting and referring members, assisting with organizational and marketing tasks, helping groups set goals and develop strategic plans, and training and supporting group leaders. Many of the skills used by counselors in working with self-help groups are equally appropriate in consulting with profit and non-profit organizations.

CONSULTING WITH ORGANIZATIONS AND THEIR EMPLOYEES

Consulting gives counselors a chance to have an impact on adults' everyday environment. Consulting can take many forms. In their Introduction to two special issues of the *Journal of Counseling and Development* on consultation, editors Kurpius and Fuqua noted that there is no universally accepted definition of consulting. However, most agree that "consultation is a process for helping individuals, groups, organizations, and communities function more effectively and efficiently, with greater satisfaction" (Kurpius & Fuqua 1993a, p. 596). When counselors are involved as consultants they have an opportunity to assist adults in transition indirectly rather than directly.

A major difference between consulting and counseling is that consulting is triadic. Counselors work directly with clients; consultants work with consultees who, in turn, serve a client system. The consultee may be an individual, a group, or an organization. The form of the consultation can be varied, but, at the broadest level, writers distinguish between expert consultation and process consultation. Consultants function in the expert role when "the consultee needs some knowledge, advice, or service that the consultant can provide" (Dougherty, 1990, p. 27). While this can be a satisfactory arrangement, Dougherty noted the danger that the individual or organization may get used to having somebody else perform the service and not develop their own problem-solving abilities.

Process consultation, which has been discussed extensively by Schein (1991, 1992), casts consultants in a less directive and more interactive role with the consultee. The consultant helps the consultee examine how problems are being addressed, rather than focusing on what the problems are. "The expert mode includes heavy responsibility for the consultant for the design, implementation, and success of an intervention. The process mode emphasizes shared responsibility between consultant and consultee and provides for the consultee to internalize planned change process as an acquired capability" (Kurpius & Fuqua (1993b, p. 599). Counselors can function as consultants in either mode if they have the required skills.

Summarizing the skills that are integral parts of every counselor's repertoire, Dougherty (1990) stated:

> Effective consultants have highly refined interpersonal and communication skills built on attitudes of positive regard, empathy, and genuineness;

a large repertoire of problem-solving skills with which to help their consultees; a set of basic skills for working with organizations; and a set of ethical and professional standards that guide their actions. (p. 25)

Dougherty (1990) developed a generic model of consultation that included four stages: (1) entry, (2) diagnosis, (3) implementation, and (4) disengagement. At all stages, consultant and consultees work together. During Stage 1, the consultant enters the organization and explores organizational needs. In Stage 2, diagnosis, the focus is on gathering information, defining the problem, setting goals, and generating possible interventions. Stage 3, implementation, is the action stage of a consultation. Consultants and consultees choose an intervention, then formulate, implement, and evaluate that plan. Stage 4, disengagement, requires evaluating the consultation process, and planning for necessary follow-up. These stages relate closely to the stages of counseling identified in the Cormier and Hackney (1993) model.

As part of the action or implementation stage of a consultant relationship, counselors can teach administrators and managers about the transition model. Managers who understand the significance of adult transitions will be more understanding of their employees' behavior and better able to provide support. Sargent and Schlossberg directed the following remarks to managers to demonstrate this aspect of consultation:

As a manager, you need to know that people in transition are often preoccupied and a little confused, even if the transition is a desired one. For example, a promotion to a first supervisory job can be exciting, yet the new supervisor—whose roles, relationships, assumptions, and routines have been altered—will be disoriented while he or she figures out what is expected in the new role. In addition, the isolation from friends who were colleagues and who are now subordinates can be upsetting . . .

When adults start new jobs, for example, they find themselves suspended awkwardly between their old role and the new one. During that period, they need special help, such as new employee orientation and the rapid development of support systems . . . The move from incompetence to competence can be tortuous. Managers can help by acknowledging the rough transition rather than denying it, and by offering support and specific strategies to learn new competencies. (1988, pp. 58–60)

Consultants may also be able to help organizations set up a transition management program. For example, in response to the tremendous amount of restructuring taking place in higher education, the

American Council on Education developed a guide, *Focus on Adults: A Self Study Guide for Post-Secondary Institutions* (1991). Consultants could use such a guide to help colleges and universities examine the responsiveness of their institutions to adult learners, and suggest ways to make adult learners feel they matter.

Consultants could also help institutions design transition management programs. Such a transition program would include a system for disseminating accurate information, training for managers who have to deliver bad news about downsizing or reorganizing, and support for students, staff, and faculty affected by the changes.

Counselors, too, need to learn new competencies when they move into other realms of activity. To learn about the various roles counselors can play, we interviewed two counselors whose career paths illustrate the broadened scope of counseling. In chronicling their work biographies, both talked enthusiastically about their own career transitions, emphasizing how their basic counseling skills serve them in their new positions.

Counselor as Consultant: A Personal Story

The first counselor we interviewed, JH, is a university-based career counselor who now functions primarily as a developer of training materials and a career consultant to business and industry. Sometimes, as when she is hired to provide career counseling to employees, she functions as an expert consultant. At other times, when she meets with managers and supervisors to discuss career development opportunities within the organization, she functions in the process mode. Below is her story of how her career evolved.

My current position builds on my training and experience as a counselor and on my earlier background in business and as a volunteer. During high school and college, I worked in a clerical capacity for insurance companies. My first post-college job was as an office manager in a foundry. What can you do with an English degree?

During the 10-plus years that I stayed home to raise children, I was a fund raiser for the League of Women Voters, a writing tutor for high school students, and the president of a co-op nursery school. In that role, I learned that I liked running the school, not working directly with the children!

When I moved to a larger city and left my support system, I decided it was time for my own development. One of the nursery school mothers referred me to a women's center. After observing the peer group facilitator, I decided I'd like to try that kind of work. I did, and after advancing up the career ladder for volunteers, I enrolled in a master's program in counseling.

After graduation I worked as a mental health counselor in a family medical practice where I got my first taste of real life. These "tastes" included seeing clients who had serious problems with alcoholism and abuse. I also launched a small private practice where I learned how to market and run a small business.

As a volunteer group leader, I found the program "Careers in Transition" to be very exciting, so I was delighted to be offered a job as a career counselor. I came to prefer career counseling to strictly personal counseling because in career counseling you can have a quicker, more direct impact on people. It's a lot easier to change your career than your personality! I still use all of my mental health counseling skills, including my ability to assess people's skills and interpersonal relations, help them set goals, identify significant barriers—internal or external—and develop strategies to cope with the barriers.

As a result of a series of model project grants, my job as a career counselor expanded to include training other professional and paraprofessional career counselors, and writing training manuals for others to replicate the program. I was frequently asked to provide career counseling and consulting to various businesses and industries. In my work as a trainer and a consultant, I use all my basic counseling skills. I have to listen, size people up, give feedback, and gently confront. In developing programs, I picture the consumer of the product. This involves needs assessment.

As I see it, the major difference between counseling individuals as a private practitioner or an agency employee and as a consultant to business is that in business you have two clients—the company which is paying you and the individual employees. You are a vendor. As counselors, we are trained to do things to benefit the individual, as a consultant we must also consider what benefits the organization. In order to work effectively within a company, you must have support from management, employees, and in some cases, union leadership.

JH suggested that counselors who want to be more involved in the business world get experience outside of their usual environment, read business journals as well as counseling journals, and attend meetings of organizations such as the American Society of Training and Development. They also need to talk with other consultants and trainers and watch them work. Cosier and Dalton (1993) offered a variety of suggestions on how counselors interested in becoming consultants could plan the change, enter the new field, and promote themselves successfully. Included in their recommendations is a list of relevant professional associations.

Consultants Morin and Cabrera have designed interventions to be used with employees who lose their jobs. Thus, they are functioning primarily as expert consultants. They stated that "our business is career continuation (often called outplacement counseling), and we teach ex-employees the skills they need to continue their careers quickly and efficiently" (1991, p. xxi). Their book affirmed what JH said about having two clients, as they are typically hired and paid by organizations to provide services for their former, or soon-to-be-former, employees. Companies provide such services, partly out of concern for their employees, and partly because they have found that if former employees make a smooth transition from one job to another, it saves money in severance pay and avoids possible legal actions. Workers who remain with the company are also reassured when they see that their former co-workers have been helped.

Noer stated that many organizations do a much better job with those they are firing than with those who are staying, those who, in our terms, have experienced a non-event transition. He used the term "layoff survivor sickness" to describe an illness characterized by a variety of feelings, including fear, anger, depression, guilt, and betrayal. In his view, "only compelling multilevel interventions can affect the pathology of layoff survivor sickness" (1993, p. 2). Toward that end, he designed a model, including interventions, that clarifies the process, facilitates grieving, breaks some existing patterns, and creates new systems.

Many of those interventions are based on skills that counselors can use either directly or as consultants to company employees. The examples just discussed illustrate the use of expert consultation skills. The following story shows how a counselor used process consultation skills to help a group deal with the need to lay people off.

A Case Study of the Transition Model in Action

One of the authors (Schlossberg) had an opportunity to consult with a group of six nurse managers and a professor of nursing in a Canadian city. The problem, as they saw it, stemmed from a Canadian health care crisis. Nursing supervisors had been "ordered" to dismiss almost half of their trained nurses. As each spoke, the situation began to sound hopeless: the nurses had to be fired, they would never get other jobs in the field, it was unfair, but the supervisors had to carry out the orders.

The consultant's first step was to listen to what the clients were saying and reflect it back. She heard catastrophe, no hope, no way out of this dilemma. Therefore the goal of the consultation became (1) to help the nurse managers put this negative transition in perspective, and (2) to provide skills so they would feel competent to help those they fire learn how to negotiate transitions.

Addressing the feelings of the nurse managers was critical to helping them take control of their role as "messengers of bad news." If they felt hopeless, they would communicate this to those they had to fire. After discussing their feelings, they began to see that while the situation was negative, it was not a disaster. Joblessness can be a defeat and leave one hungry and homeless, or it can be an opportunity to think about getting different training and reshaping goals. Once they could begin to redefine it as a challenge, albeit a negative one, they were on their way.

The supervisors expressed fear that they might some day lose their own jobs. The consultant helped them see that if in fact they were fired, they did not have to give up hope of ever being a nurse again. They might have to temporarily work outside the field, or they might see this as an opportunity to explore where the economy needs workers and how their skills could be transferred.

In addition to feeling guilty about having to fire people, the managers were concerned that they did not have the skills to do it. As they were dealing with transitions, actually creating transitions in other people's lives, they needed to learn how to help people negotiate transitions. So the consultant helped them learn to teach others how to (a) approach change, (b) assess their resources for coping with change, and (c) develop action plans to take control of the change.

She suggested that in discussing ways to approach change, the managers give all those being fired an opportunity to express their views of the transition. For example, do they see it as positive, negative, or neutral? If the firings were being discussed in a group, group members might be able to suggest alternate ways to view the situation to each other. Perhaps some will see it as an opportunity to do life planning, rethink their careers, or start over.

To help the managers assist the fired nurses in assessing their resources, she taught them how to explain the 4 S's model. Managers were to help nurses identify their resources and deficits with respect to their *situation* at the time of their job loss, their *self,* their *supports* at work and at home, and their *strategies.* In teaching the managers to help nurses develop an action plan, she suggested the use of group discussions, including brainstorming, to encourage them to identify resources they could strengthen.

In describing this consultation, the counselor noted that three groups needed attention—the supervisors who had to convey the bad news, those being fired, and those not being fired. In this situation, as in many others, "survivors" may be preoccupied with a fear of impending doom. Being aware of the needs of all three groups, rather than just the person or group you are with, exemplifies what JH said earlier about one of the differences between counseling and consulting.

DEVELOPING PROGRAMS AND WORKSHOPS

Another way that counselors can expand their impact on adults in transition is through designing and presenting structured workshops and acting as program developers. We define a *program* as an array of services offered by an organization, and a *workshop* as a short-term educational or growth experience. Thus the program of any organization may include several workshops as well as other activities.

Obviously, a competent counselor can be extremely helpful to an individual suddenly conscious of being middle-aged, to a divorced person, or to a job seeker. The same counselor, however, can reach many more people by offering a workshop on midlife changes, divorce, or job-seeking skills. And the workshop may add the bonus of group support.

In addition, some adults who are reluctant to seek counseling may find it easier or more socially acceptable to attend a workshop. Participation in the workshop may be enough to help some people through the transitions. Others may find that they are now more comfortable with the idea of counseling.

Counselors involved in designing workshops or programs may find Brookfield's (1986) ideas on adult learning useful. He recommended flexible programs that build in opportunities for serendipitous learning, and he cautioned against overreliance on predetermined objectives that leave little room for such unanticipated learning. This may be particularly important in programs for adults in transition because the needs of participants may change as they learn more about them*selves* and their *situations,* and see a need to develop new sources of *support* and alternative *strategies.*

Designing Programs

Setting up a comprehensive program is a complicated procedure. It requires that program planners look broadly at the environment, and consider the needs of the individuals to be served, as well as those of the organization and the community. Typically, designing a program requires identification of specific tasks and a time line.

The National Occupational Information Coordinating Committee (NOICC) developed the useful three-stage model for program design shown below:

> *Stage One. Planning* (0–6 months)
>   Form committees
>   Conduct needs assessment
>   Establish program standards
>   Initiate evaluation planning
> *Stage Two. Development* (7–12 months)
>   Direct committees in program development
>   Review the current program
>   Revise the plan
>   Design the evaluation
>   Identify staff development needs
> *Stage Three. Implementation* (13–24 months)
>   Involve committees in program implementation
>   Conduct staff development
>   Monitor program implementation
>   Evaluate and use results for program improvement. (NOICC, 1989, p. 17)

Since formative evaluation is a continuous process, used to improve program design, discussion of evaluation procedures continues through all stages. Committees are also involved in all stages. When committees are broadly based, and include community representatives, they can assist in marketing and recruiting as well as program design.

Re-entry students are the target group for a variety of college and university programs. Jacoby (1991) developed a model for serving adult students. The four components of the SPAR Model—services, programs, advocacy, and research—can be a useful guide for counselors. According to her definitions, services are performed *for* students and must be scheduled to accommodate their multiple roles. Programs are carried on *with* students, often through adult student organizations. Advocacy on *behalf* of students is designed to see that the policies and practices of educational institutions are responsive to student needs. Research helps counselors and other professionals better understand the needs of adult students and evaluate existing programs.

Orientation courses for adult learners, like the one at the University of Maryland, College Park's Counseling Center, addresses issues of identity, comfort with academics, and concerns about balancing work, family and study. In interviews, adult learners frequently mention the sense of community that results from participation in these workshop courses (Greenberg & Goldberg, personal communication, 1994).

Designing and Presenting Workshops

By virtue of their training and experience, counselors already have many of the communications skills necessary for conducting workshops. Typically, counselors know how to listen to workshop participants, ask clarifying questions to make sure that participants understand the information, "read" the group's nonverbal language, and promote group interaction.

Effective workshop leaders must also know how to present information clearly and use examples that are appropriate for particular individuals and groups. Counselors can learn these skills. A recent study of training needs of career development facilitators revealed a significant interest in learning how to train both clients and other career development facilitators. The authors recommended that "train-the-trainer sessions emphasize training skills and that only experienced, effective trainers be used to train other personnel (Hoppin & Splete, 1994, p. 85).

Counselors interested in designing effective workshops may find Loesch's (1985) seven-step procedure helpful. The seven steps—define your goals, profile the participants, profile the setting, design your agenda, prepare your resources, prepare yourself, and practice—can be applied to almost any workshop. If, for example, you have been asked to design a workshop for dislocated workers in your community, and you know the workers are concerned about their ability to look for jobs, your goals might be to provide practical information about job-search techniques and labor-force projections, as well as build worker confidence. In designing the agenda, you might want to consult both local employers and a list of competencies needed by job seekers, such as that contained in Goodman and Hoppin (1991).

In planning workshops it is important to think of: who, what, where, and when. Who and what need to be carefully coordinated so that the content and manner of presentation fit the needs of a particular clientele. Thus a workshop for adults who have recently learned they have Attention Deficit Disorder should not be done in a straight lecture format. A variety of activities, many experiential, should be included. A workshop for returning learners needs to inform students about resources of the college or university, and give them an opportunity to express some of their concerns about their new role.

Workshop planners also need to consider the cultural background of their participants. After investigating the self-esteem of Arab adults studying English as a second language, Klee urged counselors and teachers to cooperate in tailoring programs for their special needs. She suggested that single-gender workshops might be more appropriate for this population, and also recommended that workshop participants have "opportunities for cultural and linguistic interactions with native English speakers outside of the classroom . . . [possibly through] field trips, 'pot lucks,' forums, guest speakers, or language exchange partners" (Klee, 1994, p. 31).

The time at which a workshop is offered also affects who can come. Workshops for displaced homemakers with young children can be offered during the day if child care is available. If a business wants spouses to attend a retirement planning seminar, it usually needs to be an evening program so spouses do not need to take time off from their own jobs. Workshops for older adults often have to be scheduled when transportation is available. Safety issues are also important. In their publicity, sponsors may want to mention secure, lighted parking if that is apt to be an issue. Having representatives of the targeted population involved in the planning process increases the likelihood that the right questions about who, what, where, and when will be asked.

A Sampling of Workshops

Earlier in this chapter, we identified a number of topics that could be the focus of support groups for people experiencing individual, family, and work-related transitions. Many of those topics lend themselves to a workshop format, if a more educational focus is desired. This section contains ideas for workshops counselors can conduct or promote, and descriptions of a few we considered innovative.

Women re-entering the work world can benefit from workshops that include a counseling component. For example, PROBE (Potential Reentry Opportunities in Business and Education) was designed to help divorced, separated, and widowed women enter professional and other nontraditional careers. Empowerment of women is a major goal of the program, which is "based on feminist principles . . . [and] relies heavily on women already placed in the community as role models and sources of support" (Towns & Gentzler, 1986, p. 160). Program organizers also work with potential employers to develop jobs.

A similar combination of workshops and job development is provided for older workers of both sexes by Project Able. Their programming is targeted to "dislocated workers, displaced homemakers, terminated employees, or even recipients of 'voluntary' early retirement programs" (Barclay & McDougall, 1990, p. 53).

In the Winter, 1990 issue of *Generations,* the journal of the American Society on Aging, several counselors from different parts of the country mentioned that they make speeches and present community workshops in order to introduce ideas about adult development and psychological change to older adults and their families. This often serves as a recruiting tool, as attenders may then seek counseling for themselves or refer others.

Educational experiences do not always take place in classrooms. In San Francisco, a vacant lot turned into an urban garden is the site of an innovative program for people being released from prison. People experiencing this transition may find their pre-prison support system no longer intact and their previous strategies for coping with their lives no longer appropriate. The Garden Project, founded in 1991, is a model project designed to help recently released ex-offenders re-enter their communities, learn new skills, and avoid the temptations of the street.

A press release about the program, undated and simply titled, "The Garden Project," noted, "To help achieve personal goals, 'students' in the program also fulfill requirements to participate in alcohol and drug rehabilitation programs, as well as pursue continuing education studies." An article about the project in the *New York Times* characterized the fruits and vegetables of the garden as "metaphors for what went wrong in a prisoner's troubled past . . . The simple process of weeding is a good place to start re-examining a life gone wrong. The weeds are whatever got in the way: smoking crack or whoring or stealing" (Gross,

1992). In addition to the metaphorical value of planting, cultivating, and weeding, gardeners are paid for their efforts from the revenue earned by the produce. Local businesses support the project by their purchases, and several foundations have supplied additional income.

Another San Francisco garden program, Fresh Start Farms, hires homeless people to work as organic gardeners. According to the *San Francisco Examiner*, "The homeless workers will be bused to the garden daily, paid minimum wage, then given a bonus of $5,000 at the end of the first year to help them make a go of it in the mainstream market. They can also earn $9 an hour to train other homeless gardeners" (Nakao, 1993). Although these projects are not typical workshops for adults in transition, they represent innovative efforts for which counselors can advocate.

WORKING AS ADVOCATES

Webster's defines an advocate as "one who defends, vindicates or espouses a cause" (1980). Social scientists talk about functioning as change agents, but, in lay terms, we may think of advocacy as standing up for what you believe. Whatever the definition, in this discussion we are talking about counselor efforts to make life more fair to, and more supportive of, adults in transition. Sometimes those efforts involve working to empower adults so they can act in their own behalf. In other situations, counselors may need to intervene on a broader level, urging organizations and systems to be more responsive to the needs of adults.

In our quest to be supportive of various groups of adults, we must be careful not to take over for them. McKnight contended that "more and more conditions of human beings are being converted into problems in order to provide jobs for people who are forced to derive their income by purporting to deliver a service" (1990, p. 5). Applying this idea to the needs of an older population, he suggested that scholars conducting research on "old as a deficiency... [should be asked instead] to define the competence, the skills, and the capacities of old" (p. 9). McKnight's message can serve as a reminder to counselors to direct their advocacy efforts toward empowerment, not the creation of dependency.

In many situations, counselors need to operate on more than one level. In terms of the transition model, counselors can help clients develop more effective *strategies* and counselors and clients can work together to improve available institutional *supports*. For example, counselors in college and university settings may be able to empower returning students through workshops that build self-esteem and teach assertive skills and effective study techniques. At the same time, these counselors can encourage their educational institutions to have evening advising hours, offer financial aid for part-time students, and generally be more supportive of the needs of returning learners.

As an example, the University of Maryland, College Park, has a returning student fund that offers grants to adult learners experiencing financial emergencies. These grants, ranging from $100 to $500, have enabled a number of students to stay in school and continue to provide for their families. Several of the recipients spoke of the grants as a tremendous source of motivation, in part because they made the students feel they really mattered to someone.

To assess the degree to which adult learners feel they matter to their institutions, Schlossberg, Lasalle, and Golec (1991) developed "The Mattering Scales for Adult Students in Higher Education." These easily administered scales give students an opportunity to record their perceptions about their educational environment in five different areas: administration, advising, peers, multiple roles, and faculty. Questions deal with such issues as: the degree to which students feel appreciated or missed when they are not in class, and the degree to which they find the policies of the institution cognizant of the competing demands in their lives. Data from the scales provide information for change. Administrators and student development educators can pinpoint the areas in which adult learners feel they do not matter, and then take appropriate action to create a more hospitable environment.

Counselors in the work place can also urge the employing organization to create a more supportive environment by establishing flex-time schedules and/or making dependent care available. Intergenerational day care that serves both pre-school children and older adults at the workplace may be one approach counselors can recommend (Waters, 1991).

Counselor-advocates can also work to make non-profit agencies more "user friendly" for their adult clients. At one employment office, an official of the U.S. Department of Labor heard many unemployment counselors talking among themselves about how "their hearts ached for the people who had to stand in line to collect their checks and wait to talk with them." After looking over the office, the official suggested several changes to make the environment more supportive. He recom-

mended that people take numbers and be able to sit down while retaining their place "in line." He also recommended changing the physical environment so that clients could sit in chairs rather than lean over
a counter when talking with counselors (Robinson, 1994).

Minkler (1983) reported another example of working with and on
behalf of adults. The Tenderloin Senior Outreach Project was designed
for older adults living in single-room occupancy hotels in inner-city San
Francisco. Graduate students used weekly blood pressure screening in
the hotel lobby as an opportunity to talk with residents and facilitate
interaction. As the initial discussion group became popular, residents
of other hotels expressed interest. When group discussions indicated
that crime was the worst problem, students encouraged residents to develop an interhotel coalition to fight crime. The report is full of poignant stories of the support residents provided each other. In Minkler's
view, the project led to gradual empowerment of the elderly as individuals and as a community. To see how one counselor engaged in advocacy activities in the service of empowerment, we turn to another profile.

Counselor as Advocate: A Personal Story

HG is a counselor and counselor-educator, who was interviewed when
she was working as an advocacy coordinator for the American Counseling Association. Here is her story:

> As long as I can remember I've been involved with mental health con-
> cerns. In junior high school I volunteered in a hospital and tutored those
> with developmental disabilities. When it was time for college, I got a schol-
> arship to a nursing school that was on the grounds of a psychiatric hospi-
> tal. After a short time, I realized I hated the psychiatric system, which I
> saw as anything but healing, and I didn't think that as a nurse I would
> have any power to change the system. So I left nursing school and be-
> came a psychology major, hoping at age 18 that a psych degree would
> give me a better base from which to operate.
>
> As an undergraduate I worked part time with people labeled as
> chronically mentally ill. As a graduate student, I majored in rehabilita-
> tion and community counseling and "got hooked" on working with deaf
> students with emotional problems.
>
> My first post-master's job was with a special program for deaf chil-
> dren with multiple problems, run by the Baltimore city schools. I worked
> with children, consulted with teachers and parents, and wrote curricula
> for the affective domain. It was exciting in that it combined direct service,

training, and consulting to change attitudes. I advocated for students and got those who were functioning at a high enough level to be included in developing their own educational plans.

I was in private practice for several years and consulted with non-profit organizations that had group homes for people who were developmentally disabled or chronically mentally ill. My goal was to help the staff make environments more supportive for residents, to introduce an empowerment model.

Then I worked on a regional project involving case management for adults who had mental, emotional, or developmental problems. As a case manager, I began to shift my focus from work with individuals to policy issues. I repeatedly traveled to the state capital to justify the existence of our program. I learned how to get to decision-makers and how to communicate both information and passion to them in terms they could understand. Many of the problems our clients experience can't be "fixed" just by counseling. We need to effect change on a broader level.

My counseling skills are extremely useful in my work as an advocate. Just as I need to understand a client's frame of reference before I can work with him or her, I need to be able to understand the frame of reference of legislators. I also need to figure out their goals, and decide how I can express myself in ways so an issue becomes a shared one. If you sound self-serving, they won't listen. For example, it's not a good idea to urge legislators to pass a licensure law so counselors can get reimbursement or gain credibility. If you can convince them that licensure will be a benefit or protection for their constituents, they may vote for it. In my view it's essential that counselors get involved in advocacy for their own needs and those of their clients. I firmly believe that if we don't take responsibility for policies that affect counseling-related programs, we won't be around to provide counseling services. Lobbying is very important, but there are many other ways counselors can be advocates. Getting involved with state and national counseling organizations and being credentialed is a start. When counselors are active in community organizations— whether they be PTAs or Chambers of Commerce—they represent the counseling profession. Grassroot effects of counseling professionals are essential. We have to let the world know what we do and how we do it.

Acting at the Local, State, and National Level

Counselors can apply HG's suggestions in a variety of ways. When working with an individual client, advocacy often takes the form of "running interference," often as part of the referral process. Operationally that means you do not just give your clients the name of an agency that might provide the services they need, but you call the agency yourself, verify the services they offer and the hours they provide them, and perhaps alert them to your clients' special needs. Also, adults who are apprehensive about negotiating a transition, whether it be returning to school, attending the first meeting of a widowed persons' group, or looking into AA, may need the name of a particular person to look for, or perhaps a "buddy" to accompany them. You can be of help there.

Clients may also need help in coping with bureaucracies. The thought of going for the first time to an employment (or unemployment) office, admissions office, social security building, or senior center can appear daunting to many adults in transition. Counselors can help by walking clients through the process, literally or with an in-office rehearsal. In order to make appropriate referrals, counselors need to be knowledgeable about local resources. The process of helping adults with such practical concerns may also build trust and open the door for dealing with emotional problems as well.

Dealing with bureaucracies can pose additional problems for people in certain ethnic or minority groups. Non-English-speaking adults may have particular problems if the agency staff speak only English and if the forms they must fill out are only in English. Counselors can advocate by encouraging the agency to provide translators.

A major transition for adults may come when they need to deal with the criminal justice system for the first time. Whether they are the victim of a crime or the family member of a perpetrator, the thought of going to the police can seem overwhelming. This may be particularly true for adults who come from groups that have experienced adversial relationships with the police. Counselors can intervene both to help clients reframe their views of police as potential helpers, and to work with police to help them become more receptive to clients from different ethnic backgrounds.

Sometimes, in their advocacy role, counselors see a need for a particular service and find a way to provide it. For example, the Adult Day Care Center in Ada, Oklahoma, exists because of the efforts of a counselor-educator there (B. Shelton, personal communication, 1990). The retired executive director of the Chamber of Commerce called her to seek help for a former Chamber member who had Alzheimer's disease. They discussed the value of adult day care and set up a community meeting involving potential users of the service, as well as leaders of the business community and legislators to discuss it.

In Ada, the human services people and the business people worked well together. The first group knew what a day care center could do, the business people knew how to incorporate and access funding. This coalition worked well in part because the members were powerful people. A major challenge for counselors is to assist less powerful people to explain their needs and find ways to meet them.

The words expressed by HG, above, are echoed by many others. McCrone (1991), writing to urge efforts on behalf of those with disabilities, suggested that lobbying, testifying at hearings, supporting helpful legislators, organizing witnesses, and drafting bills will enable grassroots rehabilitation professionals to participate in the evolution of disability-related federal law. Such laws can play a crucial role in the lives of adults who become disabled.

Smith gave a broader rationale for counselor involvement in public policy. In his view counselors are fulfilling only part of their professional obligation if they work with individual clients but fail to see the larger impact they can have by being involved with public policy. He stated that we "must be involved with legislation . . . regarding aid to education or career development, or the issues of accessibility for the physically disadvantaged . . . with discriminatory practices in the work place and the legislation or lack of legislation that works to eliminate that discrimination" (1994, p. 15).

Smith mentioned but a few of the many issues where lobbying may produce helpful legislation. There are a host of issues involving health care, funding for schools at all levels, security and portability of pensions, and community-based programs to provide assistance to adults experiencing temporary crises or long-term difficulties.

As HG said, counselors can advocate in many different ways. For example, they can represent the interests of adults to community organizations and educational institutions. This may mean recommending that colleges and universities schedule supportive services at convenient hours for adults, testifying at a local hearing of a planning agency about the need for additional transportation services for persons with disabilities, or urging libraries to establish in-home services.

Some advocacy efforts are best done by counselors acting individually, whether in their professional role or as a private citizen. (Politicians do pay attention to letters and phone calls from constituents.) Other times counselors can maximize their effectiveness by working with an advocacy group representing their point of view. For example, Citizens for Better Care (CBC) is an advocacy organization monitoring conditions in nursing homes. When counselors are aware of CBC's findings, they can help families locate dependable facilities with a well-trained staff and avoid those where CBC has found instances of mistreatment. When counselors have this information, they can make appropriate referrals and perhaps ease the transition of placing a family member in a nursing home.

Increasingly, professional associations of counselors are becoming involved in advocacy efforts. The American Counseling Association's Government Relations Committee, composed of association members, as well as professional staff, advocates for the interests of both clients and counselors. The Committee's mission is to identify and initiate proactive and reactive positions on public policy issues confronting professional counselors, human development professionals, and those whom they serve.

The committee urges its members to contact their legislators on a wide range of human service needs, to provide the lawmakers with information, and to express appreciation when their actions are in line with the interests of clients and counselors.

Another major benefit of counselor advocacy has been the move toward counselor credentialing. At the national level, over 20,000 counselors have opted for voluntary certification through the National Board for Certified Counselors (1995). As of 1994, 41 states had some form of licensure law. Certification and licensure serve as a way for counselors to indicate their commitment to professionalism. Certification also makes it easier for adults in transition to identify qualified counselors.

Many advocacy activities can have considerable impact on the opportunity structure for adults. In our view, that is a major reason for counselors to be involved beyond their office doors.

SUMMARY

Because adults live, work, and play in environments that encompass a broad range of possibilities, multiple interventions are typically necessary. Let us consider two different clients we might encounter and briefly discuss some of the interventions we might employ to enhance their coping resources.

A 40-year-old displaced worker who decided to return to school might benefit from individual and/or group counseling. We, as supportive counselors, can help him explore his *situation*. For example, we might find it important to evaluate his financial resources by asking him questions about whether his previous employer will cover any educational expenses, whether he has a working partner, and whether the family has health insurance. Our counseling would also provide an opportunity for him to express his feelings about two major role changes, (1) being laid off, and (2) returning to school.

Before helping him set realistic goals, we, as counselors, could also help him explore the *self* resources he brings to the transition. What is his attitude toward change and his general outlook on life? Answers to questions about both situation and self might be important in determining whether to refer him for financial aid and in helping him decide how many courses to take the first semister.

If there were a *support* group of re-entry students available at the school he plans to attend, he would be able to obtain support and tips from them. Students who had returned to school earlier than he could serve as "veterans," in Weiss's (1976) terms. If we were serving as consultants to the school, we might encourage it to engage in a self-study, and work with faculty and staff to help them become more sensitive to and supportive of the needs of returning students. As advocates, we could testify before the state legislature urging additional funding to support the establishment of special programs for students as well as retraining for faculty and staff.

If, on the other hand, our client is a 54-year-old grandmother suddenly faced with the task of raising grandchildren, she might well need counseling to help her deal with her changing roles, relationships, responsibilities, and assumptions about herself. Her life plan has probably changed dramatically. We would also want to find her a support group of other grandmothers in similar situations, with whom she could share information and support.

In our role as consultants to social agencies or school districts, we could recommend the establishment of workshops on parenting skills for grandmothers. Teachers and counselors at the schools attended by the grandchildren might need in-service training to familiarize them with appropriate ways of handling this special group of youngsters and their grandmothers. As advocates we could argue for policy changes that would provide better financial benefits for grandmothers raising their grandchildren.

We hope these two examples underline what we have been saying throughout the chapter and the book. Counseling adults in transition is an exciting and challenging job that gives us an opportunity to function at many different levels.

Afterword

This book has been predicated on a number of assumptions that we hope have been clear as well as comprehensive. In an effort to "tie it all together," we will briefly review our assumptions.

ASSUMPTION 1. PRACTICE MUST BE TIED TO THEORY

The scientist-practitioner model, so prevalent in counseling, is based on the notion that practice stems from research and theory. This book presents a theory of individuals in transition—a theory that lays the groundwork for the many practices, programs, and strategies suggested.

Transition theory posits a structure for viewing *any* change—whether it is anticipated or unanticipated, positive or negative, a success or a failure, an event or a non-event. The persons and issues vary; the structure remains the same.

Transition theory states that individuals manage transitions differently. The variability stems largely from differences in people's resources and deficits as they approach transitions. The theory categorizes potential resources as: the individual's Situation, Self, Support, and Strategies—the 4 S system. The practice details what can be done to assess these resources and compensate for deficits that may exist.

An example of the interface between theory and practice relates to coping. It was found that people cope by either changing a situation, changing the meaning of a situation, or managing their own reactions to it. Knowledge and understanding of these categories can guide counselors as they work with clients in an individual or group setting.

Leonard Pearlin and his colleagues also emphasized that no magic coping strategy exists. Effective coping involves utilizing numerous coping strategies as appropriate. Sometimes one may use humor; other times one may need to engage in confrontation; at times mediation may be necessary; and occasionally one may choose to do nothing.

To illustrate, we will share a travel story of Nancy's with you. Several years ago, she went to Denver to make a speech. When she arrived at the hotel she was perplexed. The hotel had no record of the meeting. Nancy called the conference coordinator to discover that the meeting was scheduled for November, not October. She had arrived a month early. As Nancy said:

> I cannot describe my feeling of shock and utter dismay. I immediately called my husband and started to cry. Steve was initially empathetic, but then confronted me with, "Nancy, you've got to cope. Your book, *Overwhelmed: Coping with Life's Ups and Downs,* will be out in one month and you can't fall apart in Denver." That did it. I thought, if my book has anything to offer, then I should be able to pull out some strategies to help me get through this experience. I did several things. First, I went to an elegant restaurant, and as the maitre d' was trying to seat me, I refused to sit down. I knew I needed a support system, and he was it. As I started telling him my sad saga, he ordered me a drink, sat down, and let me talk. Then (to myself) I reviewed the coping strategies discussed in the book. Could I change the situation? No, it was October, not November, in Denver. Could I change the way I saw the situation? Yes. Instead of labeling it a failure, a disaster, I decided to reframe it. I could redefine myself as someone who is able to go to Denver for lunch or perhaps San Francisco for dinner. On a more serious side, I decided that as a mental health professional, I could utilize this episode to help others. People could compare their calendar mix-ups to mine and realize theirs were not as bad. And finally, I knew I had a great opening for the speech in Denver the next month: "You have never had a speaker more eager to talk. I even came a month early."

Though this is a minor example, it illustrates what one can do in a stressful situation or at a time when spontaneous coping is necessary. One can refer to the scientific findings about coping and then decide on an appropriate strategy.

ASSUMPTION 2.
WE CAN TAKE THE MYSTERY—IF NOT THE MISERY—OUT OF CHANGE

Change is not as mysterious as it seems. By looking at the degree to which a transition changes one's roles, relationships, routines, and assumptions, counselors can help clients gauge how traumatic a transition will be. Then counselors can help clients examine their potential resources for coping and identify deficits. They can then jointly plan ways of compensating for those deficits by deciding whether to change them, change their meaning, or manage the resultant stress. One can also better understand a client's stress by looking at where the client is in the transition process.

ASSUMPTION 3.
COUNSELORS CAN FOLLOW THE THEORY-TO-PRACTICE MODEL BY ORGANIZING THEIR THINKING AROUND THREE QUESTIONS:

(1) What do counselors need to know?
(2) What are counselors likely to hear?
(3) What can counselors do with what they know and hear?

Table A.1 shows how the book is organized to answer the three questions. In order to answer the first question, "What do counselors need to know," we detailed four different theoretical perspectives examining the adult years. To answer the second question, "What are counselors likely to hear," we described the various arenas in which most transitions take place: within the individual, in relationships, and at work. These are not discrete arenas, but provide a way to organize the issues and concerns of adults. We discussed how individuals' potential resources for coping—Situation, Self, Support, and Strategy—are critical to determining how people manage transitions.

The final section focused on specific strategies and interventions that incorporate the knowledge counselors have about transitions with their counseling skills. These may be used in either individual or group counseling. Counselors will also utilize this knowledge when they work as consultants or advocates to best meet their clients' needs.

We hope this theory-to-practice book is useful as you help clients become better able to work, love, and play.

Table A.1   Counseling Adults in Transition

<u>What Do Counselors Need to Know?</u>

What adults are really like (Chapter 1)

How adults manage transitions (Chapter 2, 3)
* The transition process
* The 4 S system

<u>What are Counselors Likely to Hear?</u>

Types of Transitions:

* Individual (Chapter 4)
* Relationship (Chapter 5)
* Work (Chapter 6)

Resources for Coping:

* Situation
* Self
* Support
* Strategies

<u>What do Counselors do with What They Know and Hear?</u>

Modalities:

* Individual Counseling (Chapter 7)
* Group Counseling (Chapter 8)
* Consultation, Program
  Development, and
  Advocacy (Chapter 9)

Process Skills:

* Relationship Building
* Assessment
* Goal Setting
* Interventions
* Termination

References

Ager, S. (1994, February 3). At 40, at midday, a time for change. *Detroit Free Press,* p. F 1.

Aging Today. (n.d.). Newsletter of the American Society on Aging, *14*(3), p. 4.

American Association of Retired Persons. (1987). *A path for caregivers.* Washington, DC: Author.

American Association of Retired Persons. (1989). *Reminiscence: Finding meaning in memories. A training kit.* Washington, DC: Author.

American Association of Retired Persons. (1990). *A single person's guide to retirement planning.* Washington, DC: Author.

American Association of Retired Persons. (1991). *Focus your future: A woman's guide to retirement planning.* Washington, DC: Author.

American Association of Retired Persons (1991a, September-October). Widows overcome barriers to grieving. *Highlights, 9* (5), 1, 10. Washington, DC: Author.

American Association of Retired Persons. (1993a). *Grandparents raising their grandchildren, what to consider and where to find help.* Washington, DC: Author.

American Association of Retired Persons. (1993b). *Planning your retirement:* Washington DC: Author.

American College Testing Program. (1989). *Discover for colleges and adults.* Hunt Valley, MD: Author.

American College Testing Program. (1990). *Discover for retirement planning.* Iowa City, IA: Author.

American Council on Education, Center for Adult Learning and Education. (1991). *Focus on adults: A self study guide for post secondary institutions.* Washington, DC: Author.

Amundson, N., & Borgen, W. (1988). Factors that help and hinder in group employment counseling. *Journal of Employment Counseling, 25,* 104–114.

Anderson, D.B., & Shaw, S.L. (1994). Starting a support group for families and partners of people with HIV/AIDS in a rural setting. *Social Work, 39* (1), 135–139.

Aslanian, C. B., & Brickell, H. M. (1980). *Americans in transition: Life changes as reasons for adult learning.* New York: College Entrance Examination Board.

Astin, H. S. (1984). The meaning of work in women's lives: A socio-psychological model of career choice and work behavior. *Counseling Psychologist, 12,* 117–128.

Atchley, R.C. (1983). *Aging: Continuity and change.* Belmont, CA: Wadsworth.

Azrin, N. H., & Besalel, V. A. (1980). *Job club counselor's manual: A behavioral approach to vocational counseling.* Baltimore, MD: University Park Press.

Bandler, R., & Grinder, J. (1975). *The structure of magic I.* Palo Alto, CA: Behavior Books.

Bandura, A. (1982). Self-efficacy: Mechanism in human agency. *American Psychologist, 37* (2), 122–147.

Barclay, T., & McDougall, M. (1990). Older-worker programs. *Generations, 14* (1), 53–54.

Barnhill, W. (1994). Self-help groups bolster Alzheimer's families. *AARP Bulletin, 35*(3), 1, 15–17.

Barusch, A.S., & Spaid, W.M. (1989). Gender differences in caregiving: Why do wives report greater burden? *The Gerontologist, 29* (5), 667–676.

Beck, A. T. (1976). *Cognitive therapy and the emotional disorders.* New York: International Universities Press.

Beck, A. T., Ward, C., Mendelsohn, M., Mock, J., & Erbaugh, J. (1961). An inventory for measuring depression. *Archives of General Psychiatry, 4,* 53–63.

Beeson, D., & Lowenthal, M. F. (1975). In M. F. Lowenthal, M. Thurnher, & D. Chiriboga (Eds.), *Four stages of life.* San Francisco: Jossey-Bass.

Belenky, M. J., Clinchy, B. M., Goldberger, N. R., & Tarule, J.M. (1986). *Women's ways of knowing.* New York: Basic Books.

Bergman, G.(n.d.). Fresh currents in the stream of life. *Gray Panther Network.* Philadelphia: The Gray Panthers Newsletter.

Bergquist, W. H., Greenberg, E.M., & Klaum, G.A. (1993). *In our fifties: Voices of men and women reinventing their lives.* San Francisco: Jossey-Bass.

Berkman, L.F., & Syme, S.L. (1979). Social networks, host resistance and mortality: A nine-year follow-up study of Alameda County residents. *American Journal of Epidemiology, 1009* (2), 186–204.

Berne, E. (1964). *Games people play.* New York: Grove.

Bertaux, D. (1982). The life course approach as a challenge to the social sciences. In T. K. Hareven & K. J. Adams (Eds.), *Aging and life course transitions: An interdisciplinary perspective* (pp. 127–150). New York: Guilford.

Betz, N. E. (1989). Implications of the null environment hypothesis for women's career development and for counseling psychology. *Counseling Psychologist, 17,* 136–144.

Bi-Folkal Productions. (undated flyer). *Materials for life review.* Madison, WI: 809 William Street.

Black, C. (1987). *It will never happen to me.* New York: Ballantine Books.

Bly, R. (1990). *Iron John. A book about men.* Reading, MA: Addison-Wesley.

Bolles, R. N. (1993). *What color is your parachute?* Berkeley, CA: Ten Speed.

Boylan, R.J., & Hawkes, G.R. (1984, November). *Midlife and midcareer transitional factors: Precursors of successful aging.* Paper presented at annual meeting of the Gerontological Society of America, San Antonio, Texas.

Brammer, L. M. (1993). *The helping relationship* (5th ed.). Boston: Allyn and Bacon.

Brammer, L. M., & Abrego, P. J. (1981). Intervention strategies for coping with transition. *The Counseling Psychologist, 6*(1), 2–9.

Bratter, B., & Freeman, E. (1990). The maturing of peer counseling. *Generations, 14*(1), 49–52.

Bridges, W. (1980). *Transitions: Making sense of life's changes.* New York: Addison-Wesley.

Bridges, W. (1988). *Surviving corporate transition.* Mill Valley, CA: William Bridges & Associates.

Brim, O. G., Jr., & Kagan, J. (Eds.). (1980). *Constancy and change in human development.* Cambridge, MA: Harvard University Press.

Brim, O. G., Jr., & Ryff, C. D. (1980). On the properties of life events. In P. B. Baltes & O. G. Brim, Jr. (Eds.), *Life-span development and behavior* (Vol. 3). New York: Academic Press.

Britnell, E.S., Madill, H., Montgomerie, T.C., & Stewin, L.L. (1992). Work and family issues after injury: Do female and male client perspectives differ? *Career Development Quarterly, 41,* 145–160.

Brody, E.M. (1985). Parent care as a normative family stress. *The Gerontologist, 25*(1), 19–29.

Brody, E.M. (1990). *Women in the middle: Their parent-care years.* New York: Springer.

Brookfield, S.D. (1986). *Understanding and facilitating adult learning: A comprehensive analysis of principles and effective practices.* San Francisco: Jossey-Bass.

Brown, R. (1988). Unpublished materials distributed at a workship at Oakland University, Rochester, MI.

Brown, S.D., & Heath, L. (1984). Coping with critical life events: An integrative cognitive-behavioral model for research and practice. In S.D. Brown & R.W. Lent (Eds.), *Handbook of counseling psychology* (pp. 545–578). New York: Wiley.

Burnside, I.M. (Ed.). (1984). *Working with the elderly: Group process and techniques* (2nd ed.). Monterey, CA: Wadsworth.

Busse, W.M.O., & Birk, J.M. (1993). The effects of self-disclosure and competititvenss on friendship for male graduate students over 35. *Journal of College Student Development, 34,* 169–174.

Butler, R. (1963). The life review: an interpretation of reminiscence in the aged. *Psychiatry, 26,* 65–76.

Caine, L. (1974). *Widow.* New York: William Morrow.

Caplan, G. (1974). *Support systems and community mental health: Lectures on concept development.* New York: Behavioral Publications.

Caplan, G. (1976). The family as support system. In G. Caplan & M. Killilea (Eds.), *Support systems and mutual help: Multidisciplinary exploration* (pp. 19–36). New York: Greene & Stratton.

Capuzzi, D., & Gross, D.R. (1992). *Introduction to group counseling.* Denver: Love.

Capuzzi, D., Gross, D., & Friel, S.E. (1990). Recent trends in group work with elders. *Generations 14*(1), 43–48.

Cass, V. C. (1979). Homosexual identity formation: A theoretical model. *Journal of Homosexuality, 4*(3), 219–235.

Charner, I., & Schlossberg, N. K. (1986). Variations by theme: The life transitions of clerical workers. *Vocational Guidance Quarterly, 34*(4), 212–224.

Cherlin, C., & Furstenberg, F.F. (1992). *The new American grandparent. A place in the family, a life apart.* New York: Basic Books.

Chin, J. W. (1993, June). Letter: Multicultural education does not always include all cultures. *Guidepost,* Newsletter of the American Counseling Association, p. 2.

Chodoff, P. (1976). The German concentration camp as a psychological stress. In R. H. Moos (Ed.), *Human adaptation: Coping with life crises.* Lexington, MA: D.C. Heath.

Cohen, F. (1980). Coping with surgery: Information, psychological preparation, and recovery. In L. Poon (Ed.), *Aging in the 1980s: Psychological issues.* Washington, DC: Americal Psychological Association.

Cohen, J.Z., Coburn, K.L., & Pearlman, J.C. (1980). *Hitting our stride: Good news about women in their middle years.* New York: Delacorte.

Colgrove, M., Bloomfield, H.H., & McWilliams, P. (1991). *How to survive the loss of a love.* Los Angeles: Prelude Press.

Continuum Center, Oakland University (1978). *Paraprofessional preventive mental health programs.* Final Report to the National Institute of Mental Health. Rochester, MI: Author.

Cooke, D. (1994, October). *A multicultural look at the transition model.* Speech at the University of Maryland, College Park conference on Transition: Thriving on Change, College Park, MD.

Cooper, K.L., & Gutmann, D.L. (1987). Gender identity and ego mastery style in middle-aged, pre- and post-empty nest women. *Gerontologist, 27,* 347–352.

Corey, G. (1991). *Theory and practice of counseling and psychotherapy* (4th ed.). Pacific Grove, CA: Brooks/Cole.

Corey, G. (1995). *Theory and practice of group counseling* (4th ed.). Pacific Grove: Brooks/Cole.

Corey, G., & Corey, M.S. (1982). *Groups: process and practice.* (2nd ed.). Monterey, CA: Brooks/Cole.

Cormier, L. S., & Hackney, H. (1993). *The professional counselor: A process guide to helping* (2nd ed.). Boston: Allyn and Bacon.

Corsini, R. J., & Wedding, D. (Eds.). (1989). *Current psychotherapies* (4th ed.). Itasca, IL: F.E. Peacock.

Cosier, R.A., & Dalton, D. R. (1993). Management consulting: planning, entry, performance. *Journal of Counseling and Development, 72*(2), 191–198.

Costa, P. T., & McCrae, R. R. (1980). Still stable after all these years: Personality as a key to some issues in adulthood and old age. In P. B. Baltes & O. G. Brim, Jr. (Eds.), *Life-span development and behavior* (pp. 66–102). New York: Academic Press.

Covington, S. (1994, June 21). Treatment of women in and out of the criminal justice system. Presentation at the University of Utah School of Alcoholism and Other Drug Dependencies. Salt Lake City, UT.

Crow, M.L. (1987). Midlife crisis: A growth opportunity for women educators. *Clearinghouse, 60,* 413–415.

Cudney, M. R. (1980a). *Instructors guide for the workbook for eliminating self-defeating behaviors.* Kalamazoo, MI: Life Giving Enterprises.

Cudney, M. R. (1980b). *Workbook for eliminating self-defeating behaviors.* Kalamazoo, MI: Life Giving Enterprises.

Cutler, L. (1985). Counseling caregivers. *Generations, 10* (1), 53–57.

Dailey, R. J. (undated). *The stress resistant personality.* unpublished workshop handout. Rochester, MI: Continuum Center, Oakland University.

Dawson, T, (1993). Relatively guilty. *New Statesman & Society, 6* (278), 12–13.

Deaux, K. (1993). Reconstructing social identity. *Personality and Social Psychology Bulletin, 19* (1), 4–12.

DeMoulin, D.F. (1991). Stress be not proud: The myth of burnout. *Journal of School Leadership, 1*(2), 140–154.

DeVault Lahey, C. (1993). Case prepared. Mimeographed. University of Maryland, College Park.

Dobson, J. E., & Dobson, R.L. (1991). Changing roles: an aging parents support group. *Journal for Specialists in Group Work, 16* (3), 178–184.

Doerr, D. C. (1993, October). Existential therapy, men, and careers. Paper presented at a meeting of the Minnesota career development association, Minneapolis, MN.

Dohrenwend, B. S., Krasnoff, L., Askanasy, A. R., & Dohrenwend, B. P. (1978). Exemplification of a method for scaling life events: The Peri life events scale. *Journal of Health and Social Behavior, 19,* 205–229.

Donner, R., & Fine, G.L. (1987). A guide for developing self-help/advocacy groups for parents of children with serious emotional problems. Washington, DC: Georgetown University Child Development Center.

Douglas, J.D. (1990–91). Patterns of change following parent death in midlife adults. *Omega, 22* (2), 123–137.

Downing, N. E., & Rousch, K. L. (1985). From passive acceptance to active commitment: A model of feminist identity development for women. *The Counseling Psychologist, 13,* 695–709.

Dougherty, A.M. (1990). *Consultation: Practice and perspectives.* Belmont, CA: Wadsworth.

Drier, H. N., Kiss, M. E., Knowdell, R., Kobylarz, L. L., & Goodman, J. (1992). *Employee career development program guide.* Alexandria, VA: PAVE.

Dubin, K. (1994). *Change of Life.* Unpublished play.

Ebaugh, H.R.F. (1988). *Becoming an ex: The process of role exit.* Chicago: University of Chicago Press.

Egan, G. (1994). *The skilled helper: A problem management appproach to help-ing* (5th ed.). Pacific Grove, CA: Brooks/Cole.

Ellis, A. (1984). *Rational-emotive therapy and cognitive behavior therapy.* New York: Springer.

Elmer, V. (1994, July 11). Loyalties die as companies change, shrink. *Detroit Free Press,* p. 5A.

Erikson, E. H. (1950). *Childhood and society.* New York: Norton.

Erikson, E., Erikson, J., & Kevenic, A.Q. (1986). *Vital involvement in old age.* New York: Norton.

Farmer, H. S. (1985). Model of career and achievement motivation for women and men. *Journal of Counseling Psychology, 32,* 363–390.

Fassinger, R. E. (1991). The hidden minority: Issues and challenges in working with lesbian women and gay men. *The Counseling Psychologist, 19,* 157–176.

Fassinger, R. E., & Schlossberg, N. K. (1992). Understanding the adult years: Theoretical advances in life span development. In S.D. Brown & R.W. Lent (Eds.), *Handbook of counseling psychology* (pp. 217–250). New York: John Wiley & Sons.

Fiske, M. (1980). Changing hierarchies of commitment in adulthood. In N. J. Smelser & E. H. Erikson (Eds.), *Themes of work and love in adulthood* (pp. 238–264). Cambridge, MA: Harvard University Press.

Fiske, M., & Chiriboga, D.A. (1990). *Change and continuity in adult life.* San Francisco: Jossey-Bass.

Fitzgerald, L. F., & Weitzman, L. M. (1992). Women's career development: Theory and practice from a feminist perspective. In H. D. Lee & Z. D. Leibowitz (Eds.), *Adult career development: Concepts issues and practices* (2nd Ed., pp. 124–160). Alexandria, VA: National Career Development Association.

Folken, M.H. (1991). The Importance of group support for widowed persons. *Journal for Specialists in Group Work, 16* (3), 172–177.

Folkman, S., Chesney, M., McKusick, L., Ironson, G., Johnson, D.S., & Coates, T. J. (1991). Translating coping theory into an intervention. In J. Eckenrode (Ed.), *The social context of coping* (pp. 239–260). New York: Plenum.

Fouad, N., & Fahje, N. (1989). An exploratory study of the psychological correlates of infertility on women. *Journal of Counseling & Development, 68,* 97–101.

Fowler, J. (1981). *Stages of faith: The psychology of human development and the quest for meaning.* San Francisco: Harper & Row.

Fox, C., & Halbrook, B. (1994). Terminating relationships at midlife: a qualitative investigation of low income women's experiences. *Journal of Mental Health Counseling.* In press.

Frey, D. (1993, March/April). Play therapy can be a tool in working with adults. *The National Psychologist, 21.*

Friedan, B. (1963). *The feminine mystique.* New York: Norton.

Gazda, G. M. (1989). *Group counseling: A developmental approach.* (4th ed.). Boston: Allyn and Bacon.

Gelatt, H. B. (1991). *Creative decision making: Using positive uncertainty.* Los Altos, CA: Crisp.

Gelatt, H. B. (1993, November). *Career development in organizations.* Paper presented at the California Career Conference, San Diego.

Gendlin, E. T. (1981). *Focusing.* New York: Bantam.

Generations, Journal of the American Society on Aging, *14*(1).

George, L. K., & Siegler, I. C. (1981). *Coping with stress and coping in later life: Older people speak for themselves.* Durham, NC: Center for the Study of Aging and Human Development and Department of Psychiatry, Duke University Medical Center.

Gilligan, C. (1982). *In a different voice.* Cambridge, MA: Harvard University Press.

Gilligan, C. (1988). Remapping the moral domain: New images of self in relationship. In C. Gilligan, J. V. Ward, & J. M. Taylor (Eds.), *Mapping the moral domain* (pp. 3–19). Cambridge, MA: Harvard University Press.

Gladding, S.T. (1991). *Group work: a counseling specialty.* New York: Merrill.

Gooden, W. E. (1989). Development of Black men in early adulthood. In R. L. Jones (Ed.), *Black adult development and aging* (pp. 63–90). Berkeley, CA: Cobb & Henry.

Goodman, J. (1992). The dental model for counseling. *American Counselor, 1* (3), 27–29.

Goodman, J., & Hoppin, J. M. (1990). *Opening doors: A practical guide to job hunting* (2nd Ed.). Rochester, MI: Continuum Center, Oakland University.

Goodman, J., & Hoppin, J.M. (1991). *Leader guide for opening doors: A practical guide for job hunting* (2nd Ed.). Rochester, MI: Continuum Center, Oakland University.

Goodman, J., & Waters, E.B. (1985). Conflict or support: Work and family in middle and old age. *Journal of Career Development, 12*(1), 92–98.

Gordon, A. (1990). *Safe at home.* Toronto, Ont., Can.: McClelland & Stewart.

Gross, J. (1992, September 3). A jail garden's harvest: Hope and redemption. *The New York Times.*

Gutek, B. A., & Larwood, L. (1989). *Women's career development.* Newbury Park, CA: Sage.

Gutmann, D. C. (1977). The cross-cultural perspective: Notes toward a comparative psychology of aging. In J. E. Birren & K. W. Schaie (Eds.), *Handbook of the psychology of aging.* New York: Van Nostrand Reinhold.

Gutmann, D. (1987). *Reclaimed powers: Toward a new psychology of men and women in later life.* New York: Basic Books.

Gwyther, L. (1986). Family therapy with older adults. *Generations, 10,* (3), 42–45.

Hagestad, G.O. (1986). Dimensions of time and the family. *American Behavioral Scientist, 29* (6), 679–694.

Hagestad, G.O., & Burton, L. M. (1986). Grandparenthood, life context, and family development. *American Behavioral Scientist, 29* (4), 471–484.

Hagestad, G. O., & Neugarten, B. L. (1985). Age and the life course. In E. Shanar & R. Binstock (Eds.), *Handbook of aging and the social sciences* (2nd ed.). Mimeograph.

Haley, J. (1976). *Uncommon therapy.* New York: Norton.

Hall, D.T. (1986). *Career development in organizations.* San Francisco: Jossey Bass.

Halstead, R.W. (1991). Career counseling and culture: The case of Ebo. *Career Development Quarterly, 40,* 24–35.

Hanna, F. J. (1992). Reframing spirituality: AA, the 12 steps and the mental health counselor. *Journal of Mental Health Counseling, 14* (2), 166–179.

Hansson, R.O., Jones, W.H., Carpenter, B.N., & Remondet, J.H. (1986). Loneliness and adjustment to old age. *International Journal of Aging and Human Development, 24,* (1), 41–53.

Hareven, T. K. (1992). Family and generational relations in the later years: A historical perspective. *Generations, 16* (3), 7–12.

Harvard Mental Health Letter (1993). Self-help groups—Part I. *9,*9,(1–3). Boston: Harvard Medical School.

Hassan, G. (1992). No holds barred. *New Statesman & Society, 5* (215), 15–27.

Hatcher, M.A. (1988). What happens to the early retiree? *Career Development Quarterly, 37,* 184–190.

Hedberg, A. (1989, October). Caring for your aging parents. *Money*, 136–145.

Helms, J. E. (1985). Cultural identity in the treatment process. In P. Pedersen (Ed.), *Handbook of cross-cultural counseling and therapy* (239–246). Westport, CT: Greenwood.

Helms, J. E. (1990). *Black and white racial identity: Theory, research and practice.* New York: Greenwood.

Hennig, M., & Jardim, A. (1977). *The managerial woman.* New York: Doubleday.

Hill, R. (1949). *Families under stress.* New York: Harper.

Hill, R. (1965). Generic features of families under stress. In H. J. Parad (Ed.), *Crisis intervention: Selected readings.* New York: Family Service Association of America.

Hiner, N. R. (1985). Adults in historical perspective. In N. K. Schlossberg et al (Eds.), *The adult years: Continuity and change* (pp. 47–53). Columbia, MD: International University Consortium and Ohio University.

Hines, M. (1992). Group counseling with couples and families. In D. Capuzzi & D.R. Gross (Eds.), *Introduction to group counseling* (pp. 205–218). Denver: Love.

Hof, L. (1993). The elusive elixir of hope. *The Family Journal: Counseling and Therapy for Couples and Families, 1*, 220–227.

Hoffman, E. (1990). *Lost in translation: A life in a new language.* New York: Penguin Books.

Holmes, T. H., & Rahe, R. H. (1967). The Social Adjustment Rating Scale, *Journal of Psychosomatic Research, 2*, 213–218.

Hoppin, J., & Splete, H. (1994). *Training needs of career development facilitators.* Rochester, MI: Career Development Training Institute at Oakland University.

Hopson, B. (1981). Response to the papers by Schlossberg, Brammer, & Abrego. *The Counseling Psychologist, 9* (2), 36–39.

Hornby, G. (1988). Launching parent to parent schemes. *British Journal of Special Education, 15* (2), 77–78.

House, R.M., & Tyler, V. (1992). Group counseling with gays and lesbians. In D. Capuzzi & D.R. Gross (Eds.), *Introduction to group counseling* (pp. 183–204). Denver: Love.

Howard, J. (1978). *Families.* New York: Simon & Schuster.

Hudson, F.M. (1991). *The adult years: Mastering the art of self-renewal.* San Francisco: Jossey-Bass.

Hughes, A., & Graham, S. (1990). Adult life roles. *Journal of Continuing Higher Education, 38* (2), 2–8.

Isenhart, M.W. (November 10–13, 1983). *Passages: Rafting the Green River as an analogy to the mid-life transition.* Paper presented at the annual meeting of the Speech Communication Association. Washington, DC.

Ivey, A. E. (1994). *Intentional interviewing and counseling: Facilitating client development in a multicultural society.* Pacific Grove, CA: Brooks/Cole.

Jacoby, B. (1991). Today's students: Diverse needs require comprehensive responses. In T.K. Miller & R.B. Winston, Jr. (Eds.), *Administration and leadership in student affairs,* (pp. 281–307), Muncie, In: Accelerated development.

Jepsen, D. (1992, March). *Career as narrative.* Paper presented at the annual meeting of the American Counseling Association, Baltimore, MD.

Johnson, M.E., Fortman, J.B., & Brems, C. (1993). *Between two people: Exercises toward intimacy.* Alexandria, VA: American Counseling Association.

Johnson, R. P. (1990). The Serenity prayer. *Co-op Networker.* Newsletter from the family practice center, St. John's Mercy medical center, St. Louis County, Mo. 6 (1), p.2.

Johnston, L. (February 17, 1994). For Better or Worse. Comic strip in the *Detroit Free Press,* p. 6F.

Joseph, J. (1987). *Warning.* In S. Martz (Ed.), *When I am an old woman I shall wear purple* (2nd ed.). Watsonville, CA: Papier-Mache. p. 1.

Josselson, R. (1987). *Finding herself: Pathways to identity development in women.* San Francisco: Jossey-Bass.

Kagan, J. (1980). Perspectives on continuity. In O. G. Brim & J.Kagan (Eds.), *Constancy and change in human development.* Cambridge, MA: Harvard University Press.

Kahn, R. L. (1975). Memorandum to SSRC Committee on Work and Personality in the Middle Years. Ann Arbor, MI: June 2.

Kahn, R.L., & Antonucci, T.C. (1980). Convoys over the life course: Attachment, roles, and social support. In P.B. Baltes & O. C. Brim (Eds.), *Life-span development and behavior* (pp. 383–405). New York: Academic Press.

Kalish, R.A. (1985). *Death, grief and caring relationships* (2nd ed.). Monterey, CA: Brooks/Cole.

Kaminer, W. (1992). *I'm dysfunctional, you're dysfunctional.* Reading, MA: Addison-Wesley.

Kanter, R. M. (1977). *Men and women of the corporation.* New York: Basic Books.

Kantrowitz, B. (1994, May 16). Men, women, and computers. *Newsweek,* pp. 48–55.

Kapes, J. T., Mastie, M. M., & Whitfield, E. (1994). *A counselor's guide to career assessment instruments* (3rd ed.). Alexandria, VA: The National Career Development Association.

Kastenbaum, R. (1985). When aging begins: A lifespan developmental approach. *Research on Aging, 6* (1), 105–117.

Katz, M. R. (1975). SIGI: A computer based system of interactive guidance information. Princeton, NJ: Educational Testing Service.

Kelley, H. H., & Michela, J. L. (1980). Attribution theory and research. In *Annual review of psychology* (Vol. 31). Palo Alto, CA: Annual Review, Inc.

Kessler, R.C., Foster, C., Webster, P.S., & House, J.S. (1992). The relationship between age and depression in two national surveys. *Psychology and Aging, 7,* 119–126.

Kidder, T. (1993, October–November). Inside Linda Manor. *Modern Maturity.* 55–56.

Kiersey, D., & Bates, M. (1984). *Please understand me: Character and temperament types.* Del Mar, CA: Prometheus Nemesis.

Kimmel, D.C. (1990). *Adulthood and aging: An interdisciplinary developmental view* (3rd ed.). New York: John Wiley & Sons.

Kincade, S. (1987). *A delegation workshop.* Toledo, OH: Unpublished.

Kivlighan, D., Johnsen, B., & Fretz, B. (1987). Participants' perceptions of change mechanisms in career counseling groups: The role of emotional components in career problem solving. *Journal of Career Development, 14,* 35–44.

Klee, K. B. (1994). Self-esteem among Arab adults: Studying English as a second language. *Michigan Journal of Counseling and Development,* 22(2), 27–32.

Kobasa, S.C. (1980, September). *Alienation and illness.* Paper presented at the meeting of the American Psychological Association, Montreal, Canada.

Kobasa, S.C., Maddi, S.R., & Kahn, S. (1982). Hardiness and health: A prospective study. *Journal of Personality and Social Psychology, 42,* 168–177.

Kohlberg, L. (1970). Stages of moral development as a basis for moral education. In C. Beck & E. Sullivan (Eds.), *Moral education.* Toronto, Canada: University of Toronto.

Kohn, M. L. (1980). Job complexity and adult personality. In N.J. Smelser & E. H. Erikson (Eds.), *Themes of work and love in adulthood*, (pp. 193–210). Cambridge, MA: Harvard University Press.

Krumboltz, J. D. (1991). *Career beliefs inventory* Palo Alto, CA: Consulting Psychologists Press.

Krumboltz, J. D., & Hamel, D. A. (1977). *Guide to career decision-making skills*. New York: Educational Testing Service.

Kübler-Ross, E. (1969). *On death and dying.* New York: Macmillan.

Kurpius, D.J., & Fuqua, D.R. (1993a). Introduction to the special issues. *Journal of Counseling and Develolpment, 71* (6), 596–597.

Kurpius, D.J., & Fuqua, D.R. (1993b). Fundamental issues in defining consultation. *Journal of Counseling and Development, 71*(6), 598–600.

Land, G., & Jarman, B. (1992). *Breakpoint and beyond: Mastering the future—today.* New York: Harper Collins.

Lange, A.J., & Jakubowski, P. (1976). *Responsible assertive behavior.* Chammpaign, IL: Research Press.

Layton, P.L. (1984). *Self efficacy, locus of control, career salience, and women's career choice.* Unpublished doctoral dissertation, University of Minnesota.

Lazarus, A. A. (1981). *Behavior therapy and beyond.* New York: McGraw-Hill.

Lazarus, R. S. (1980) The stress and coping paradigm. In L. A. Bond & J. C. Rosen (Eds.), *Competence* and coping during adulthood. Hanover, NH: University Press of New England.

Lazarus, R.S., & Delongis, A. (1983). Psychological stress and coping and aging. *American Psychologist, 38*(3), 245–254.

Lazarus, R. S., & Folkman, S. (1984). *Stress, appraisal, and coping.* New York: Springer.

Lee, H.D., & Leibowitz, Z.B. (Eds.), (1992). *Adult career development: concepts, issues and practices* (2nd ed.). Alexandria, VA: National Career Development Association.

Leibowitz, Z., Schlossberg, N.K., & Shore, J.E. (February 1991). Stopping the revolving door. *Training and Development Journal,* 43–49.

Leibowitz, Z., Schlossberg, N. K., & Shore J. (1992). *The joining up process: A guide for new employers.* Silver Spring, MD: Conceptual Systems.

LeMasters, E. E. (1957). Parenthood as crisis. *Marriage and Family, 19,* 352–355.

Lent, R.L., & Hackett, G. (1987). Career self-efficacy: Empirical status and future directions. *Journal of Vocational Behavior, 30,* 347–382.

Levine, S. V. (1976). Draft dodgers: Coping with stress, adapting to exile. In R. H. Moos (Ed.), *Human adaptations: Coping with life crises.* Lexington, MA: D.C. Heath.

Levinson, D. J. (1978). *The seasons of a man's life.* New York: Ballantine.

Levinson, D. J. (1986). A conception of adult development. *American Psychologist, 41,* 3–13.

Levinson, D.J. (1989 May). Speech at University of Maryland, College Park, national conference, new options for adult counselors.

Lewin, K. (1943). In D. Cartwright (Ed.), *Field theory in social science* (pp. 43–59). New York: Harper.

Lewin, T. (1993, Nov. 8). Conflict for working couples: When he retires, must she? *The New York Times,* pp. A1, B.9.

Lewis, P.H. (March 8, 1994). Strangers, not their computers, build a network in time of grief, *New York Times,* pp. A1 & C18.

Lieberman, M. A. (1975). Adaptive processes in late life. In N. Datan & L. H. Ginsberg, (Eds.), *Life-span developmental psychology* (pp. 135–159). New York: Academic Press.

Lieberman, M.A. (1990). A group therapist's perspective on self-help groups. *International Journal of Group Psychotherapy, 40,* 252–278.

Lieberman, M. A., & Snowden, L. R. (1993). Problems in assessing prevalence and membership characteristics of self-help group participants. *Journal of Applied Behavioral Science, 29* (2), 166–181.

Lindeman, B. (1987, July). Nana, I can't visit you. *50 Plus,* p.4.

Lindemann, E. (1965). Symptomology and management of acute grief. In J. J. Parad, (Ed.), *Crisis intervention: Selected readings* (pp. 7–21). New York: Family Service Association of America.

Lipman, A. (1986). Homeosexual relationships. *Generations, 10* (4), 51–55.

Lipman-Blumen, J. (1976). A crisis perspective on divorce and role change. In J. R. Chapam, & M. Gates (Eds.), *Women into wives: The legal and economic impact of marriage.* Safe Yearbook in Women's Policy Studies (Vol. 2). Beverly Hills, CA: Safe Publisher.

Lipman-Blumen, J., & Leavitt, H. J. (1976). Vicarious and direct achievement patterns in adulthood. *Counseling Psychologist, 6,* 26–32.

Livneh, H., & Pullo, R.E. (1992). Group counseling for people with physical disabilities. In D. Capuzzi & D.R. Gross (Eds.), *Introduction to group counseling* (pp. 141–164). Denver: Love.

Livneh, H., & Sherwood-Hawes, A. (1993). Group counseling approaches with persons who have sustained myocardial infarction. *Journal of Counseling & Development, 72* (1), 57–61.

Locke, D. C., & Parker, L. D. (1994). Improving the multicultural competence of educators. In P. Pederson & J. Carey (Eds.), *Multicultural counseling in schools: A practical handbook* (pp. 39–58). Needham Heights, MA: Allyn & Bacon.

Loesch, L. C. (1985). Guidelines for conducting workshops. Unpublished manuscript prepared for Contining education in aging for professional counselors, a project of the American Association for Counseling and Development.

Loevinger, J. (1976). *Ego development: Conceptions and theories.* San Francisco: Jossey-Bass.

Loevinger, J. (1993). Ego development: Questions of method and theory. *Psychological Inquiry, 4* (1), 56–63.

Lopata, H.Z. (1987). Widows and their families. In C.S. Chilman, E.W. Nunnally & F.M. Cox (Eds.), *Variant family forms* (pp. 133–149). Newbury Park, CA: Sage.

Louis, M. R. (1980). Newcomers as lay ethnographers: Acculturation during organizational socialization. In B. Schneider (Ed.), *Organizational climate and culture* (pp. 85–129). San Francisco: Jossey-Bass.

Lowenthal, M. J., & Weiss, L. (1976). Intimacy and crises in adulthood. *The Counseling Psychologist, 6* (1), 10–15.

Lustbader, W. (1994, March). Presentation on caregiving. Annual Convention of American Society on Aging. San Francisco.

Lustbader, W., & Hooyman, N.R. (1994). *Taking care of aging family members: a practical guide.* New York: The Free Press.

Markides, K.S., & Mindel, C.H. (1987). *Aging and ethnicity.* Newbury Park, CA: Sage.

Martin, W.E., Jr. (1991). Career development and American Indians living on reservations: Cross-cultural factors to consider. *Career Development Quarterly, 39,* 273–283.

Maslow, A. (1954). *Motivations and personality.* New York: Harper & Row.

Mawson, D. L., & Kahn, S.E. (1993). Group process in a women's career intervention. *Career Development Quarterly, 41*(3), 238–245.

Mayer, K. U., & Schoepflin, U. (1989). The state and the life course. *Annual Review of Sociology, 15,* 187–209.

McCarn, S. R., & Fassinger, R. E. (1991, September). *Embracing our diversity: An inclusive model of lesbian development.* Paper presented at annual convention of Association for Women in Psychology, Hartford, CT.

McCrone, W.P. (1991). The federal legislative process for rehabilitation counselors. *Journal of Applied Rehabilitation Counseling 22* (3), 16–20.

McEwen, M., Komives, S., & Schlossberg, N. K. (1990). *A pilot study of college presidents leaving the presidency.* College Park, MD: The University of Maryland. Unpublished.

McKnight, J.L. (1990, July). The need for oldness. Unpublished paper presented at a meeting of the elderly cluster of W.K. Kellogg Foundation grantees, Minneapolis. Author affiliated with Center for Urban Studies, Northwestern University.

Meichenbaum, D. H. (1977). *Cognitive-behavior modification: An integrative approach.* New York: Plenum.

Merton, R. K. (1957). *Social theory and social structure.* Glencoe: The Free Press of Glencoe.

Mihovilovic, M.A. (1968). The status of former sportsmen. *International Review of Sport Sociology, 3,* 73–96.

Minkler, M. (1983, November). Building supportive networks in a "gray ghetto": The tenderloin senior ourtreach project. Paper presented at the annual meeting of the Gerontological Society of America, San Francisco.

Minuchin, S., & Fishman, H. C. (1981). *Family therapy techniques.* Cambridge, MA: Harvard University Press.

Mirabella. (February, 1994). Beauty News section.

Moody, H.R. (1988). Twenty-five years of the life review: Where did we come from? where are we going? In R. Disch (Ed.), *Twenty-five years of the life review: theoretical and practical considerations* (pp. 7–21). New York: Hawarth.

Moody, R.A. (1978). *Laugh after laugh: The healing power of humor.* Jacksonville, FL: Headwater.

Moore, D., & Haverkamp, B.E. (1989). Measured increases in male emotional expressiveness following a structured group intervention. *Journal of Counseling and Development, 67* (9), 513–517.

Moos, R. H., & Tsu, V. (1976). Human competence and coping: An overview. In Moose, R. H., (Ed.), *Human adaptation: Coping with life crises.* Lexington, MA: D.C. Heath.

Morin, W.J., & Cabrera, J.C. (1991). *Parting company: how to survive the loss of a job and find another successfully.* San Diego: Harcourt Brace Jovanovich.

Mosak, H. H. (1987). *Ha ha and aha: The role of humor in psychotherapy.* Muncie, IN: Accelerated Development.

Myerhoff, B. (1984). "Rites and signs of ripening and intertwining of ritual, time and growing older." In D. Kertzer & J. Keitch (Eds.), *Age and anthropological theory* (pp. 305–330). Ithaca, NY: Cornell University Press.

Myerhoff, B. (1985). "Rites of Renewal." Film, Owings Mills, MD: International University Consortium and Ohio University.

Myers, I.B. (1980). *Gifts differing.* Palo Alto, CA: Consulting Psychologists Press.

Myers, J.E., & Perrin, N. (1993). Grandparents affected by parental divorce: A poulation at risk. *Journal of Counseling and Development, 71* (1), 62–66.

Myers, J.E., Poidevant, J.M., & Dean, L.A. (1991). Groups for older persons and their caregivers: a review of the literature, *Journal for Specialists in Group Work, 16* (3), 197–205.

Nakao, A. (1993, November 2). New roots from tender shoots. *San Francisco Examiner,* pp. B1, B7.

National Board for Certified Counselors. (1995). *NBCC General Practice Counselor Certification Information 1995.* Greensboro, NC: Author.

National Occupational Information Coordinating Committee. (1989). *The national career development guidelines (Trainer's manual).* Washington, DC. Author.

Neugarten, B. L. (1968). The awareness of middle age. In B.L. Neugarten (Ed.), *Middle age and aging* (pp. 93–98). Chicago: University of Chicago Press.

Neugarten, B. L. (1976). Adaptation and the life cycle. *The Counseling Psychologist, 6* (1), 16–20.

Neugarten, B. L. (1979). Discontinuities in the study of aging. In T. K. Hareven & K. J. Adams (Eds.), *Aging and life course transitions: An interdisciplinary perspective* (pp. 55–74). New York: The Guilford Press.

Neugarten, B. L. (1982, August). *Successful Aging.* Paper presented to the annual meeting of the American Psychological Association, Washington, DC.

Neugarten, B. L., & Neugarten, D. A. (1987). The changing meanings of age. *Psychology Today, 21,* 29–33.

Nevill, D. D., & Schlecker, D. I. (1988). The relation of self-efficacy and assertiveness to willingness to engage in traditional/non-traditional career activities. *Psychology of Women Quarterly, 12*(1), 91–98.

Nevill, D. D., & Super, D. E. (1988). Career maturity and commitment to work in University students. *Journal of Vocational Behavior, 32,* 139–151.

Newlon, B.J., & Arciniega, M. (1992). Group counseling: Cross-cultural considerations. In D. Capuzzi and D.R. Gross (Eds.). *Introduction to group counseling* (pp. 285–306). Denver: Love.

Newsbrief (1994, Winter). Newsletter of the Southwest Detroit Community Mental Health Services, Inc. pp. 4–5.

(1993, November 8). *The New York Times,* p. A12.

Niemela, P. (1987). The significance of the 50th birthday for the woman's individuation. *Hot Flash, 6,* 2, 3.

Noer, D.M. (1993). Leadership in an age of layoffs. *Issues & Observations. 13*(3), 1–5. Greensboro, NC: Center for Creative Leadership.

Occupational Outlook Handbook (1990). Washington, DC: U.S. Department of Labor.

Okun, T. (1992). They should be our people. *Social Policy, 23* (2), 44–49.

Parkes, C. M. (1971). Psycho-social transitions: A field for study. *Social Science and Medicine, 5,* 105–115. London: Pergamon.

Parkes, C. M. (1982). Attachment and the prevention of mental disorders. In Parkes, C. M., & Stevenson-Hinde, J. (Eds.), *The place of attachment in human behavior* (pp. 295–309). New York: Basic Books.

Pearlin, L. I. (1980). Life-strains and psychological distress among adults. In N. J. Smelser & E. H. Erickson (Eds.), *Themes of work and love in adulthood* (pp. 174–192). Cambridge, MA: Harvard University Press.

Pearlin, L. I. (1982). Discontinuities in the study of aging. In T. K. Hareven & K. J. Adams (Eds.), *Aging and life course transitions: An interdisciplinary perspective* (pp. 55–79). New York: Guilford.

Pearlin, L. I., & Lieberman, M. A. (1979). Social sources of emotional distress. In R. Simmons (Ed.), *Research in community and mental health* (Vol. 1) (pp. 217–248). Greenwich, CT: JAI Press.

Pearlin, L. I., & Schooler, C. (1978). The structure of coping. *Journal of Health and Social Behavior, 19,* 2–21.

Pearsall, P. (1987). *Superimmunity: Master your emotions, improve your health.* New York: McGraw-Hill

Pearson, R.E. (1990). *Counseling and social support: Perspectives and practice.* Newbury Park, CA: Sage.

Pearson, R.E., & Petitpas, A.J. (1990). Transitions of athletes: Developmental and preventive perspectives. *Journal of Counseling and Development, 69,* 7–10.

Pearson, R.E.(1992). Group counseling: Self-enhancement. In D. Capuzzi & D.R. Gross (Eds.), *Introduction to group counseling.* Denver: Love.

Peck, T. A. (1986). Women's self-definition in adulthood: From a different model? *Psychology of Women Quarterly, 10,* 274–284.

Peluso, E., & Peluso, L.S. (1988). *Women and drugs: Getting hooked, getting clean.* Minneapolis: CompCare.

Perosa, S.L., & Perosa, L.M. (1984–85). The mid-career crisis in relation to Super's career and Erikson's adult development theory. *International Journal of Aging and Human Development, 20* (1), 53–68.

Personnel Decisions, Inc. (1994). *Transition coping guide.* Minneapolis, MN: Author.

Peter, L. J. (1978). *Peter's quotations: Ideas for our time.* New York: Bantam Books.

Peterson, C., & Austin J. T. (1985). Review of Coopersmith self-esteem inventories. In J. Mitchell (Ed.), *The ninth mental measurement yearbook* (pp. 396–397). Lincoln, NE: Buros.

Peterson, G., Sampson, J., & Reardon, C. (1991). *Career development and services: A cognitive approach.* Pacific Grove, CA: Brooks/Cole.

Plath, D.W. (1980). Contours of consociation: Lessons from a Japanese narrative. *Life-span Development and Behavior. 3.* pp 287–305.

Random House Dictionary of the English Language. (1987). New York: Random House.

Raphael, L. (1994, February). Journey through menopause. *Hers, 1*(6), p. 10.

Remondet, J.H., Hansson, R.O., Rule, B., & Winfrey, G. (1987). Rehearsal for widowhood. *Journal of Social and Clinical Psychology, 5,* 285–297.

Riessman, F., & Bay, T. (1992). The politics of self-help. *Social Policy, 23* (2), 28–39.

Riordan, R.J., & Beggs, M.S. (1987). Counselors and self-help groups. *Journal of Counseling and Development, 65,* 427–429.

Ritter, K. Y. (1985). The cognitive therapies: An overview for counselors. *Journal of Counseling and Development, 64,* 42–45.

Rodin, J. (1990). Control by any other name: Definitions, concepts and processes. In J. Rodin, C. Schooler, & K. W. Schaie (Eds.), *Self directedness: Cause and effects throughout the life course.* Hillsdale, NJ: Lawrence Erlbaum Associates.

Roberts, P., & Newton, P. M. (1987). Levinsonian studies of women's adult development. *Psychology and Aging, 2,* 154–163.

Robinson, J. (1994, August). *Making informed labor market choices: the right tools, the right times.* Presentation at national conference of State Occupational Information Coordinating Committees. Danvers, MA.

Rogers, C. R. (1957). The necessary and sufficient conditions of therapeutic personality change. *Journal of Counseling Psychology, 21,* 95–103.

Rosen, J. L., & Bibring, G. L. (1968). Psychological reactions of hospitalized male patients to a heart attack: Age and social class differences. In B. L. Neugarten (Ed.), *Middle Age and Aging* (pp. 201–211). Chicago: University of Chicago Press.

Rosenbaum, J. E. (1979). Tournament mobility: Career patterns in a corporation. *Administrative Science Quarterly, 24,* 220–241.

Rosenberg, M., & McCullough, B.C. (1981). Mattering: Inferred significance to parents and mental health among adolescents. *Research in community and mental health* (Vol. 2). R. Simmons (Ed), Greenwich, CT: JAI Press.

Ross, D. B. (1984). A cross-cultural comparison of adult development. *Personnel and Guidance Journal, 62,* 418–421.

Rotter, J. (1966). Generalized expectancies for internal versus external control of reinforcement. *Psychological Monographs, 80* (1), Whole No. 609.

Rounds, K.A., Galinsky, M.J., & Stevens, L.S. (1991). Linking people with AIDS in rural communities: The telephone group. *Social Work, 36* (1), 13–19.

Rubin, L. (1981). *Women of a certain age: The midlife search for self.* New York: Harper & Row.

Rubin, L.B. (1986). On men and friendship. *The Psychoanalytic Review, 73,* 1, 165–181.

Ruffin, J. E. (1989). Stages of adult development in Black professional women. In R. L. Jones (Ed.), *Black adult development and aging* (pp. 31–62). Berkeley, CA: Cobb & Henry.

Sagaria, M.A. (1989). Toward a woman-centered perspective of careers: The quilt metaphor. *Journal of Employment Counseling, 26* (1), 11–115.

Sand-Pringle, C., West, J. D., & Bubenzer, D. I. (1991). Family counseling rituals: A case study. *Journal of Mental Health Counseling 13* (4), 500–505.

Sargent, A.G., & Schlossberg, N.K. (1988). Managing adult transitions. *Training and Development Journal, 41*(12), 58–60.

Satir, V. (1972). *Peoplemaking.* Palo Alto, CA: Science & Behavior Books.

Savickas, M.L., Passen, A.J., & Jarjoura, D.G. (1988). Career concern and coping as indicators of adult vocational development. *Journal of Vocational Behavior, 33* (1) 82–98.

Schein, E.H. (1991). *Process consultation, Vol. 1: Its role in organization development* (2nd ed.). Reading, MA: Addison-Wesley.

Schein, E.H. (1992). *Process consultation, Vol. 2: Lessons for managers and consultants.* Reading, MA: Addison-Wesley.

Scheier, M.F., Matthews, K.A., Owens, J.F., Magovern, G.J., Lefebvre, R.C., Abbott, R.A., & Carver, C.S. (1989). Dispositional optimism and recovery from coronary artery bypass surgery: The beneficial effects on physical and psychological well-being. *Journal of Personality and Social Psychology, 57* (6), 1024–1040.

Schlossberg, N. K. (1981). A model for analyzing human adaptation to transition. *The Counseling Psychologist. 9*, (2), 2–18.

Schlossberg, N. K. (1991). *Overwhelmed: Coping with Life's Ups and Downs.* Lexington, MA: Lexington Books.

Schlossberg, N.K., Lassalle, A. & Golec, R. (1991). The Mattering Scales for Adult Students in Higher Education. College Park, MD: University of Maryland.

Schlossberg, N. K., & Leibowitz, Z. B. (1980). Organizational support systems as buffers to job loss. *Journal of Vocational Behavior, 18*, 204–217.

Schlossberg, N.K., Lynch A.Q., & Chickering, A.W. (1989). *Improving higher education environments for adults.* San Francisco: Jossey-Bass.

Schlossberg, N.K. & Robinson, S.P. (1993). Non-events: Another name for heartbreak. *American Counselor, 2* (4) 21–25.

Scofield, M. (1993, June 6). About men: Off the ladder. *The New York Times Magazine,* p. 22.

Seligman, M. (1990). *Learned Optimism.* New York: Alfred A. Knopf.

Shapiro, C. (1982). The impact of infertility on the marital relationship. *Social Casework: The Journal of Contemporary Social Work, 82*, 387–393.

Sharf, R. S. (1992). *Applying career development theory to counseling.* Pacific Grove, CA: Brooks/Cole.

Sharify, N. (1988, June). Views of an educator. In S. Karkhanis (Ed.), *How to avoid dead end in your career: An Asian American perspective, and library services for the Asian/Pacific American Librarians Association.* Papers of the 1987 Program of the Asian/Pacific American Librarians Association, San Francisco.

Sherman, E., (1987). Reminiscence groups for community elderly. *The Gerontologist, 27*, (5), 569–572.

Siegel, B. S. (1986). *Love, medicine, and miracles: Lessons learned about self healing from a surgeon's experience with exceptional patients.* New York: Harper & Row.

Silverman, P.R. (1980). *Mutual help groups: organization & development.* Beverly Hills, CA: Sage.

Silverman, P.R. (1986). *Widow to Widow.* New York: Springer.

Silverman, P., Mackenzie, D., Pettipas, M., & Wilson, E. (1974). *Helping each other in widowhood.* New York: Health Sciences.

Silverstone, B. (1994, March). You and your aging parent revisited: A 20–year retrospective on family caregiving. Lecture presented at the 40th annual meeting of the American Society on Aging. San Francisco.

Singer, V.I., Tracz, S.M., & Dworkin, S.H. (1991). Reminiscence group therapy: A treatment modality. *Journal for specialists in group work. 16*, (3) 167–171.

Smelser, N. K., & Erikson, E. H. (1980). *Themes of work and love in adulthood.* Cambridge, MA: Harvard University Press.

Smith, H. (1994). Rationale for counselor involvement in public policy. *Quest, 27* (1), 15. St. Johns, MI: Michigan Counseling Association.

Sparks, S.M. (1992). Exploring electronic support groups. *American Journal of Nursing, 92* (12), 62–66.

Spencer, S.A., & Adams, J.D. (1990). *Life changes.* San Luis Obispo, CA: Impact.

Spierer, H. (1977). *Major transition in the human life cycle.* New York: Academic Press for Educational Development.

Spokane, A.R. (1991). *Career intervention.* Englewood Cliffs, NJ: Prentice-Hall.

Stachow, D.M. (1993, November). Beyond Awareness: The key to designing a non-biased model for counseling individuals over sixty. Presentation made at conference of the Association for Adult Development and Aging. New Orleans.

Stephan, N. (1989). *Finding your life mission.* Walpole, NH: Stillpoint.

Sue, D-W., & Sue, D (1990). *Counseling the culturally different: Theory and practice* (2nd. ed.). New York: John Wiley & Sons.

Super, D.E. (1980). A life-span, life-space approach to career development. *Journal of Vocational Behavior, 16* (3), 282–298.

Super, D.E. (1985). *New dimensions in adult vocational and career counseling. Occasional Paper No. 106.* Columbus, OH: The National Center for Research in Vocational Education.

Super, D.E. (1992). Adult career development in an uncertain future. In H. D. Lee & Z. D. Leibowitz (Eds.), *Adult career development: Concepts issues and practices* (2nd ed, pp. 417–425). Alexandria, VA: National Career Development Association.

Super, D.E., & Knasel, E.G. (1979). *Development of a model, specifications, and sample items for measuring career adaptability (vocational maturity) in young blue collar workers.* Cambridge, England: National Institute for Careers Education and Counselling, and Ottawa Canada: Canada Employment and Immigration.

Super, D.E., & Knasel, E.G. (1981). Career development in adulthood: Some theoretical problems and a possible solution. *British Journal of Guidance & Counselling, 9* (2), 195–201.

Super, D. E., & Nevill, D.D. (1984). Work role salience as a determinant of career maturity in high school students. *Journal of Vocational Behavior, 25,* 30–44.

Super, D. E., & Nevill, D. D. (1985). *The salience inventory.* Palo Alto, CA: Consulting Psychologists Press.

Sussman, M. B. (1972). An analytic model for the sociological study of retirement. In F. M. Carp (Ed.), *Retirement.* New York: Human Sciences Press.

Szapocznik, J., & Kurtines, W. N. (1993). Family psychology and cultural diversity: Opportunities for theory, research, and application. *American Psychologist, 48* (4), 400–407.

Tannen, D. (1990). *You just don't understand: Women and Men in conversation.* New York: William Morrow.

Taylor, S. E. (1989). *Positive illusions: Creative self-deception and the healthy mind.* New York: Basic Books.

Temes, R. (1984). *Living with an empty chair.* New York: Irvington.

Terry, A. (1992). Group counseling: Career and lifestyle issues. In D. Capuzzi & D.R. Gross (Eds.), *Introduction to group counseling.* Denver: Love.

Toffler, A. (1970). *Future Shock.* New York: Bantam.

Towns, K., & Gentzler, R. (1986). Empowering reentry women: An organizational case study: The story of PROBE. *Women and Therapy, 5* (2–3), 159–66.

Trupin, S. (1993). Moral support for "grandparents who care": A nursing success story. *American Journal of Nursing, 93*(4), 52–57.

Tubesing, N.L., & Tubesing, D.A. (undated) Structured exercises in stress management (Vols. 1–4). Duluth,MN: Whole Person Associates.

Update. (1988). Newsletter of the Government Relations Committee, Alexandria: VA: American Counseling Association.

U.S. Department of Commerce, Bureau of the Census (1993). *Statistical abstract of the United States* (113th ed.). Washington, DC: Author.

Vaillant, G. E. (1977). *Adaptation to life.* Boston: Little, Brown.

Vaillant, G. E. (May 1982). *Maturity over the life cycle.* Paper presented at the meeting of the Helpers of Adults conference, College Park, MD.

Van Gennep, A. (1960). *The Rites of Passage.* Chicago, IL: The University of Chicago Press.

Vernon, A. (1992). Group counseling: Loss. In D. Capuzi & D. R. Gross (Eds.), *Introduction to group counseling* (pp. 263–281). Denver: Love.

Viorst, J. (1976). *How did I get to be forty . . . and other atrocities.* New York: Simon & Schuster.

Walter, J., & Peller, J. (1992). *Becoming solution-focused in brief therapy.* New York: Brunner/Mazel.

Wapner, S. (1981). Transactions of persons-in-environments: Some critical transitions. *Journal of Environmental Psychology, 1*, 223–239.

Waters, E. B. (1990). The life review: Strategies for working with individuals and groups. *Journal of Mental Health Counseling, 12* (3), 270–78.

Waters, E., McCarroll, J., & Penman, N. (1987). *Training mental health workers for the elderly.* Rochester, MI: Oakland University Continuum Center.

Waters, E. B., & Goodman, J. (1990). *Empowering older adults: Practical strategies for counselors.* San Francisco: Jossey Bass.

Waters, E. B., & Samson, J. (1993). *Strengthening your team: A training program for volunteers and staff who work with older adults.* Rochester, MI. Oakland University Continuum Center.

Waters, R. (1991, October). Intergenerational day care/ Young and old alike. *Parenting* 74–79.

Waters, R. (1994, October 12). Women who make a difference: Help for grandparents. *Family Circle, 106,* (14), 17–18.

Wax, J. (1985). Self-help groups. *Journal of Psychosocial Oncology, 3* (3), 1–3.

Webster's new collegiate dictionary (1980). Springfield, MA: G & C Merriam.

Weenolsen, P. (1986, August). *Life and self meaning: The process of their creation.* Paper presented at the 94th Annual Convention of the American Psychological Association, Washington, DC.

Wegscheider, S. (1981) *Another chance: Hope and health for the alcoholic family.* Palo Alto, CA: Science and Behavior Books.

Weiss, R. S. (1973). *Loneliness: The experience of emotional and social isolation.* Cambridge, MA: MIT Press.

Weiss, R. S. (1976). Transition states and other stressful situations; their nature and programs for their management. In G. Caplan & M. Killilea (Eds.), *Support systems and mutual help: Multidisciplinary explorations* (pp. 17–26). New York: Grune & Stratton.

Whitbourne, S. (1985). The psychological construction of the life span. In J. E. Birren & K. W. Schaie (Eds.), *Handbook of the psychology of aging* (2nd ed., pp. 594–618). New York: Van Nostrand Reinhold.

White, B. (1992) "Me - the Helpee." *Feedback.* Newsletter of the Continuum Center, Oakland University, *20* (3), pp. 7–8.

White, R. (1976). Strategies of adaptation: An attempt at systematic description. In R. Moos (Ed.), *Human adaptation: Coping with life crises.* Lexington, MA: D.C. Heath.

Widowers overcome barriers to grieving (1991, September-October). *Highlights 9* (5), 1, 10. Washington, DC: American Association of Retired Persons.

Wilcoxon, S.A., & Puleo, S.G. (1992). Professional development needs of mental health counselors: results of a national survey. *Journal of Mental Health Counseling. 14*(2), 187–195.

Worden, J.W. (1991) *Grief counseling and grief therapy* (2nd ed.). New York: Springer.

Wuthnow, R. (1994). *Sharing the journey: support groups and America's new quest for community.* New York: Free Press.

Yalom, I.D. (1985). *The theory and practice of group psychotherapy* (3rd ed.). New York: Basic Books.

Yang, J. (1991). Career counseling of Chinese American Women: Are they in limbo? *Career Development Quarterly, 39,* 350–358.

Young, C. I. (1983). *Inscape: A search for meaning.* Rochester, MI: Continuum Center, Oakland University.

Young, P. R. (1988, June). Experiences of an Asian/American librarian. In S. Karkhanis (Ed.), *How to avoid dead end in your career: An Asian American perspective, and library services for the Asian/Pacific American Librarians Association.* Papers of the 1987 Program of the Asian/Pacific American Librarians Association, San Francisco.

You, Seung-Woo (undated). *Understanding and managing a transition: New immigrants from Korea.* unpublished class paper.

Zaleznik, A., & Jardim, A. (1967). Management. In P. F. Lararsfeld, W. H. Sewell, & H. L. Wilensky (Eds.), *The uses of Sociology* (pp. 193–234). New York: Basic Books.

Zimpfer, D.G. (1990). Groups for divorce/separation: A review. *Journal for Specialists in Group Work, 15* (1), 51–60.

Zunker, V.G. (1994). *Career counseling: Applied concepts of life planning* (4th ed.). Pacific Grove, CA: Brooks/Cole.

Index

A

Adaptability, work transition and, 148–150
Adult development theories, 3–24
adulthood, theoretical approaches to, 4–19
age, 20
development based on, 8–10
concepts, of adult experience, 20
context, 4–8, 20
development, 8–15, 20
domain-specific development, 12–13, 20
issue resolution, 11–12, 20
life span, 16–18, 20
overview, 24
perspectives, theoretical, application of, 19–23
transition, 18–19, 20
Advocacy, 241–268
Age, and adult development theories, 20
development based on, 8–10
Altruism, group counseling, 205–206
American College Testing Program, 90
Anxiety reduction techniques, individual counseling, 198
Appraisal, of transition, 49–51
Assertiveness training
group counseling and, 238–239
individual counseling and, 197–198
Assessment
in individual counseling, 171, 175–184
of transition, 57

Assets, transition and, 76–77
liabilities, balancing, 48-49
Autonomy, and individual transition, 93–94

B

Balance, work transition and, 145–148
Bandura, A., 97, 150, 182
Behavioral interventions, individual counseling, 196–198
Belenky, M.J., 12, 113
Belonging, and relationship transition, 127–128
Brammer, L.M., 37, 246
Bridges, W., 40, 110
Brody, E.M., 121

C

Caplan, G., 133
Career planning programs, group counseling, 229–232
Career-related transitions, groups for people facing, group counseling, 227–232
Caregivers, groups for, group counseling, 225–226
Catharsis, group counseling and, 208
Cautions, about group counseling, 208–209
Cohesiveness, group counseling and, 207
Combination interventions, individual counseling, 198–201

Consultant, counselor as, 252–254
Consultation, 241–268
Context
    of adult development theories, 4–
        8
    transition and, 31–33
Control
    source of, and individual
        transition, 54–55, 90–91
    and work transitions, 54–55, 143,
        144
Coping
    effectiveness training, group
        counseling, 237–238
    resources, 48
    responses, 75–76
    strategies, list of, and relationship
        transition, 136
    transition and, 48, 75–76
Corey, G., 209
Cormier/Hackney model, and four
    "S" transition model,
    combination of, individual
    counseling, 175
Counseling
    group, 203–240. *See also* Group
        counseling
    individual, 169–202. *See also*
        Individual counseling
Counselor
    as advocate, 263–264
    as consultant, 252–254
Couples, groups for, 221–222
Cultural diversity, group counseling,
    211
Curative factors, group counseling,
    204–208

D

Demographic characteristics,
    transition and, 58–62
Denial, selective, and individual
    transition, 101–102
Disputation, individual counseling,
    194
Distracting, individual counseling,
    193
Divorce
    groups, 222–223

relationship transition and, 112–
    113
Domain-specific development, and
    adult development theories,
    12–13, 20
Duration, of transition, 56, 89–90

E

Egan, G., 100, 104, 246
Eldercare, relationship transition
    and, 120–122
Erikson, E.,11, 91, 92, 126, 217
Existential factors, group counseling,
    208
Experience
    and adult development theories,
        20
    previous, with similar transition,
        work transition and, 56–57,
        144
Explanations, alternative, seeking,
    individual counseling, 194

F

Factors that influence transition, 47–
    80
Family
    groups for, 221–222
    relationship transitions, groups for
        people facing, 219–226
Fassinger, R.E., 4, 8, 14, 15
Fiske, M., 18, 48, 55, 57, 60, 61, 66,
    126
Folkman, S., 100, 237
Follow-up, individual counseling,
    173–174
Four "S" model
    group counseling, 232–239
    transition and, 47–52
Friendship, relationship transition
    and, 123–124

G

Gazda, G.M., 208, 209, 232
Gelatt, H.B., 158, 200

Gender differences, work transition and, 163–166
Gilligan, C., 13, 18, 93, 113, 127
Goal
    self, related to, individual counseling, 185
    situation, related to, individual counseling, 184–185
    strategies, related to, individual counseling, 186
    support, related to, individual counseling, 185–186
Goal setting in individual counseling, 172, 184
Goodman, J., 130, 154, 166, 173, 190, 192, 232, 234, 259
Grandparenting, relationship transition and, 117–119
Group counseling, 203–240, 213–219, 227–229
    action/decision model, mastery, 226
    altruism, 205–206
    assertiveness training, 238–239
    career
        planning programs, 229–232
        transitions, groups for people facing, 227–232
    caregivers, groups for, 225–226
    catharsis, 208
    cautions about, 208–209
    cohesiveness, 207
    coping effectiveness training, 237–238
    couples, groups for, 221–222
    cultural diversity, 211
    curative factors in, 204–208
    divorced people, groups for, 222–223
    effective groups, characteristics of, 211–213
    existential factors, 208
    family
        groups for, 221–222
        relationship transitions, groups for people facing, 219–226
    four "S" model, 232–239
    groups/techniques, illustrative, for intrapersonal transitions, 214–219

hope, instillation of, 204–205
identity, investigation into, 214–215
illnesses, groups for persons with, 216–217
imitative behavior, 206
information, imparting, 204
interpersonal learning, 206–207
intrapersonal transitions, bringing clients to groups, 213–214
job search groups, 232
life mission, 216
life review groups, 217–219
as modality, 204–213
programs/techniques
    career-related transition, 229–232
    illustrative, 221–226
recapitulation, of primary family group, corrective, 206
self, 234
separated people, groups for, 222–223
situation, 233
socializing techniques, development of, 206
strategies, 236–239
stress management programs, 238
summary, 239–240
support, 234–236
transitions, common, bringing clients to groups, 219–220
types of groups, 209–210
universality, 205
widowed persons, groups for, 223–224
women, in midlife, 215–216
Groups, effective, characteristics of, 211–213

H

Hackney, H., 169, 173–201, 246, 251
Hagestad, G.O., 6, 8, 109, 110, 118
Hardiness, individual counseling, 180
Helms, J.E., 14, 15
Hope
    and individual transition, 102–106
    instillation of, group counseling, 204–205
Hudson, F.M., 86, 126

I

Identity
  and individual transition, 91–92
  investigation into, group
      counseling, 214–215
Illnesses, groups for persons with,
      216–217
Imagery training, individual
      counseling, 196–197
Imitative behavior, group counseling,
      206
Impact, of transition, 33–35
Individual counseling, 169–202
  anxiety reduction techniques, 198
  assertion training, 197–198
  assessment, 171, 175–184
  behavioral interventions, 196–198
  case study, 186–187
  combination interventions, 198–
      201
  Cormier/Hackney model, and
      four "S" transition model,
      combination of, 175
  decatastrophizing, 194
  disputation, 194
  distracting, 193
  explanations, alternative, seeking,
      194
  follow-up, 173–174
  goal
      self, related to, 185
      setting, 172, 184
      situation, related to, 184–185
      strategies, related to, 186
      support, related to, 185–186
  hardiness, 180
  imagery training, 196–197
  intervention, 172–173, 187–201
      affective, 188–191
      cognitive, 191–196
  model, 196
      Cormier/Hackney, 170–174
  overview, 201–202
  play therapy, 200–201
  problem-solving interventions,
      198–200
  rehearsal, 196
  relationship-building, 170–171
  rituals, developing, 201
  role play, rehearsal, 196

self
  assessing, 179–182
  efficacy of, 182
situations, assessing, 176–179
solution-focused brief counseling,
      200
strategies, assessing, 183–184
supports, assessing, 182–183
termination, 173–174
Individual transition, 81–106
  autonomy and, 93–94
  control, source of, 90–91
  denial, selective, 101–102
  duration, 89–90
  hope, 102–106
  identity and, 91–92
  meaning-making and, 94–97
  optimism, 102–106
  reframing, 100–101
  self, 91–97
      efficacy and, 97
  situation and, 82–91
  spirituality and, 99–100
  strategies and, 100–106
  support, 98–100
      types of, 98–99
  timing and, 86–88
  triggers, 83–86
  stress, concurrent, 57
  support, 67–70
      functions of, 68–69
      overview, 69–70
      social
          convoy of, 72
          measurement of, 69
      types of, 67–68
  timing, 54
  trigger, 53–54
Information, imparting, group
      counseling, 204
Integration, model of transition, 44–
      45
Interpersonal learning, group
      counseling, 206–207
Interventions
  affective, individual counseling,
      188–191
  behavioral, individual counseling,
      196, 198
  cognitive, individual counseling,
      191–196

individual counseling, 172–173, 187–201
Intimacy, relationship transition and, 125–127
Intrapersonal transitions, bringing clients to groups, 213–214
Issue resolution, and adult development theories, 11–12, 20

J

Job search groups, group counseling, 232

K

Kahn, R.L., 68, 69, 133, 134, 182, 235
Kimmel, D.C., 117
Krumboltz, J.D., 179, 182, 199

L

Lazarus, R.S., 19, 31, 49, 70, 74
Leibowitz, Z., 41, 156
Lesbian mother, case study, adult development theories, 22–23
Levinson, D.J., 8, 9, 93
Liabilities, transition and, 48–49
Life
    mission, group counseling, 216
    review groups, group counseling, 217–219
    span, and adult development theories, 16–18, 20
Lipman-Blumen, J., 36, 164
Local level, acting at, 264–267

M

Mattering, relationship transition and, 129
Meaning
    ability to establish, and individual transition, 94–97
    establishment of, work transition and, 152–153
Midlife male, case study, adult development theory, 21–22
Model
    Cormier/Hackney, individual

counseling, 170–174
transition, overview of, 26–27
work transition, 159
Modeling, individual counseling, 196
Multicultural view, options, 51-52
Myerhoff, B., 43, 201

N

National level, acting at, 264–267
Neugarten, B.L., 7, 16, 61, 113
Neutral zones, transition and, 39–40
Non-event, transition and, 29–31

O

Optimism, and individual transition, 102–106
Organizations, and employees, consulting with, 250–256

P

Parent, death of, relationship transition and, 122–123
Parenting, relationship transition and, 116–117
Partnering relationships, relationship transition and, 110–112
Pearlin, L.I., 16, 29, 32, 62, 70, 183
Pearson, R.E., 88, 98, 126, 206, 210, 235, 236
Personal characteristics, 58–62
Personnel Decisions, Inc., 77
Perspective
    of adult development theories, 8–15
    theoretical, application of, and adult development theories, 19–23
    of transition, and adult development theories, 18–19
Play therapy, individual counseling, 200–201
Previous experience, with similar transition, and transition, factors influencing, 56–57
Problem-solving
    individual counseling, 198–200
    relationship transition and, 136

Program
  career-related transition, group
      counseling, 229–232
  designing, 257–258
  illustrative, group counseling,
      221–226
Program development, 241–268,
    256–261
Psychological Resources, 62–66

R

Reappraisal, of situation, relationship
    transition and, 136
Recapitulation, of primary family
    group, corrective, group
    counseling, 206
Recurring issues, relationship
    transition and, 125–129
Reframing process, individual
    transition and, 100–101
Rehearsal, individual counseling, 196
Relationship transition
  belonging, 127–128
  coping strategies, list of, 136
  divorce, 112–113
  eldercare, 120–122
  friendship, 123–124
  grandparenting, 117–119
  intimacy, 125–127
  mattering, 129
  parent, death of, 122–123
  parenting, 116–117
  partnering relationships, 110–112
  problem-solving behaviors, 136
  reappraisal of situation, 136
  recurring issues, 125–129
  remarriage, 115–116
  resources, assessment of, 130–137
  self, 131–132
  situations, 130–131
  strategies, 135–137
  stress, reactions to, 136
  summary, 137
  support, 132–135
  types of, 110–124
  widowhood, 113–115
Relationship-building, individual
    counseling and, 170–171
Relativity, and transition, 31

Remarriage, relationship transition
    and, 115–116
Resilience, work transition and, 148–
    150
Resources, assessment of,
    relationship transition and,
    130–137
Retirement, 55, 97, 100, 159–162,
    227–232, 251–252
Rituals, developing, individual
    counseling, 201
Role play, individual counseling, 196

S

"S" system, the four, transition and,
    47–52
Salience, work transition and, 145–
    148
Schein, E.H., 250
Schlossberg, N.K., 4, 19, 36, 40, 41,
    42, 89, 92, 117, 129, 156,
    159, 161, 188, 262
Self
  assessing, individual counseling,
      179–182
  group counseling, 234
  individual counseling, 182
  individual transition and, 91–97
  issues related to, work transition
      and, 145–153
  relationship transition and, 131–
      132
  work transition and, 150–152
Self-help groups
  advantages of, 243–244
  how counselors relate to, 244–247
  limitations of, 243–244
  summary, 249
  working with, 242–249
Seligman, M., 63, 104, 182
Silverman, P.R., 224
Separated people, groups for, 222–
    223
Situation, individual transition and,
    82–91
Socializing techniques, development
    of, group counseling, 206
Solution-focused brief counseling,
    individual counseling, 200

Spirituality, individual transition and, 99–100
Strategies
assessing, individual counseling, 183–184
group counseling, 236–239
individual transition and, 100–106
issues related to, work transition and, 155–156
relationship transition and, 135–137
Stress
concurrent, timing, work transition and, 142–143
management programs, group counseling, 238
reactions to, relationship transition and, 136
Sue, D-W., 14
Super, D.E., 145, 146, 147, 148, 149, 158, 179
Support
assessing, individual counseling, 182–183
group counseling, 234–236
individual transition and, 98–100
types of, 98–99
issues related to, work transition and, 153–155
relationship transition and, 132–135

T

Termination, individual counseling, 173–174
Theories, of adult development, 3–24, 20
age, development based on, 8–10
concepts, of adult experience, 20
context, 4–8, 20
development theories, age, 20
domain-specific development, 12–13, 20
experience, adult, perspectives, 20
issue resolution, 20
development based on, 11–12
life span, 16–18, 20
overview, 24
perspective of, 8–15

perspectives, theoretical, application of, 19–23
transition, 18–19, 20
understanding, theoretical approaches to, 4–19
Timing, and individual transition, 86–88
Transition
anticipated, 29
approach to, 27–35
beginnings, 40
bringing clients to a career-related group, 227–229
common, bringing clients to groups, 219–220
context and, 31–33
endings, 38–39
factors influencing, 47–80, 53–76
appraisal of, 49–51
assessment, 57
assets, 76–77
liabilities, balancing, 48–49
control, 54–55
coping
resources, 48
responses, 75–76
demographic characteristics, 58–62
duration, 56
experience, previous, with similar transition, 56–57
four "S" system, 47–52
liabilities, 76–77
multicultural view, options, 51–52
personal characteristics, 58–62
psychological resources, 62–66
role change, 55–56
self, 58–67
review of, 67
situation, 53–58
strategies, 70–76
stress, concurrent, 57
support, 67–70
functions of, 68–69
overview, 69–70
timing, 54
trigger, 53–54
impact of, 33–35
individual, 81–106. *See also* Individual transition

integrative model, 44–45
model
  in action, case study of, 254–256
  and Cormier/Hackney model, 174–201
  overview of, 26–27
neutral zones, 39–40
non-event, 29–31
perspective of, and adult development theories, 18–19
process, 27, 35–44
relationship transition, 107–137. *See also* Relationship transition
relativity and, 31
summary, 35, 46
as theoretical framework, 25–46
types of, 29–31
types of groups for, 247–249
unanticipated, 29
work, 139–168. *See also* Work transition
Triggers, individual transition, 83–86
Types of groups, group counseling, 209–210

U

Unanticipated, 29
Universality, group counseling, 205

W

Waters, E.B., 130, 166, 217, 218
Weiss, R.S., 124, 212, 228, 268
Widowhood
  groups for, 223–224

relationship transition and, 113–115
Women, in midlife, group counseling, 215–216
Work transition, 139–168
  adaptability, 148–150
  balance, 145–148
  control, 143–144
  experience, previous, with similar transition, 144
  gender differences, 163–166
  meaning, establishment of, 152–153
  model, 159
  movement around, 156–163
  resilience, 148–150
  salience, 145–148
  self
    efficacy, 150–152
    issues related to, 145–153
  situation, issues related to, 141–145
  strategies, issues related to, 155–156
  stress, concurrent, timing and, 142–143
  summary, 144–145, 153, 166
  support, issues related to, 153–155
  triggers, 141–142
Workshops
  developing, 256–261
  presenting, 258–259
  sampling of, 259–261

Y

Yalom, I.D., 204

1996